INSTITUTE OF MEDICINE

Ethics
of
Health
Care

Papers of the Conference on
Health Care and Changing Values, *Institute of Medicine, 1973.*
November 27-29, 1973

LAURENCE R. TANCREDI
Editor

NATIONAL ACADEMY OF SCIENCES
WASHINGTON, D.C. 1974

Library of Congress Cataloging in Publication Data

Conference on Health Care and Changing Values, Institute of Medicine, 1973.
   Ethics of health care.

   Includes bibliographical references.
   1. Medical ethics–Congresses. 2. Medical care–United States–Congresses. 3. Medical
policy–United States–Citizen participation–Congresses. 4. Medical education–United
States–Congresses. I. Tancredi, Laurence R., ed. II. Institute of Medicine. III. Title. [DNLM:
1. Ethics, Medical–Congresses. W50 C742e 1973]
   R724.C62   1973   174'.2   74-28130
   ISBN 0-309-02249-5

R724
C62
1973

Conference on Health Care and Changing Values
supported by Health Services and Mental Health
Administration, Department of Health, Education,
and Welfare, Contract No. HSM 110-72-209

Available from

Printing and Publishing Office, National Academy of Sciences
2101 Constitution Avenue, N.W., Washington, D.C. 20418

Printed in the United States of America

Preface

Abortion, euthanasia, organ transplantation, and the potentials for genetic engineering are contributing to a growing awareness of the social and ethical features of medical research and care. Until relatively recently, attention to ethical considerations was directed mostly toward human experimentation. This was due in large part to the Nazi "medical" atrocities during World War II and the subsequent decision of the United States Military Tribunal at Nuremberg in 1949, which introduced the requirement of "informed consent," the first formal control by the patient over the actions of the researcher or physician. Since that time there has been much debate on the effectiveness of any existing instrument, including informed consent, for protecting the patient. Many feel that the power of decision still heavily rests with the medical profession; the complexities of modern technology can make virtually impossible a real informing of the patient, and the special relationship of trust between a patient and his physician induces patients to accept any recommended medical procedure.

In the context of medical experimentation, human value issues have assumed increasing importance in recent years, finding expression in many proposed regulations, such as the establishment of protection committees and national ethics review boards. But these concerns are no longer limited to medical experimentation. They are being carried

iii

01980

well beyond the Hippocratic Oath tradition of medical ethics that was focused on the responsibilities of the individual practitioner for his patient. The issues have been expanded to encompass the ethical implications of a broad variety of health-related decisions, including not only decisions affecting individuals but also the effects of societal actions in the health field. Issues of a social justice nature, especially where they entail economic decisions of resource allocation, are becoming particularly prominent.

There are several major reasons for this expansion in the scope of ethical concerns. First, expansion of medical capabilities has added greatly to the possibilities for intervention against disease, disability, and even death. The complexity of many of these interventions and their implications for the welfare of individuals and of society as a whole have greatly complicated medical decision making, which in the past could be carried out on the single criterion of extended life or reduced disability for the individual. Second, because of the tremendous growth in the capability of medicine to treat a variety of diseases, health care has become a significant consumer of society's resources. As the total volume of resources devoted to health has grown, there has been a sharper awareness of resource constraints and the need to make choices. Choices that deny the availability of certain resources or services, despite the existence of technical capability, are becoming more explicit and open, often conflicting with society's value judgments. Third, we are moving into an era in which health care is perceived as a concern of society as a whole rather than as an individual matter only of arrangements between the patient and health care providers. Fewer decisions are being made by individuals, and more are being made by the collective actions of public officials, consumers, and health professionals. Society's welfare and society's value judgments are entering into an ethical picture once dominated by the simpler concern of what was good for the individual patient. There is little precedent in our medical–ethical tradition for the way in which these important social contributions should be considered in defining medical responsibility and in resolving such questions as *what* care should be available to *which* segments of the population.

Recognizing the shift in responsibility for health decisions and the attendant emerging ethical problems, the Institute of Medicine, with support from the Department of Health, Education, and Welfare, established a committee to examine the broader social–ethical issues of health care and to delineate these issues into topics that could be the subject of analytical papers. The committee was asked to develop a classification of ethical issues in health care that could serve as the framework for ordering and analyzing such issues in the future. The committee was constituted of experts in law, clinical and administrative medicine, ethics and religion, the social sciences and economics, and psychiatry. Its attention was centered on analysis of the operational values underlying the larger social structural issues in health care. These issues range from determining how "consciousness" of an abstraction such as health is shaped in society and in its institutions to what is meant by the "right to health care" and how controlling institutions regard this social principle of care. Because many of the broader social–ethical problems of health care are connected with the economic capacities of the health sector, issues of the distribution and allocation of limited resources were paid particular attention by the committee.

After several months of reflecting on these broader ethical concerns, the committee concluded that the issues fall within six general categories, within which specific topics were identified for development into major analytical works. Scholarly papers on these topics were commissioned and presented in November 1973 at the Institute-sponsored Conference on Health Care and Changing Values. In addition to the major presentations, scholars were invited to prepare and present critical comments on the major topics.

The first of the six general categories is concerned with establishing the theoretical framework for ethical issues in health. To achieve this, as explained in the first paper, it is essential to relate medical conflicts of a human values character to the fundamental principles of philosophical ethics. The authors of this paper, Albert Jonsen and Andre Hellegers, see three principal theories that assist in determining how men should in fact behave, particularly in the medical care system. These three theories are a theory of virtue, a theory of duty, and a theory of common good. The authors relate medical–ethical problems to these theories and suggest the importance of shifting the emphasis of ethical analysis toward the theory of common good.

The second general category is concerned with how decisions are made in the society regarding the preciousness of life. The author of the second paper, Kenneth Arrow, focuses on government's role in shaping the way decisions are made with regard to life and death decisions. He views the government's role as one part, and not necessarily the major part, of decisions that determine the final social outcome in matters of life and death. Issues that are perhaps more significant to Arrow concern the extent to which information about medical care is disclosed by the health care provider to the patient.

The consumer's perception of health as a value is the subject of the third general category developed by the committee. Within this category, three topics were considered particularly important. The first of these, presented by David Mechanic at the conference, is the conflict of values between consumers and health providers. This analysis emphasizes the main determinants of values in the two groups and the political and cultural changes that have brought these values into conflict.

The second topic attends the emergence of what Peter Schuck of the Consumers Union calls "the medical empires," which seem to be dominating the health care field and have created a need for the organization of consumer power. He assesses the underlying values of the consumer movement and the manner in which power is distributed and shared among various segments of the population with regard to health and welfare as well as the relative effectiveness of various kinds of existing mechanisms for expressing consumer interest and power. In his paper, Schuck discusses what he considers to be several major structural defects of the health care market and recommends ways that the system should be restructured to allow greater consumer involvement in critical decisions regarding health care.

The third topic under the general category of consumer evaluation of health care is the effects that mass communication, in particular television, are having on the shaping of consumer and provider values in health. Because of medically centered TV programs like "Dr. Welby," information that was previously the province of the physician is being conveyed to the consumers of health care. On one level such information might be valuable for instructing people how to protect themselves from illness and disease, but on another level it might induce them to engage in activities that are potentially harmful or damaging. In addition, the mass media influence the expectations that people have about the goods that can be delivered in the health care system. These aspirations or demands cannot necessarily be equated with the needs of people and may in fact be contributing to both overuse of health care and discouragement about what can be achieved by modern medicine.

The fourth general category developed by the committee is concerned with professional values. More specifically, how are these values determined by both the process of selection into medical schools and the educational experience? The first topic presented deals explicitly with the selection process. When determining who should be accepted into medical, nursing, or dental schools, committees inevitably are influenced by their own perceptions of qualities important for the health professional. These values may be quite inflexible, preventing some from entering the system who could contribute significantly to the practice of medicine. John Wellington, an assistant dean involved in the selection of medical students, examines the criteria frequently used by admission committees in deciding who should be accepted into medical schools.

In their comments on Wellington's paper, Anne Kibrick and Clifton Dummett relate these factors in the selection process to their experience in nursing and dental education.

The second topic in the category of professional socialization is the effects of the educational process on the shaping of professional values. Renée Fox examines the values as they are affected both by professional education and such current societal concerns as the philosophical problems of life and death, suffering and evil, and justice and equity.

In their evaluation of organizational medical care as against fee-for-service, Michael Halberstam and Carl Stevens discuss the values that underlie alternative settings for the delivery of care. Care settings and values, the fifth broad category, introduces particularly sensitive ethical issues at a time when the health care system appears to be undergoing radical change. Halberstam maintains that the fee-for-service setting provides the best incentives for quality of care to the individual patient. He recognizes that government has an important role in medical care but not at the expense of continuing with the fee-for-service system. Stevens approaches the issue of appropriate care settings for delivery and health from the standpoint of assessing which settings respond best to consumer preferences. He founds his analysis on the proposition that access by everyone to adequate health care is a basic right.

The last general category covers the ethical problems of treating the chronically ill and the aged. Because of the limited resources being channeled into the health care system, these patients often are neglected in favor of younger people who may be returned to productive lives in the community. Jerome Kaplan, administrator of a chain of nursing homes, analyzes the value implications of social policy regarding health care to this expanding segment of the population.

The Committee on Human Value Issues in Health Care sees these broad categories as setting the theoretical framework for many specific ethical issues now arising in medical care. The topics discussed at the Conference on Health Care and Changing Values represent some—but not all—of the important specific issues in each of these categories. In no case have the ethical concerns been resolved, nor was this expected in a first effort. Instead, the presentations and comments highlight the conflicts that exist among various value systems—those of consumers, the health care providers, the society, and all as reflected in government decisions on resource allocation—and lay the groundwork for future discussions, evaluations, and research on these issues.

Laurence R. Tancredi, M.D., J.D.
Institute of Medicine

COMMITTEE ON HUMAN VALUE ISSUES IN HEALTH CARE

F. C. REDLICH, M.D., *Chairman;* Professor of Psychiatry, Yale School of Medicine

THEODORE COOPER, M.D., Director, National Heart and Lung Institute

PAUL B. CORNELY, M.D., Assistant to Executive Medical Officer, United Mine Workers Association—Welfare Retirement Fund

CLARK C. HAVIGHURST, J.D., Professor of Law, Duke University School of Law

ANDRE E. HELLEGERS, M.D., Director, Kennedy Institute for Bioethics, Georgetown University Medical School

ALBERT R. JONSEN, S.J., Ph.D., Adjunct Associate Professor of Bioethics, School of Medicine, University of California, San Francisco

JEROME KAPLAN, M.D., Adjunct Associate Professor of Sociology, The Ohio State University

ROBERT MICHELS, M.D., Associate Professor, Department of Psychiatry, College of Physicians & Surgeons, Columbia University

EDMUND D. PELLEGRINO, M.D., Chancellor of the Medical Units, Vice President for Health Affairs, University of Tennessee

PAUL RAMSEY, Ph.D., Professor of Religion, Princeton University

W. RICHARD SCOTT, Ph.D., Professor and Chairman, Department of Sociology, Stanford University

RICHARD J. ZECKHAUSER, Ph.D., Professor of Political Economy, Kennedy School of Government, Harvard University

Contents

x

I

Conceptual Foundations

Ethical problems emerging from modern medical technology have been evaluated on an issue-by-issue basis. Clearly, there is a need for a framework in medical ethics that allows for the establishment of broad principles on the basis of which individual ethical conflicts can be assessed. The papers in this category, relying to a great extent on traditional notions of philosophical ethics, take a major step toward the development of a conceptual foundation of medical ethics.

ALBERT R. JONSEN, S.J., Ph.D.
*Adjunct Associate Professor of Bioethics, School of Medicine,
University of California, San Francisco*

ANDRE E. HELLEGERS, M.D.
*Director, The Joseph and Rose Kennedy Institute for the Study of
Human Reproduction and Bioethics, Georgetown University*

Conceptual Foundations
for an Ethics of Medical Care

I

Medical ethics is currently in a muddle. Many questions are asked, but
few answers are offered. Many anxieties are aired, but few are assuaged.
Worst of all, the diversity of subjects discussed and the variety of arguments propounded makes one wonder whether there is any proper subject matter or proper methodology deserving the name, "medical
ethics."

During July 1973, when this essay was first conceived, the newspapers
carried three major, and many minor, stories about "medical ethics." In
New York, a respected physician was accused of injecting potassium
chloride into his dying cancer patient. In Chicago, the American Medical Association commented on the standards governing the ownership
of stock in pharmaceutical companies by individual physicians and by
the Association itself. In Aiken, South Carolina, three obstetricians refused, for what they called "social reasons," to deliver the babies of
welfare mothers unless the mothers submitted to sterilization. All three
stories were headlined "medical ethics." Euthanasia, financial investments, sterilization for social reasons: all three concern behavior by
physicians, all three pertain, immediately or remotely, to the practice
of medicine. This may justify use of "medical," but what justifies the
"ethics?"

3

The title of this essay, while rather grandiose, refers to the modest task of stating the propriety of denominating certain sorts of considerations as medical "ethics" or the "ethics" of medical care. This essay is designed as a road map for this conference on Health Care and Changing Values. It will, hopefully, provide to its participants the main features of the topography of that ancient realm of the mind called ethics, through which modern medicine must travel.

Popularly, ethics seems to mean any body of prescriptions and prohibitions, do's and don'ts, that people consider to carry uncommon weight in their lives. When their lives are deeply involved in certain activities, ethics can refer to the rules that guide those activities. The *Lexicon* of the Sydenham Society[1] defined "ethics, medical" as "the laws of the duties of medical men to the public, to each other and to themselves with regard to the exercise of their profession. In this purview, euthanasia, financial investments in drugs, and sterilization for social reasons obviously belong to the family of ethics.

However, ethics, at least for most ethicians, means much more than a body of prescriptions and prohibitions. Ethics means the critical assessment and reconstruction of such bodies in the context of a comprehensive theory of human morality. By "morality" the present authors mean the actual behavior of human beings, involving judgments, actions, and attitudes, constructed around rationally conceived and effectively based norms whereby that behavior can be judged right or wrong and around values whereby states effected by that behavior are judged good or bad. By "ethics" the authors mean an academic discipline, a systematic set of propositions that constitute the intellectual instruments for the analysis of morality.

This discipline seeks to elucidate how the norms and values are established and perceived and how the actions are justified. It inquires how one argues or should argue from norms and facts to decisions. It tries to show how values and norms are related to purposes and results. To accomplish such analyses, a theory must be elaborated, within which these elements are comprehensively described and coherently articulated. It provides, when rightly done, not only a descriptive discipline of morality, but a normative one as well, for its analysis purports to reveal the roots of obligation and value appreciation, thereby exposing not how men do *in fact* behave, but how *in principle* they should behave. Ethics, then, is the normative discipline of morality.[2]

An adequate ethics would be a theoretical system capable of suggesting some answers to the sorts of questions arising about morality. The authors believe that since there are at least three sorts of questions, an adequate ethics would consist of at least three principal theories, which we call, in reverence to the traditions of the discipline, the theory of virtue, the theory of duties, and the theory of the common good.

In response to questions like, "What sort of person can rightly be called a morally good man?," the theory of virtue will expatiate on the character of moral agents, like attitudes, habits, affections, and motives. In response to questions like, "What ought I to do in this situation?," the theory of action will discuss the nature of action, its objectives, goals, intentions, consequences, and conditions for freedom, and voluntariness. In response to questions like, "What is the best form of human society?," the theory of common good seeks to understand not the good man alone nor his right actions but the social institutions that make and are made by good men acting rightly.

Medical ethics is, we believe, a species of the genus *Ethics*. It should, then, be constructed out of the three essential theories of ethics. In this essay we contend that, traditionally, medical ethics has dwelt mostly within two of those three theories, namely, the theories of virtue and of duty. Both of these theories, while in need of refurbishing and modernization, remain indispensable to medical ethics. But the nature of contemporary medicine demands that they be complemented by the third essential theory—the common good. We shall review two traditional forms of medical ethics, indicating their relationship to the classical ethical theories. We shall then state the condition of modern medicine that calls for the theory of the common good. We suggest that this does not merely add an appendix to medical ethics but that it can be the source of a new concept of the discipline that can profoundly affect the more traditional theories of virtue and duty.

II

The term "medical ethics" is frequently applied to those statements of professional standards that are set forth in "codes." There are many such codes, but we shall select the *Ethical Principles of the American Medical Association* as a paradigm. We believe that our analysis applies generally to what is sometimes called "code ethics."[3]

The AMA code, adopted in 1847 and revised four times (1903, 1912, 1947, 1955), now consists of ten sections in which such subjects as consultations and precedence, scientific competence, professional courtesy, cooperation with nonphysician health personnel, solicitation of patients, fees, conditions of practice, and confidentiality are treated. Some of these subjects are discussed at length but, for the most part, the principles are succinctly expressed. For example, "It is unethical . . . for a physician to provide or prescribe unnecessary services or unnecessary

ancillary facilities" (Section 4). "The acceptance of rebates on appli-
ances and prescriptions or of commissions from those who aid in the
care of patients is unethical" (Section 7). The preamble states that
"these principles . . . are not immutable laws to govern the physician,
for the ethical practitioner needs no such laws; rather they are standards
by which he may determine the propriety of his own conduct." The
substance of the code, which comes to 67 pages in its latest edition,
consists of these standards that serve to "standardize" the more common transactions, social and economic, between physicians, between
physicians and patients, and between physicians and third parties, such
as legal authorities, insurance providers, and the press. We call these
standards "pragmatic directions."[4]

Interspersed among these pragmatic directions are occasional exhortations to cultivate certain virtues considered proper to the physician. A
citation from the Hippocratic literature opens Section 1: The physician
"should be modest, sober, patient, prompt to do his whole duty without anxiety; pious without going so far as superstition, conducting himself with propriety in his profession and in all the actions of his life."
Physicians are expected, notes Section 2, "in their relationship with patients, with colleagues and with the public, to maintain under God, as
they have down the ages, the most inflexible standards of personal
honor." At various points, the virtues of fearlessness, benevolence, pa-
tience, and delicacy are recommended. The Preamble notes that, while
"interpretation of these principles by an appropriate authority will be
required at times . . . as a rule . . . the physician who is capable, honest,
decent, courteous, vigilant, and an observer of the Golden Rule, and
who conducts his affairs in the light of his own conscientious interpretation of these principles will find no difficulty in the discharge of his
professional obligations."[5]

Pragmatic standards for common transactions predominate; exhortations to virtue are sparse and, one might cynically say, perfunctory. The
predominance of the pragmatic directions has prompted many to refer
to the codes as an "etiquette" rather than an "ethic." One of the first
codes is *Decorum,* more literally the *Etiquette,* found in the Hippocratic
corpus; during the nineteenth century medical codes were frequently
called "etiquettes." Dr. Chauncey Leake[6] writes in the preface to his
edition of *Percival's Medical Ethics,* which served as exemplar for the
early A M A codes:

The term "medical ethics" introduced by Percival is a misnomer. Based on Greek
traditions of good taste . . . it refers chiefly to the rules of etiquette developed in
the profession to regulate the professional contacts of its members with each

other . . . medical etiquette is concerned with the conduct of physicians toward each other and embodies the tenets of professional courtesy. Medical ethics should be concerned with the ultimate consequences of the conduct of physicians toward their individual patients, and toward society as a whole, and it should include consideration of the will and motive behind this conduct.

The concept of etiquette is enticing because it sidesteps the pitfalls of having to define morality. An etiquette is a set of conventional rules, usually quite arbitrary, that reflect behavior in polite society. With obvious repugnance, but impeccable *noblesse oblige,* Lord Chesterfield admonished his son, "Without hesitation, kiss the Pope's slipper or whatever else the etiquette of that court requires." An etiquette is hardly susceptible to ethical analysis, for it is seldom possible or profitable to attempt to justify its precepts, which are either simply "just done" or devised with a clear view to avoiding arguments about precedence, confusion over procedures, etc.

Etiquette is then a set of rules for external behavior that may be presumed to come from an internally virtuous man. Obviously, the external behavior may not reflect the internal man. Yet this is not sufficient to become cynical about the rules of etiquette. At best, they will truly reflect virtue. At worst, they are likely to keep the individual on his *qui vive.*

However, the word "etiquette" is a misleading discription of the codes. They do consist predominantly of pragmatic and arbitrary standards of behavior. But the sparse, almost perfunctory, exhortations to virtue in the modern codes are the faded tokens of their ancestry as ethics. The immediate progenitor of the American codes, Percival's *Medical Ethics*, is a treatise on the "Gentleman Physician." In the eighteenth century, "gentleman" denoted much more than a polite, gracious, considerate man with *savoir faire.* It was a synonym for the virtuous man. A century earlier, Isaac Walton[7] had written, "I would rather prove myself a Gentleman, by being learned and humble, valiant and inoffensive, virtuous and communicable than by a fond ostentation of riches." The long tradition of medicine, from the Hippocratic corpus through the Admonita and Epistulae of the Middle Ages, the *Medicus Politicus* of the Renaissance and the eighteenth century treatises on *Duties* and *Character of the Physician* is replete with exhortations to virtues proper to those who would practice medicine. This whole tradition mingles these exhortations with pragmatic directions about bedside manners, consultations, and fees; but the vision of the "upright man instructed in the art of healing" predominates.

These exhortations to virtue tend to dwindle, almost disappear, in more recent codes. Apparently, they seem to some superfluous, for they

belabor the obvious. To others, they seem futile, for they cannot be enforced. Again, they seem vacuous, for they offer no practical guidance
for action. Finally, they might seem embarrassing, for they smack of
posturing for public consumption.

However, we suggest that these exhortations to virtue constitute the
heart of code ethics. Indeed, they are the justification for calling the
codes "ethics" at all. They give to the pragmatic directions a moral substance without which they are, indeed, merely etiquettes. Their dis-
appearance in current codes is not merely a mildly deplorable withering
of a charming, but rather quaint, affirmation of the good, the true, and
the beautiful. It reflects fundamental uncertainty about the character
desired in the person who would practice medicine.

The theory of virtue is a treatise about moral character. It has always
been recognized that moral judgments bear not only on the rightness or
wrongness of discrete actions but also upon the goodness or badness of
rather fixed states of persons who perform actions. Although "virtue"
and "vice" are words with Victorian tone, great ethicists from Aristotle
through Kant to Hartmann have used them to describe rationally intended, effectively rooted attitudes whereby persons consistently seem
to incline toward certain sorts of behavior. Terms such as benevolence,
honesty, trustworthiness, and sobriety described particular modes of
these states of character.[8]

The great ethicists have always noted that while a spectrum of virtues
should adorn the good man, particular dispositions were proper to certain roles: courage to the soldier, fairness to the judge, discretion to the
ruler. A theory of virtue in medical ethics must explore that disposition
most proper to the relationship between physician and patient—trust.

The patient approaching the physician suffers from more than his illness; he suffers from significant social disadvantages. He enters a mysterious domain, where arcane knowledge and rare skills rule. He is ner-
vous, fearful, and perhaps even terrified. He places himself in the hands
of a fallible human being. The novelist Kurt Vonnegut writes sardon-
ically in *Goodbye, Mr. Rosewater,* "The most exquisite pleasure in the
practice of medicine comes from nudging a layman in the direction of
terror, then bringing him back to safety again." The potential for such
sadism, which does lie within any physician's power, must be countered
by the bond of trust. This bond—or as Paul Ramsey aptly titles it, covenant—arises from more than a contract; it is nourished by the evident
trustworthiness of the physician.[9]

Codes do not create virtue. Their pragmatic directions establish certain regularities of procedure that elicit public confidence. But confidence elicited is fulfilled and confirmed only in the personal relation-

ship that Pedro Lain Entralgo[10] calls "the medical friendship," a delicate alliance that must simultaneously encourage confidence and discourage dependency. The apparent fading of this friendship, under the cold exigencies of scientific skill, technical expertise, harried services, and, frankly, cupidity, has been blamed by many as the major cause of the "dehumanization" of care.

In sum, code ethics, as they now exist, might be called the archeological ruins of a doctrine of medical virtue. The codes are, in their present form, collections of pragmatic directions that mark the outer walls of the physician–patient covenant. Their inspiration and the inner confirmation of this covenant require the virtue of trustworthiness. Restoration of exhortations to virtue in the codes would not, of course, ensure the actual existence of virtue in physicians. This comes from the manner in which the profession selects and socializes its members, from exemplarity, and from exercise. Nonetheless, the theory of virtue in medical ethics requires serious reflection on the virtues proper to the physician and on the obstacles to their realization in contemporary settings and in contemporary men. Multiplication of codes, regulations, statutes, and standards, particularly if they are expected to be self-enforcing, as are most professional codes, is futile unless those to whom they are addressed comprehend and possess the virtues of the physician.

III

Virtue is the inner spirit of morality; action is its outer manifestation. The virtuous physician without skill may be comfort, but cold comfort, to one seeking cure. Medicine is a practical science: theory and experience evoked in clinical decision and action. Medical ethics, then, must be as concerned about the rightness of acts as about the goodness of the agent. A theory of virtue is a necessary, but not sufficient, part of medical ethics.

Ethics provides a second complementary theory, often called theory of duty, that defines the criteria whereby actions are judged right or wrong. It analyzes the relationship between intentions and consequences, motivations and circumstances. It studies the conditions of freedom and responsibility underlying imputation of guilt and innocence.

The need for an ethical analysis of actions comprising clinical practice is demonstrated in daily news articles on euthanasia, transplantation, and experimental trials. Serious efforts have been made to provide such an analysis. Jewish medical ethics is predominantly a doctrine of duties. Joseph Fletcher's pioneer work in medical ethics applies utilitarian theory of action to clinical acts. The present authors wish to use as an example the natural law theory of duties as it is found in Roman Catholic medical ethics. A volume on medical ethics in the Catholic tradition contains lengthy discussions of specific clinical actions such as euthanasia, abortion, transplantation, obstetrical techniques, and cosmetic surgery. Pope Pius XII had intense interest in questions of medical ethics and his frequent statements, delivered before distinguished medical societies, lent authoritative tone to the theologians' efforts.[11]

The medical ethics of this tradition is, in a very proper sense, a doctrine of duties. Medical interventions and procedures are analyzed in light of an explicitly formulated ethical system of principles and argumentation that can be broadly described as natural law.

The first affirmation of the system is that God has dominion over his creation, the human body, while man is granted a derived dominion over his body that he must exercise in view of the divinely appointed finality of his body and its functions. Because he is ultimately not his own, man has an obligation to preserve his life and health. Any mutilation of his body is an abuse of the derived dominion, unless that mutilation contributes to the good of the whole body. This affirmation, entitled the principle of totality, is the proximate governing principle of Catholic medical ethics.[12]

Other carefully defined principles allow the Catholic moral theologian to thread a precise path through the complexities of medical procedures. The principle of double effect can be invoked when an intervention involves the problem of finding moral justification for both the physical evil of mutilation and some other evil such as the death of a fetus removed in a salpingectomy done for ectopic pregnancy. The distinction between ordinary and extraordinary means of sustaining life, elaborated within the context of the principles of divine dominion and totality, provide to physician and patient thoughtfully defined ethical grounds for making painful ultimate decision about life and death.[13]

The theory of duty elaborated in Roman Catholic ethics describes an act in terms of (1) the *object,* that is, the objective design of the act and its immediate consequences; (2) the *end,* that is, the intention of the agent; and (3) the *circumstances,* that is, time, place, office, and other relevant concrete conditions of the act. In this approach, all three elements of an act must be right before the act is considered objectively moral. Criteria for evaluating the rightness of the action and its elements are such principles as divine and derived dominion and, more directly, the principle of totality.

In this scheme, a surgical intervention in the case of an ectopic pregnancy, described in terms of its objective, might be called a salpingectomy. The circumstances are advanced erosion of the fallopian tube, the presence of a fetus, and the absence of any therapeutic possibilities other than radical resection. The surgeon intends the removal of the eroding tube and tolerates the inevitable death of the developing fetus. The act would be judged morally right, for in its object, in the intention of the surgeon, and in the given circumstances, it effects the restoration of the integrity of the patient. The abortion is neither intended nor is it the principal objective of the act. It is, in the technical language of this school, an "indirect" abortion.

The purpose of this description and evaluation of actions is to enable the agent to discern actions that are morally right from those that are morally wrong. Morally right actions must or may be performed. Morally wrong action must be avoided. Thus, this doctrine of duties contains a doctrine of obligation, grounded in the principle of divine and derived dominion, which distinguishes between obligatory, permissible, and forbidden actions. There is an absolute moral obligation to refrain from morally wrong acts and a conditional moral obligation to perform right acts. The purpose of the theory of duties is to guarantee the moral rectitude of medical intervention. Almost every medical procedure of diagnosis and therapy requires an invasion of the sphere of the patient's physical and psychological independence.

Two points are particularly noteworthy about this example of a theory of duties. First, the principle of totality is defined in terms of the integrity of the *physical* organism of an individual person. Efforts have been made, from time to time, to extend its range to *social* or *interpersonal* totality, but these have never been enthusiastically adopted. Thus, early discussions of homographs, such as renal transplants, tended to disapproval because of the nonbeneficial mutilation of the donor. The suggestion that the bond of charity could thereby be strengthened between donor and recipient won little favor and the transplantation was finally justified on grounds more consonant with traditional doctrine of totality, namely that donation of one of paired organs did not absolutely impair functional integrity. Similarly, attempts to defend contraception by means other than periodic abstinence on the basis that hormonal alteration or tubal ligation would, ultimately, improve the psychological and physical well-being of a woman or benefit the total family situation were met with disfavor. The principle of totality remains tightly linked to physical integrity of single persons, rather than their psychological or social integrity.[14]

This problem has been framed in terms of the traditional Roman Catholic use of the principle of totality. However, it is not a problem unique to that particular form of the theory of duties. Most efforts to formulate a theory of duties, in particular, those influenced by Kantian ethics, have a tendency to thrust the single act or the isolated agent onto center stage and leave the interrelationships of acts and agents in the shadows.

Second, any theory of duties issues prescriptions, prohibitions, and permissions. The physician committed to this moral reasoning must refrain from prohibited interventions. Even though certain concessions are made for unwilling and compelled cooperation in immoral acts, the physician's moral duty is quite clear. Direct abortion, direct sterilization, positive euthanasia are clearly forbidden. Refusal to perform these actions assures the moral integrity of the physician's conscience. However, from the point of view of those who do not share the physician's conscience, his refusal to perform an act is perceived as denial of a benefit to the petitioner. While any single petitioner might seek that benefit elsewhere, could it be that the conscientiously acting physician, by accumulation of his decisions and by his efforts to effect public policy in favor of his conscience, might impede some public good? And what if all physicians were of identical mind on the issue and all patients of opposite mind?[15]

Both of these problems, the restriction of the principle of totality to the *physical* integrity of single persons and the possibility of disagreement between adherents of this theory of duty and the possible demands of a broader public, suggest that a theory of duties, while necessary, may not be sufficient for adequate ethics. To the extent that such theories concentrate on discreet acts and individual intentions, they neglect the ethical issues arising from the intersection of multiple actions in institutions and society. Thus, an adequate ethics calls for an explicit reflection on the morality of institutions and on the relationship, and possible clash, between social values and individual values. Classical ethics has made such a reflection. It can be conveniently called a theory of the common good.

IV

The ethical theories of virtue and of duty are complemented by a theory of the common good. A theory of the common good seeks to elucidate the nature of human communities. These are the institutional forms that human actions create and human virtues sustain and, in their turn, should become the objective conditions nurturing virtue and sustaining action. This theory should treat two principal questions: First, what is the "common" good or goods? Second, how should they be distributed? The first question inquires about the goods and values that are necessary for individuals and for the society. In the present context, "health and health care" might be discussed as common goods. This is a crucial discussion for ethics of medical care. However, the second question, properly called the problem of social justice, will be the problem to which we shall attend in the remainder of this paper.[16]

Before considering this problem, it is important to realize that the theory of the common good is not merely a separate third chapter of ethical concepts that should be glanced at from time to time whenever a "social question" arises. Properly conceived, the theory of the common good is a third dimension in which virtues and actions take on a depth and tone that they do not have in isolation. The very meaning of a virtue or an action depends on its social or institutional setting. For example, lying and deception can be viewed and analyzed as a private interaction between two individuals, as in the recent drama "Sleuth." But when they are considered within the structures of public trust, authority and responsibility that constitute an institution, for example government, quite different issues arise. In what sense, for example, does the problem of National Defense Security morally qualify an act of deception? And, analogously, would a National Health Security be sufficient warrant to deceive patients, or experimental subjects, about the nature of what was being done to them?

It must be clear that considerations of the common good do not *ipso facto* override considerations of individual rectitude of action. Rather, the purpose of the doctrine of the common good is to consider how conflicts may be avoided, reconciled or, more importantly, how the institutional structure can be designed so as to avoid conflict, how to reconcile discord, and how to compensate unjust harm.

There is little or nothing that can be identified as a doctrine of the common good in contemporary ethics of medical care. There is, of course, a conviction on the part of most professionals that they do serve the common good in a significant way. Yet there is, further, a contention on the part of many professionals that the practice of medicine involves significant social injustices. The authors do not intend to argue either conviction or contention. Neither of them, however valid, constitutes a theory of the common good. Such a theory must consist of a comprehensive description of the exigencies of medical care and the institutional forms that serve these exigencies at present. It must propose criteria whereby these institutional forms can be analyzed and criticized, not only in terms of the exigencies of care, but in light of certain exigencies of human moral existence. These latter exigencies, when seen in the light of social institutions, have been most clearly expressed by the great ethicists in terms of a doctrine of justice.

Justice, while a virtue, or personal characteristic, of individuals, is

above all the "virtue" of institutions.[17] An institution may be judged
ethically "good" if it exhibits in its organizational structure and in its
procedures the characteristics of justice. The establishment of a just society, for the great ethicists, required not merely the assembling of many
just men but the design of social institutions, laws, policies, and economics in which the habits, inclinations, and intentions of just men
could be realized in public policy and practice. It is curious that while
we often speak of just laws, just courts, just taxes, just contracts, we do
not often speak of just medicine.

If, however, justice is pre-eminently the virtue of institutions, our
failure to apply the criteria of justice to medicine may result from our
failure to recognize that medicine has become, in fact, an institution.
Medicine has, in recent years, evolved from a practice, a private technical interaction between two parties, through a profession, a socially coherent, publicly recognized group that defines the conditions under
which those private transactions take place, to an institution.[18]

By an institution, we mean a complex interaction of professionals,
paraprofessionals, and the public, on informational, economic, and occupational levels, in identifiable physical environments, whose coordinated
decisions and actions have magnified public impact and is recognized culturally and legally as affecting the public welfare in a significant way.
Law enforcement, the free market, religion, higher education are institutions in this broad sense.

Just as the free market once consisted simply of a solo producer ex-
changing his product for consideration by a single buyer (and still, in
essence, consists of that) so the medical transaction once was, and still
essentially is, a solo physician diagnosing and treating a single patient.
But that essential transaction has gradually been surrounded by the
indispensable cooperation of other people, by accessory producers, by
physical environments, by customary and legal prescriptions. The face-
to-face decisions made in the private transaction have magnified public
impact since they now engage the attention of multiple other parties,
nurses, druggists, insurance carriers, etc. The coordinated decisions and
actions of the institutions have magnified public impact because accepted
forms of diagnosis and treatment, research, and prevention engage the
manufacture of products, the construction of buildings, and the enact-
ment of laws.

Modern medicine, then, is an institution that incorporates a profession
that practices a technique and an art. The practice remains, indeed, at
the heart of the institution, but it cannot be adequately performed or
understood outside of it. Doctrines of virtue and action supply ideals
and norms and pragmatic directions for the profession and for the prac-

titioner; a doctrine of the common good must be added to provide an ethics for the institution.

It must be emphasized again that a doctrine of the common good does not supplant the other two modes of ethical analysis. All three doctrines are required for an adequate ethics. The practice of medicine, once conceived as the relief of the suffering of one person by another properly qualified person, was adequately analyzed in ethical terms by the two doctrines of virtue and of duty. Today, however, the institutionalization of practice and profession calls for an institutional ethic. On the other hand, the possibility that misjudgments about the ethical exigencies of virtue and duty might be propagated throughout the institution, still demands a careful ethical scrutiny of quality of individual character and rectitude of single actions.

Institutions are vehicles for the distribution of the benefits and burdens of social life, and it is the function of the principles of justice to determine fair and equitable assignment of rights and duties and fair and equitable distribution of benefits and burdens.[19]

An institution possesses an identity, an organization, and resources that enable activities performed by its members to have an extensivity and perpetuity that they otherwise could not have. By extensivity, we mean that activities can have effects on a broad contemporary population. By perpetuity, we mean that they can be prolonged in time by affecting future populations. It may be argued that medical actions always factually had effects that fulfilled these definitions of extensivity and perpetuity. However, the development of epidemiology and biostatistics has made the dimensions of this extensivity and perpetuity vividly evident in contemporary medicine.

Only the institutional form provides the exchange of information, the continuity and cooperation, the designation of qualified participants and the utilization of physical and financial resources to support extensivity and perpetuity. A profession may have an identity based on possession of similar knowledge and techniques and may cooperate to share and assure possession of them, but a professional, as such, did not deliberately utilize information and resources to effect extensivity and perpetuity. Medicine has, in the last 100 years, by virtue of certain scientific and technical accomplishments, evolved from a profession with knowledge of limited effects in time and space to an institution with knowledge of extensive and perpetuated effects.

The most pressing ethical issues of modern medicine arise from the potential for extensivity and perpetuity inherent in its new institutional status. At one time a medical intervention was perceived as a transaction between a physician and a patient. The benefits and the costs were, for the most part, thought to be quite strictly limited to that transaction. Today, benefits and costs are known to be distributed broadly in many ways. Financial costs of medical research and education are borne by an extensive public. Costs of care are borne by insurance purchasers and tax payments. Resource allocation distributes benefits of research to certain afflicted populations at a cost to others. Certain treatment modalities impose burdens on those other than the treated. The effects of certain medical interventions can be perpetuated into future generations, for example, the burden of heredity of certain genetic diseases such as diabetes and hemophilia. Formerly, these patients often did not live long enough to reproduce and hence the defective gene was eliminated from the pool. Techniques for genetic diagnosis and control are directed toward modification of inheritable characteristics.

Where benefits and burdens can be so distributed, the problem of justice arises. Some who will benefit will not bear costs; some who will bear costs will not benefit. When this situation depends not on chance or accident but on planned and conscious decisions about the structure of the institution, it is necessary to ask, "What justifies the imposition of a burden, a cost, a risk, on any single individual?" Why should one individual benefit at the apparent cost to another? These are the questions at the heart of each of the serious ethical issues of medicine as they are of justice.

The problem of access to medical care is the most obvious field for the application of the concept of justice. This appears to be, on its face, a problem of distributive justice. A subset of this problem is the allocation of scarce resources, such as renal dialysis. However, many other problems that are not usually considered in terms of justice involve deliberate distribution of costs and benefits. Randomized clinical trials, particularly when one of the alternatives is a proven therapeutic agent, involves costs without compensating benefit to certain individuals. An increasing number of therapeutic modalities lay burdens of risk on others than the beneficiaries such as drugs administered to pregnant mothers. In the near future, nuclear-powered artificial hearts—and, perhaps in the further, but real future, DNA therapy through viral agents— will have this effect. The entire realm of genetic control, whether it utilizes elimination of births or elimination of defective genomes, raises the question of justice to future generations. Psychosurgery and psychoactive drug therapy, while they may be conceived as interventions beneficial to the individual, have the potential to impose stringent limitations on that individual's freedom from which others may benefit socially, politically, and economically. The classical problem of euthanasia is aggravated by the institutionally supported potential for prolonging dying at great cost, emotional and financial, to survivors.

JONSEN & HELLEGERS / Conceptual Foundations

Finally, the nagging, but ill-defined, problem of dehumanization of medical care may obtain clarity within the concepts of justice. The great jurisprudent, Georgio del Vecchio, wrote, "The ideal criteria of justice. . . demand the equal and perfect recognition . . . of the quality or personality in oneself as in all others for all possible interactions among several subjects."[20] Dehumanization is, at bottom, unequal and imperfect recognition of the quality of personality, an entity most difficult to quantitate under the criteria required for a just theory of the common good.

Many of the moral problems of medicine appear to be problems of justice. Many of the old problems of medicine, placed in the modern setting, seem to have been transmuted from problems of virtue or duty, into problems of justice. Yet, the theories of justice long familiar to ethics have not been fully mined for their relevance to the moral problems of medicine. The authors are not so naïve as to suppose that the ancient conflicts of individual versus institution and personal duty versus social good will be resolved by yet another invocation of the doctrine of justice. Still, to the extent that considerations of justice contribute to the design of institutions of medicine and to policies governing its practice, many moral problems may be either avoided or ameliorated.

The traditional definition of justice is "giving to each his due." The problem of justice is defining what is "due" to each. This is done, first, by recognizing that the "each" of the definition is both everyman (with a basic humanness shared by all), and the single person, different in ability, merit, and need from all others. Justice thus requires an impartiality resting on the fundamental similarity of all persons and an equity that allows for different treatment justified by different conditions of ability and merit. Effecting justice becomes the continual process of critical scrutiny of the reasons proposed for different treatment of persons. This scrutiny must measure particular considerations against universal characteristics, the claims of ability, merit, and need against the claims of equality of liberty, consideration, and treatment. So stated, the conundrum is not vastly different than the problem of reconciling the age-old precept to give to each according to his need with that of giving to each according to his merit.[21]

The requirements of a theory of justice are not satisfied by the proposition that an act or institution is ethically justified when it produces the "greater good for the greater number." This thesis, called Utilitarianism, has been much disputed by ethicists and its inherent defects revealed. Nonetheless, it appears to be the dominant ethic for many policymakers in scientific medicine.[22] The problem of the lesser number, disadvantaged for the sake of the greater, remains unsolved.

In medicine, this problem can be particularly pressing, for traditionally medicine has favored the good of individuals, while the law has favored the common good. Today, the realization of extensivity and perpetuity of modern medicine place many medical interventions directly within the sphere of the common good. Whether the problems thus raised can be "justly" solved depends on how deeply modern medical practitioners and policymakers reflect on the profound moral dilemmas and theses of the theory of justice. They must refuse to relax those dilemmas either by a facile appeal to the "inestimable social benefits of medicine," on the one hand, or to the "inviolable individual rights of patient or practitioner," on the other. Neither assertion can stand alone; both must be comprehended within an adequate theory of justice. Above all, public policy relative to the shape of institutions, the flow of money and people through them, the regulation of their powers, and vigilance over their performance must be devised with the requirements of justice foremost in mind.

Several final points should be made about "just" medicine. First, the cynical often say, "Ethics is no more than the simulation of good intentions." Doctrines of virtue, because virtue can be so easily simulated by scoundrels, are most susceptible to this pessimistic criticism. Doctrines of duty can take refuge in excuses and protestations of ignorance. But doctrines of justice rest on different ground. Their concern is the fair and equitable structure and function of institutions. In this theory of ethics, we are concerned about the institutional forms that set up problems in certain ways and restrict or expand the alternatives for their solution. We do not limit our attention to good intentions alone or to the outcome of single actions. We are concerned about the assignment of rights and duties, the design of offices and tasks, the currents of resources, and support that can best eliminate problems of unfair distribution of burdens and benefits and can best enable virtuous character and right action.

Second, the advent of institutions heralds the appearance of laws. Medicine has always been governed, to a greater or lesser degree, by civil law. Medicine has seldom been happy under that governance. "Just" medicine raises the menacing threat of medical practice cribbed, cabined, and confined by statute and regulation. This need not necessarily be the case. Justice and law are not synonymous. A theory of justice is concerned basically with the design of institutions. Institutional design can be created and effected by innumerable agencies other than the state. The profession, related professions and industries, interested and impartial groups, organized and unorganized consumers can, if allowed and enabled, assist in institutional design. However, to the extent that civil law and regulations are advisable, a doctrine of justice is indispensable. It alone can provide the vision of just and equitable distribution that the enacted law should, imperfectly, piecemeal, but steadily, seek to realize.

Without a doctrine of just medicine, laws and regulations will be haphazard, aimless, and for this reason frustrating to professional and consumer alike.

In conclusion, then, the thesis of this essay might be restated in terms of an ancient Roman definition of the entire field of ethics: *Honeste vivere, nemini laedere, suum cuique tribuere*—live uprightly, hurt no one, give to each his due. The authors have attempted to state the conceptual foundations for an ethics of medical care under similar titles. It must consist, they maintain, of three essential theories of ethics applied to the unique enterprise of medicine and health care. The theory of virtue concerns those dispositions and qualities that define uprightness of life for those who practice medicine and engage in care. The theory of duties concerns criteria that enable the practitioner to recognize acts that ultimately harm those who seek his help. The theory of justice concerns the establishment of fair and equitable institutions for the practice of medicine and the provision of care. It is the authors' impression that in discussions of medical ethics these questions are often jumbled, that their theoretical bases are unrecognized, and that their intellectual history is unknown. They contend that fruitful progress might be made if future discussions acknowledge the distinction and the interrelation of these three theories of ethics and undertake their careful application to the difficult moral problems of modern medicine. This will make, they hope, for better medicine, for better ethics, and for a better ethics for medical care.

REFERENCES AND NOTES

1. Lexicon of Medicine and Applied Sciences. London, The Sydenham Society, 1881–1889.
2. Frankena W: Ethics. Englewood Cliffs, Prentice-Hall, 1963, pp 1–10.
   Wallace G and Walker A (ed): The Definition of Morality. London, Methuen, 1970.
3. Opinions and Reports of the Judicial Council. Chicago, American Medical Association, 1969. On the ethical nature of codes, see Veatch R: Medical ethics: professional or universal? Harvard Theolog Rev, 65: 531–559, 1972. On the history of the AMA code, see Konold D: A History of American Medical Ethics. Madison, University of Wisconsin, 1962.
4. Our intention is to give an *ethical* analysis of codes. A sociological analysis can be found in Freidson E: The Profession of Medicine. New York, Dodd-Mead, 1970.
5. This echoes an early critique of the AMA code: "Were the great rule of Christian ethics present to the mind of the physician, 'do unto others as ye would that they would should do unto you,' there would be but little necessity for societal codes." Duglison R: On the present state of medicine in the United States. Br Foreign Med Rev 3: 227, 1837.
6. Leake C: Percival's Medical Ethics. Baltimore, Williams & Wilkins, 1927, pp 1–2;

Leake C: Theories of ethics and medical practice. J Am Med Assoc 208: 842–847, 1969. On the term "etiquette," see Jones WHS: The Doctor's Oath. Cambridge, University Press, 1924; and Ancient medical etiquette, Hippocrates II. Cambridge, University Press, 1923.

7. Compleat Angler 1:13, 1653. See King LS: The Medical World of the Eighteenth Century. Chicago, University of Chicago Press, 1958, p 256.
8. Klubertanz G: Habits and Virtues. New York, Appleton, Century, Crofts, 1965.
9. Ramsey P: Patient as Person. New Haven, Yale University Press, 1970, preface.
10. Lain Entralgo P: Doctor and Patient. New York, McGraw-Hill, 1969.
11. Pius XII: The Human Body. Boston, St. Paul Press, 1960. See Healy E: Medical Ethics. Chicago, Loyola Press, 1959; Kelly G: Medico-Moral Problems. St. Louis, Catholic Hospital Association, 1958; Paquin J: Morale et Médecine. Montreal, L'Immaculee-Conception, 1960.
12. Aquinas T: Summa Theologica II–II, q. 65, a.1.
13. Kelly G: On the duty of using artifical means to preserve life, Theolog Stud 11: 203–220, 1950; 12: 550–556, 1951.
14. Nolan M: Principle of totality in moral theology, Absolutes in Moral Theology. Edited by C Curran. Washington, Corpus, 1968; Curran C: Medicine and Morals. Washington, Corpus, 1970.
15. This problem is reflected in the debate over the Code of the Catholic Hospital Association. See Catholic hospital ethics: report of the Commission on Ethical Directions for Catholic Hospitals. Linacre Q 39, Nov 1972; Brennan J: Quicksands of compromise. Reich W: Policy vs. ethics. McCormick R: Not what the Catholic hospitals ordered. Linacre Q 39, Feb 1972.
16. Our use of the terms "common good" and "social justice" may be elucidated by the following: "Social justice [is] the equal treatment of all persons except as inequality is required by relevant, that is, just-making, considerations . . . it takes equality of treatment to be a *prima facie* requirement of justice, but allows that it may on occasion be overruled by other principles of justice . . . the differences in treatment are not justified simply by arguing that they are conducive to the general good life, but by arguing that they are required for the good lives of the individuals concerned. It is not as if one must first look to see how the general good is best subserved and only then can tell what treatment of individuals is just. Justice entails the presence of equal *prima facie* rights prior to any consideration of utility." Frankena W: The concept of social justice, Social Justice. Edited by R Brandt. Englewood Cliffs, Prentice-Hall, 1962, pp 13, 15.
17. Rawls J: Theory of Justice. Cambridge, Harvard University Press, 1971, Ch 2.
18. Mechanic D: Medical Sociology. Glencoe, Free Press, 1968, Ch 10–11.
19. Rawls: *op. cit.*, p 55.
20. del Vecchio G: Justice. Edinburgh, University Press, 1952, p 116.
21. del Vecchio G: *op. cit.;* Perelman C: Justice. New York, Random House, 1967; Friedrick, C,Chapman J (ed): Nomos VI: Justice. New York, Atherton Press, 1963.
22. ". . .the dicta of that school [Utilitarianism] . . . are still used as part of the language of men of science." Singer C, Underwood EA: A Short History of Medicine. New York, Oxford Press, 1962, p 208. For critique of Utilitarianism, see, among others, Lyons D: Forms and Limits of Utilitarianism. Oxford, Clarendon Press, 1965.

PAUL RAMSEY, Ph.D.
Professor of Religion, Princeton University

Commentary

I must first indicate my extensive agreement with Jonsen/Hellegers (J/H) concerning the need for general ethical analysis as the framework for discussing any problems in medical ethics and with the clear and weighty things they have said on that subject. For a reason our authors do not state, the overriding need is to enliven and articulate the genus *Ethics* in which to locate medical ethics. If there are moral dilemmas in modern medicine, if, as some would say, there is a moral crisis in the ethics of the medical profession, this does not result from recent triumphs in medical research or the great promise and grave risks stemming from medical technology. The fundamental reason is the continuing moral crisis in modern culture that generally reverberates throughout all professions. It can no longer be assumed in the human community that we are agreed on moral action guides, the practice of virtue, the premises and principles of the highest, most humane, most bracing ethics, or what a moral agent owes to anyone who bears a human countenance. In the present day, nonutilitarian requirements in morality are eroded in society generally and can no longer be counted on silently to inform the physician's conscience. As a result, physicians and medical ethics generally must become more literate and establish explicit communication with the writings and reflections of ethicists. That conclusion I regret, since medical

21

ethics worked better when moral consensus was intact and there was less need for ethical reflection and analysis.

Nevertheless, I am not altogether persuaded by J/H that exhortations to virtue constitute the heart of code ethics. Is it not equally evident that an ethics of action or duties constitutes the heart of code ethics? Perhaps I ought instead to say that our authors have not demonstrated more than a provisional distinction between character and deeds and that in this they faithfully record the nature of moral experience.

Of course, with the aid of Luther one can resolve all good works into some condition of the moral agent: Good works do not make a good man, while a good man spontaneously (i.e., without much of a theory of action) does good works. Or with a number of contemporary philosophers, one can try to resolve states of the soul of moral agents altogether into descriptions of sets of observable actions. Since J/H and the codes of medical ethics contain better moral philosophy than either of those extremes, I suggest that not only the moral character of the ethical physician (i.e., his "steady state" for acting in commendable ways) but also an ethics of right and wrong behavior are—indifferently—the moral background of code ethics, the dual reason for calling them "ethics" at all.

In the belief that "medical ethics" is a species of "general ethics," Jonsen and Hellegers have placed before us an account of a theory of virtue, a theory of action, and a theory of the common good that they believe any adequate ethics must give attention to. I would describe their view as a threefold canopy of general ethics; "threefold" suggests that although its component parts can be distinguished, they cannot be separated.

In the main, they mean to exhibit a reciprocal three-in-oneness of general ethics: character, action, and the common good. I hear them saying that these three ingredients of ethics are co-equal accounts each needing the others for completeness' sake, interrelated and interacting aspects, none claiming primacy or sovereignty over the others. These are interpenetrating interpretations that, should one be absent or diminished, would impoverish our apprehension of the full human good. Virtue, right action, and social justice are the three foci of the field of ethics and, thus, of medical ethics also.

Of course, at any time or place in the moral history of mankind, one can see a need for greater emphasis to be placed on one or another of these modalities, e.g., on personal moral character, the rectitude of actions, or the common good. Such seems to be our authors' program when they tell us that, "Traditionally, medical ethics has dwelt mostly within two of those three theories [namely, virtue and duties]" and when they pronounced that, "The nature of contemporary medicine demands that

they be *complemented* by the third essential theory, the common good"
[italics added]. The prominence to be given to the common good comes
as a corrective of a past deficiency. The contingent conditions of modern
medicine call for the proposed redress. However, final justification of
these three ingredients of medical ethics derives from general ethical
theory itself.

Then it may be that when we bring the common good into view, personal "virtues and actions take on a depth and tone that they do not
have in isolation," as J/H claim. For we can also affirm, in the alternative, that when true virtue and right action are given their full weight,
the common good also takes on a quality and tone it does not have in
isolation. But J/H surely err when they write that "the *very meaning* of
a virtue or an action depends on its societal or institutional setting"
[italics added]. Again, we can reverse that and say that the very meaning
of the common good or a proper societal or institutional setting depends
on the kind of virtue or action inculcated therein.

This brings me to the first of three criticisms or complementary comments I wish to make on this paper.

1. Jonsen/Hellegers have not directly and clearly addressed the problem of a lexical ordering, or some other value-ranking, among the three
modes of ethical analysis. The simple observation that our times call for
greater stress on the common good raises no theoretical issues for ethics.
Our authors, however, mean more than this. They have appealed to the
contours and logic of general ethics to determine the specific shape medical ethics should take and its modes of reasoning.

But within the amplitude or richness of general ethics, they fail to
address clearly and rigorously the issue: Which of these moral claims has
priority (e.g., in case of conflict)? Therefore, the shape of medical ethics
and the weights to be assigned to its constitutive norms are left undeter-
mined.

After all, even the assumption that ideals of good character, the requirements of right action, and the claims of the common good are in
mutual parity is a kind of ordering that needs to be sustained by rational
ethical argument. Departure from that similarly requires cogent warrant.
A lexical order or any other weights to be given to theory of virtue,
theory of action, and theory of the common good would seem to be a
major task of general ethics. Whatever else it may be, medical ethics cannot claim to be a species of general ethics (i.e., it would be not ethics at
all) if it claimed to incorporate norms for the physician as moral agent,
norms governing his clinical action, and norms pertaining to justice in
medical practice for the common good, while at the same time ranking

elements in medical practice in an order indefensible in general ethics or indefensible in terms of the examined morality of a wider human community. For all the amplitude of the ethical framework our authors have provided, they have not helped us on this matter of the ordering of spheres of ethical reasoning, or on the matter of the primacy to be assigned to the corresponding spheres of medical-ethical justification.

Our authors also avoid addressing the issue of determining a lexical or some other order among one's norms or principles of ethical appraisal at a crucial point within their consideration of a theory of the common good. Just as an "unseen hand" ensures that mutual parity among moral virtue, right actions, and service of the common good will always endure and that these assessments never come into open conflict, so it is in the matter of social justice. Here again J/H rely on an "unseen hand" to avoid conflict. Enjoining medical practitioners and policymakers to reflect on the profound dilemmas and theses of the theory of justice, our authors' assumption seems to be that such reflection will not lead to the need to establish a lexical or some other ordering among the elements in which justice consists, or any priority among its tests or claimants.

J/H write that as we reflect profoundly on a theory of justice we "must refuse to relax those dilemmas either by a facile appeal to the 'inestimable social benefits of medicine,' on the one hand, or the 'inviolable individual rights of patient or practitioner,' on the other. Neither assertion can stand alone; both must be comprehended within an adequate theory of justice."

Granted. But *how* those moral appeals are to be comprehended may entail a decision within the ethical system itself (of which medical ethics is one species) as to which justification must first be satisfied before the other good or claim is taken up. (That is the meaning of lexical order.) Or it may require some other principle of adjudication or defendable weighing of the claims. What is or is not a "facile" appeal to overriding social benefits, or to inviolable individual rights, depends on foreseeing the possibility of conflict between justifications, and the need for some priorities or principles for resolving such conflicts first in the canopy of general ethical theory and the need, therefore, for similar modes of moral decision making in specifically medical ethics.

Doubtless, it is the purpose of a theory of the common good to discover how to avoid such conflicts. One of its chief tasks is to try to reconcile competing moral claims. But when J/H add to that the task of discovering "how to compensate *unjust* harm" [italics added], they reach the point where most ethicists have been forced to assign weights, priorities, and some order among ethical justifications. It is one thing to devise schemes for compensating for acceptable and accepted risks of injury and for any actual harm to "normal volunteers"—no injustice done. It is quite another thing to speak of compensating "unjust harm." That shows, rather, that one ought not to have done that harm in the first place and that a theory of right action claims priority over a theory of the common good, unless the "very meaning" of the latter is dependent on the former. It may be that "the problem of the lesser number, disadvantaged for the sake of the greater, remains unsolved" because it is unsolvable without a clear choice in case of conflict between some individual harms and some social benefits. Again, the smooth equivalence of all moral claims threatens to come apart when J/H speak of costs without compensating benefits to certain individuals in randomized clinical trials "particularly when one of the alternatives is a proven therapeutic agent." Some would view the withholding of a proved remedy from a control group to be an instance of "unjust harm" that no medical research benefits could justify even when redressed by extrinsic benefits to those less well treated.

2. Under the heading of theory of action, Jonsen and Hellegers discuss the theory of natural law. That, indeed, is a worthy example of how ethics generally addresses the justification for praising or blaming certain sorts of actions reasonably.

However, at risk of being pedantic, I want to say that if the tradition of natural law is deemed to have had its day and ceased to be, there are alternative theories of action in the writings of contemporary philosophers—indeed, since Kant—that are quite credible candidates for the role "natural law" plays in J/H's paper. From most of these less traditional, philosophical theories of action, it is possible to derive some rather firm action guides, perhaps a number of unexceptionable action directives. It is important that an alternative theory of action of this order be made known to physicians and policymakers for the following negative reason: It is commonly supposed that otherwise reasonable people hold to firm action guides only because of their adherence to natural law. If we could absent the relics of natural law, the furniture of our minds would consist solely of that footstool, situation ethics, or that love seat, social utilitarianism, or both. Nothing could be further from the truth, as any, even limited, acquaintance with ethical writing today should make abundantly evident. We live, indeed, in an era of broken-down intellectual discourse, and I do not want anyone to go away with the impression that natural law is the only theory of action whose adherents believe can supply some certainties about the morality of human actions and, therefore, about physicians' actions.

One can simply begin in his ethical reflection with a moral agent or community of moral agents in interface with some cherished value. One

can begin, in religious ethics, with "hesed" or steadfast fidelity to the
covenant of life with life or with Christian love or compassion. Those
standards in the Hebrew Bible and the Christian Scriptures root, of
course, in conviction as to God's steadfast love for his created people;
but the point to be made here is that those ethical outlooks need not
incorporate any articulation of "natural law." Or one can begin with
"respect for life" or "respect for persons" (the outstanding philosophical proponents today of this standard expressly disavow what they
understand "natural law" to mean). Or one can begin with the term
"care" or loyalty as the requirement upon moral agents in their relation
to anyone who bears a human countenance. I do not mean "care" in the
sense of specific actions in a medical context, but "care" as a strong,
ethical expression, the source of all particular obligations and one's
court of final appeal for deciding the features of actions and practices
that make what we do right or wrong in any context. That, then, would
be a general ethics of actionable duties, the norm governing what anyone should do in his relations with others. Or finally one might begin
with what is called in the title of another paper, "The Preciousness of
Life" (unless that turns out to mean "price").

Let me take at this point "the preciousness of manuscripts" as a standard governing a scholar's conscience to show how, from any of the
foregoing (allegedly and historically), nonnatural law systems of general
ethics can and may and must be derived from some firm, perhaps exceptionless action guides. Anyone using manuscripts in the Beinecke Rare
Book and Manuscript Library at Yale University is ask·d to read and sign
in order to indicate his understanding and acceptance of them, a set of
"rules governing the use of manuscripts." Among other things, this codi-
fication of the principles of scholarly behavior states that "the use of
any kind of pen is prohibited. Manuscripts may not be leaned on, written on, folded anew, traced, fastened with rubber bands, or handled in
any way likely to damage them. Eating and smoking are prohibited in
manuscript reading rooms." No mention is made of qualifications or
exceptions allowed to anyone because he cherishes the preciousness of
manuscripts only on the whole or in the long run, even though one can
construct such justifiable sorts of exceptions in outlandish, unlikely examples. (Someone with a precious manuscript in hand, the whole build-
on fire, may need to pop some pep pills or salt or vitamin pills to bolster
his failing strength and, therefore, may make direct appeal beyond the
rules to his need to "eat" in the manuscript room in order to act out
successfully his true cherishing of that manuscript!) Recently when I
read this "code of scholarly ethics" and signed the card indicating I
understood and meant to abide by those rules, I placed the card on top

of a manuscript of Jonathan Edwards and signed in pen, to the conster-
nation of all the librarians! That was a lesson to me that there can be
practically exceptionless rules stemming simply from the preciousness
of manuscripts and an upright conscience in the moral agent in relation
to that value.

Let us take "care" as a standard in the strong sense explained above
and "the preciousness of life"; and let us ask, What does care or the
preciousness of life require of moral agents generally and of physicians
in particular? That question breaks down into two sorts of questions
productive of two sorts of answers.

One can say, first, that we are to tell what we should do in a particular dilemma by making sure we know the facts of that situation and the
options it affords and then asking which specific action takes most care
of human life—present lives and (in the case of research) future lives. In
more or less discrete decisions in the face of more or less unique problematic cases, we are to ask, "What singular deed or design of ours is
most likely to embody or convey care or respect for human life?"

This first form of our question is productive of balancing decisions
to operate or not to operate in particular cases. It is also productive of
the second Article of the Nuremberg Medical Code, which states that an
experiment on human subjects "should be such as to yield fruitful results for the good of society," etc. These are essentially prudential decisions concerning what care is required, which only the physician or researchers are competent to make and which they decide in case after
case, from protocol to protocol.

The second form of the question, however, leads to answers of a different order. One can say in medical ethics that we are to tell what we
ought to do, not only by asking which particular action or research design is most caring, but also by asking which rules of practice, what
principles of action, what moral institutions or "covenants of loyalty"
(as I prefer to call them) would, if maintained or established in the regulations of the medical profession, prove generally most caring for the
dignity of man in patients or research subjects? Some contemporary
philosophers call answers to this question "rules of the game"; and I suggest that there are some universal rules of the game called caring.

This sort of ethical reasoning from the ultimate norm "caring" or "the
preciousness of life" is productive, for example, of the first Article of
the Nuremberg Medical Code, which requires a free and informed consent in human experimentation. Now, the physician must also make
prudential judgments in applying that principle in medical care and research. For this reason some physicians are under the impression that
they are engaged in the same sort of activity when they judge a patient's

or subject's consent to be an understanding, voluntary one as they are
when they make balancing judgments to operate or not.

In this I believe they are mistaken. In the latter case, the physician
tries to respond aptly to a particular situation. In the former, he is asking the applicable meaning of a principle of medical ethics, a rule of
professional practice. He is exploring the requirements of a governing
"moral notion." He asked what he should do in order to apply a moral
principle.

Objection will be forthcoming to the more strenuous of these conclusions, to the view that professional medical ethics, like any other ethics,
consists also of universally binding obligations. The objection will be
that there are always "exceptions." But every ethicist knows that "exceptions" to rules of practice are themselves implied by the standard
(the "care") in question. Furthermore, "exceptions" themselves are
"universals," only more specifically defined.

An "exception" indicates a class or sort of case having relevant moral
features in common. The "exception" is a "moral notion," not a particular. The relevant moral features of cases are as universal as was the original rule before the exception was added. A chief exception to the need
for consent—if such it is—still tells us, as a guide to action, that similar
agents should do likewise in similar situations. One who is a physician,
for example, not just I who am, nor just because that is a socially worthy
individual over there by the side of the road, should stop to help in
emergencies even if he had no contract with me to be his physician. The
moral judgment remains intact, even if all personal pronouns are removed (who I am or who he is, except for the relation of care). Even if
suddenly there were no more crushed bodies along the highways, that
would still in principle be the "right" thing to do. Even if never repeated
again, what was done is essentially repeatable. In stopping to help without prior patient consent, the physician wills what he does to be a universal moral law governing medical practice. He prescribes for himself
and all men a moral institution. When the personal pronouns are removed, any idiosyncratic or situationally unique features are removed;
yet the moral judgment remains intact. Such decisions are clearly not
like deciding to operate or not to operate. In the latter case, one decides
what care requires in a particular situation. In the former, one decides
what actions fall under a rule of care and loyalty to the dignity of any
person in need.[1]

3. An important conclusion from the foregoing in criticism of the J/H
paper is as follows: There are "rules of practice" and not only singular,
particular duties to be derived from a proper theory of action. Of course,
this is true also for natural law as a theory of action. It is strange that
J/H do not take note of this fact when discussing the common good. In-

stead, too wide a gulf exists between the general justice of institutions and a physician's virtues and his actions in one-to-one relation to his patient's needs. Forgotten is the fact that the physician has a moral role in relation to that patient, a role having universal features and not particular features only. Justice is first of all a virtue of the physician's role and professional practice vis-à-vis patients. That justice is therefore compatible with the justice that is "pre-eminently the virtue of institutions."

I understand J/H to say that medicine as a "practice" means only one-to-one physician-to-patient relations having few if any generalizable features. They define a "practice" as "a private. . .interaction between two parties." Only an ethics of institutional forms seems not to "limit our attention to good intentions alone or to the outcome of single actions." So they say, "Modern medicine, then, is an institution that incorporates a profession that practices a technique and an art. The practice remains, indeed, at the heart of the institution, but. . . ." There can be no objection to that statement, except to say that it bridges a gulf that ought not to have been so wide. For with the backing and appraisals of a proper theory of action, a physician's practice of his technique and art already entails "rules of practice." These are as close to institutionalization under a theory of the common good as a physician's habitual aptitudes of character are to a theory governing the appraisal of his clinical actions.

Granted, in appraising the relief of the suffering of one person by another properly qualified person, one does not perceive that situation or evaluate it primarily in terms of the action's external "major effects in extensivity perpetuity" upon those "not now suffering or even not yet born." But in that situation of one qualified practitioner in relation to one suffering other human being, one should abstract also from all personal pronouns, letting what "care" requires remain intact; one should also treat similar cases similarly; one also universalizes the right action to other like cases. There is already a "design of offices and tasks," roles and relations, in a theory of blameworthy and praiseworthy individual action. Universalizable principles governing the practice of medicine do not arise alone when considerations of the common good come into view. There should be "just medicine" before ever the question of a just society is raised, or else there is not likely to be "just medicine" after that.

REFERENCE AND NOTE

1. A more extensive elaboration and demonstration of these points can be found in Ramsey P: The nature of medical ethics. Edited by RM Veatch, W Gaylin, Councilman Morgan. The Teaching of Medical Ethics. Hastings Center Publication, 1973, pp 14–28.

II

Government Decision Making and the Preciousness of Life

The passage last year of the renal disease provision of of the Social Security Amendments of 1973 highlights the government's growing role in health care decisions involving life and death. The government appears to be assuming more and more the role of a giver of life itself. The main presentation and comments examine the implications of this function of government from the standpoint of human value issues and the distribution of limited medical services.

KENNETH J. ARROW, Ph.D.

Professor of Economics, Harvard University

Government Decision Making and the Preciousness of Life

I

The economist and the decision analyst address themselves to the coherence of means with ends, to the implementation of values among feasible alternatives. As part of that analysis it is sought to clarify the structure of values. No economic or decision analysis can define values as such, but by providing a suitable language they can go some distance toward removing inconsistencies and assisting decision makers in achieving clarification of their own underlying value structure.

It is not surprising that the decision theorists' wonted elegance and consistency are somewhat marred when faced with a value that in some sense is more basic than any other, one whose satisfaction is a precondition for having any values at all. (This remark should make clear that my starting point is a presupposition of human, thus worldly, values. I leave to others with greater confidence their interpretations of higher sources of value.)

My discussion therefore will not be highly systematic and deductive in nature; instead, I shall freely intersperse personal value judgments among the useful lessons we can still draw from general economic theory and decision analysis. I must indeed stress, after my initial disclaimer, that our general principles are still full of considerable clarificatory use, as will be made clear, I hope, in my application.

33

The starting point in assessing the role of government decision making with regard to life and death, or for that matter any other social end, is the recognition that the government's role is merely part, and not necessarily the major part, of the decisions that jointly determine the final social outcome. The individual members of the society make many decisions—their use of medical care, their highway driving habits, their food consumption, their concern for each other in risky situations—all of which powerfully affect the mortality statistics. (Of course, forces beyond control of any decisions, social or individual, set ultimate bounds on the possibilities of change. But we are concerned here only with the effects of decisions, and so with life and mortality as they can be affected.)

Economic analysis has most typically started with a world in which all decisions are made by individuals (mediated, however, through a market) and then sought to analyze the effects of introducing a certain amount of government influence on a final allocation of resources. The government has been typically thought of as marginal to the main social decision-making force, the multitude of individual decisions, each one a very small scale compared with the total. This point of view serves tolerably well for large areas of the economic system, although it certainly fails for analysis of wars that are not without important consequences for both economic welfare and mortality. In the present context the existence of a large sphere of competence in individual decisions is also a useful starting point. Thus the issues can be clarified by asking why, and in what way, do we need to depart from a laissez-faire model of decision making.

To anticipate objections let me state immediately that I am not an advocate of unrestricted laissez-faire, either in the discussion of lifesaving or in that of economic allocation of resources. Nevertheless, I find that starting with the laissez-faire formulation is the clearest way of putting the issues of governmental intervention in proper perspective to give us a guide as to where it is most important and useful.

No doubt one of the chief impulses for starting with the laissez-faire policy is a basic value criterion, which we may term libertarian: The government has as its aim the improvement of the welfares of its individual citizens. There is no separate room for a social aim above and beyond that.

Let me hasten to add that this criterion is by no means unambiguous. I will enumerate some of the difficulties involved shortly, but clearly it strongly suggests the desirability of a laissez-faire policy, of the absence of any governmental decision making. If the aim is to maximize the individual's welfare, the simplest and most effective procedure would seem to be to let the individual make his own decisions. However, logically the libertarian criterion does not, without further argument, imply the laissez-faire policy. One has to show under what circumstances individual decisions really achieve their highest welfare. Clearly, if individuals are completely independent of each other in the sense that measures that improve the life chances of any one individual have no effect on those of others, it would sound reasonable to argue that the libertarian criterion implies a laissez-faire policy. But even in this very simple case, there are complications. One, which I shall not pursue further, is the idea of redistribution or redress for inequality: If life chances are greatly unequal, should there be some public intervention to equalize them or to equalize welfare in some other way? For the moment, I have assumed that independence of mortality among individuals; presumably, therefore, there is no social policy that can help anyone even by hurting someone else. One might, however, argue that compensation should be made to those with higher death risks, in order to equalize their welfares. This point has certainly been argued by recent writers but it is perhaps outside our general text.

The second reservation is widely pervasive but certainly has a special force with regard to the stated theme. It is the discrepancy, real or fancied, between the decisions an individual would reach on his own and those that he should reach to increase his own welfare. In short, he may be ill informed about what is good for him. We have here, of course, the classic paternalistic argument.

An individual after all may very well be ill informed. He may believe in the quacks and nostrums that abound or he may have an excessive belief in the efficiency of orthodox medical care. He may not be aware that cigarette smoking is dangerous. He may fail to fasten his seat belt. He may be excessively careful to protect his life, not realizing the horrors of the invalid life for which he has prepared himself.

I am raising here a problem that seems to me to have received insufficient attention in both decision theory and ethical literature: i.e., the role of knowledge in choice. Issues of life and death perhaps sharpen the questions, but the difficulties are more pervasive. Basically, the situation is that information, knowledge, or whatever other similar term is desired is unequally distributed. By virtue of superior ability or simply by virtue of specialization of function, some individuals have access to more of some kinds of information than others. Laissez-faire policy is based on the general presupposition that an individual is more informed about his own wants and needs than anyone else. Hence, there is a presupposition that he should specialize in making decisions about himself. But in fact this assumption is clearly not universally valid. The whole concept of medicine as a specialized profession raises a contrary presupposition. With respect to diagnosis and treatment of illnesses, the physician is expected to know more about a patient than the patient does himself. There is no mystery about the origins of this special role. There is a body of knowledge, valid for human beings at large, that must be acquired in order to analyze and prescribe for illness. There is a considerable cost in time and other scarce resources in the acquisition process. But information, though acquired at a cost like other economic commodities, is not used like them, for it is not used up when it is used. It can be employed repeatedly without loss, indeed, like some cutting tools, with gain due to practice. Hence, from the point of view of an efficient allocation of resources, it pays to have some small group of individuals in the economy specialize in this profession, rather than have everyone acquire the knowledge for his own use.

This kind of specialization might occur even if everyone had equal ability; it is indeed one of the points stressed by Adam Smith in his famous encomium of the efficiency virtues of division of labor. In addition, specialization of function may be socially efficient in concentrating knowledge and skills, say in medicine, in the hands of those most capable and most motivated.

The arguments for specialization in skills are widely applicable in the economy. Medicine, along with the other professions, is distinctive in that the specialization is in sheer information. What the client is buying from a lawyer, physician, or a teacher is primarily a specific piece of knowledge, a small part of his total.

The causes of an unequal distribution of information are clear enough, though not simple to analyze in detail; but the implications for the practical and ethical problems of decision making are more complex. In fine, the problem is that there is a conflict between an individual's deciding his own course of action and his dependence on others for the information he needs. Even if we accept the individual's own welfare as the sole criterion for action concerning him, we find that the evaluation of some aspects of his welfare are better done by others. His autonomy as a decision maker becomes impaired.

The decision-making machinery for an individual is now enlarged to include other individuals. One could try to treat this relation as one does the acquisition of ordinary commodities. Just as one may try to solve a transportation problem by buying the services of a train or airplane or a psychological problem by buying alcohol or narcotics, so one tries to solve a medical problem by buying information from a physician. But the very definition of the problem is now in someone else's hands or mind. The provision of the information by the physician is not costless to him; it requires time and effort. Hence, he may have an incentive to economize on effort, to do less than the best possible job. Further, the decisions as to further treatment are based on the physician's information; his incentives to proceed optimally from the patient's viewpoint conflict with possibilities for gain in other directions. Nor need the conflict be entirely a question of selfish motives; the physician may want to learn something of value in treating patients. Indeed, he may be a medical researcher whose main motive is developing new knowledge. In that case, there can easily be a conflict between his obligations to the particular patient and his obligations to use this case to try new methods and find out if they are in fact useful.

The difference in information between the patient and the physician implies that the former has relatively little check on the latter. He may never be in a position to know whether the physician did as well as he could; if the patient knew that much, he would be a physician. Thus, the usual reasons why the market acts as a check to ensure quality operate here with very weak force. It is for this reason that ethical indoctrination of physicians is of such crucial importance. The control that is exercised ordinarily by informed buyers is replaced by internalized values.

But there is a still more subtle problem that arises in the medical field, and it is one that begins to come close to the topic of this paper. To what extent should information be conveyed by the physician to the patient? Let us waive the incentive issues of the previous two paragraphs. Let us suppose that the physician is fully motivated to maximize the welfare of the patient as the physician perceives it. If there is an illness with a straightforward cure, there is no problem. But let me pose a few dilemmas in increasing order of seriousness from the patient's viewpoint. (1) Suppose there are two possible treatments, both effective, but one is speedier but more expensive than the other. Should the physician inform the patient of his choice or simply choose? (2) Suppose there are two possible treatments, neither certain; one is more probably effective but more expensive than the other. (3) Suppose there are two possible treatments, neither certain and equally expensive; one is more probably effective but has a higher probability of dangerous side effects. (4) Suppose that death will follow in a predictable period of time in the absence of treatment, while with treatment there is a probability of recovery and a probability of a much sooner death. [This is basically a more dramatic version of (3).] (5) Suppose that the patient will certainly die of the illness. Should the physician inform him? Does it matter if the date of death is relatively certain or not? Does it matter if the illness will be painful or not?

If we can assume that the physician is capable and motivated to supply all the information possible, then I suppose the laissez-faire answer to each of these questions would be to supply the information and, at least in cases (1)–(4), let the patient make the decision. In general, an inequality of information would be met by transmitting all the needed information to the individual decision maker. Yet one can envisage objections by those not convinced *a priori* of the virtues of laissez-faire. A general kind of argument would be something like the following: The physician knows, from his superior knowledge of the consequences and from past experience with other patients, what the correct decision is. Why waste time in conveying information instead of simply making the decision? Further, because the patient's informational background is so low, it might be difficult to convey the choices meaningfully and credibly; he might not understand or might not believe he is being told the truth and so he might make the wrong decision. If he does understand and believe, the patient will be trusting the physician to be accurate; why not trust him to make the right decision?

An additional argument presents itself when the consequences are possibly serious, for example, death. The patient now has an anxiety about the future, a disutility; he would have been better off not knowing.

With these arguments and counterarguments, let us re-examine each case. Case (1) shows clearly the superiority of the laissez-faire case. Each individual has his own trade-off between recovery time and cost of treatment that will depend on economic opportunities, wealth, and personal tastes. About none of these is the physician more knowledgeable than the patient; the patients differ among themselves very much, and the physician has only the obligation to present the facts. There may be some cost in his time; it would seem that both superior efficiency in tailoring decisions to individual differences and the value of autonomy, of self-determination, to the individual outweigh the cost in physician's time and effort.

Case (2) is very much like (1). Now, however, the relevant trade-off of the individual is between risk avoidance and cost. Again, these depend on individual circumstances. The more subtle issue is the information to be conveyed; it is a set of probabilities. Neither the physician nor the patient think in numerical terms about probabilities, and they are usually not such well-defined objective facts anyway. Good statistics are rarely kept on these matters, and those that are are not completely relevant. In an ideal situation, enough records may have been kept to say that 75 percent of all patients recover with treatment A and only 60 percent with treatment B. But the particular patient is not a random patient, either in his eyes or in that of the physician. He may be judged more likely to benefit from either treatment, or possibly it may be felt that he will benefit more than the normal from A but not from B. Implicit in any decision is a set of probabilities, but these may reflect judgment which can differ among equally informed individuals. Clearly, the physician's probabilities are to be preferred (usually); but unless he can express himself well, it may be difficult for him to articulate his information well enough to convey it meaningfully to the patient.

In (3), the case for the physician's choice is certainly stronger. The trade-off is now between two probabilities, both of which can be apprehended better by the physician than by the patient. No doubt, individual preferences as between the effects of the illness itself and the side effects of the treatment are relevant to the choice. Since the patient has not usually previously experienced either, his preferences can hardly be very meaningful. But here is a situation in which the responsibility of the physician has to be given a social dimension. In any concrete case, the physician may be wrong; that is what we mean by speaking of "probabilities." Now we must recall our provisional abstraction with regard to incentives. A fire in a house may have been either plain bad luck or the result of carelessness or arson, and an insurance company will reserve the right to investigate. Similarly, the incorrect choice in any given case may be the bad result that must occur if success is only probable, or it may be the result of laziness, greed, or incompetence on the part of the physician. In the situation of informational inequality, the patient will not really know the answer. To have confidence in the physician's decisions, he must have the social assurance of a recourse mechanism, whether it be malpractice suits, peer review, or a general confidence that the social ethics and enforcement codes of organized medicine ensure a pressure for good decisions.

Thus we see that society as a whole plays a significant guaranteeing role in ensuring the viability of shifting decisions from a principal to his more knowledgeable agent. I should perhaps make clear that the need for guarantees arises even when only information is being transmitted; assurance is needed that the information is accurate. But clearly the need for placing the responsibility on the physician or other agent is both more acute and more easily enforceable when it concerns specific decisions.

It is really not necessary at this stage that it be the government that intervenes here as the guarantor. All that has been brought out is the need for some social entity. However, the trend of a century or more has been to make the government the one ultimate social authority. It may accomplish its aims by delegation to private groups, though this has been less and less true. As the role of the government in the financing of medical care becomes more important, the tendency for the government itself to arrange the standards by which crucial medical decisions are validated will increase.

The trend toward the increasing role of the government is not one with which I am happy. The impersonality and remoteness of government, at its best, and its liability to irresponsibility, at its worse, are serious drawbacks. On the other hand, the record of participatory control by smaller groups, particularly by consumer groups, in other fields is hardly satisfactory. Professional groups have had much greater success and have played a large part in the establishment of standards. However, they have not avoided either the fact or the reputation of using their position for promotion of their own interests. I would judge that professional peer review in a generalized form will always be the ultimate safeguard, but I think it essential that it be modified to include lay participation to keep it from deteriorating into control of entry and other forms of promoting the interests of the profession at the expense of the public.

The particular area of medical research and the decision problems that arise there have been taken over, at least formally, by the government. The doctrine of informed consent is an attempt to use governmental authority to impose a laissez-faire ideal, a paradox that is inherent in any attempt to preserve freedom of choice in a world of unequal information.

Case (4) is, in a sense, an extreme version of (3). The absence of treatment can be thought of as a form of treatment (not always the worst). The choice then is between two forms of treatment, one of which reduces the overall probability of death but increases the probability of an earlier one. (In view of the high stakes here, the cost of treatment may be thought of as a negligible factor.) But by sharpening the statement to include the question of life and death, I think other considerations begin to emerge. Most specifically, we begin to consider the question of anxiety. When faced with the choice, the information conveyed to him may reveal that either alternative is worse than he thought before. Also, and some would add this, a stress has been added for the interval of time left to him—the anticipation of early death. Whether or not this is a loss additional to the general worsening of one's life prospects is unclear to me. If the decision is made by the physician, the individual need not know the predictions.

This raises a deep issue for the evaluation of an individual's welfare over a period into the future. Do we consider his current subjective feelings, which may be unrealistically euphoric? Or do we consider what will in fact occur? This difficulty occurs in any welfare judgment extended into the future; but clearly it occurs with special piquancy in the case of death. Are we to consider that an individual is better off for a false expectation of continued life? Or, conversely, is a false expectation of death a punishment, a reduction in welfare? Certainly, the czarist officials who sentenced Dostoevski and his friends to death, with no intention of carrying the sentence out, must have thought so.

The English economist A. B. Atkinson* has raised the same point with regard to information about the relation between lung cancer and smoking. The information decreases the individual's subjective probability of survival and therefore decreases his expected welfare as he sees it.

The possible loss of welfare by improved information is brought out even more clearly in case (5). Here, unlike (4), the information about death cannot help the patient to make a better decision. (Actually, this is not entirely accurate. The patient may make some financial decisions differently, or indeed he may wish to dispose of his own life differently in the knowledge of his coming death.) One might argue even more strongly for concealment of the truth here.

But I am not convinced in either (4) or (5) that the truth should be withheld. One point of view is that which I have already suggested; that is, what will be will be, and the evaluation of the individual's welfare is based on what will happen, not what he believes will happen. *Ex post*, all will be known; present planning for the future should be an anticipation of what will be, not a present feeing of illusions.

This view, which is an axiom rather than a deduction from other principles, is reinforced by another consideration. In some sense, it is impossible to deceive individuals. One must consider the implications of a policy of withholding information, not merely the withholding on any particular occasion. Suppose no one is given a prediction, neither those expected to die soon nor those expected to recover. Then each individual will, if rational, estimate his chances according to some standard mortalities, perhaps adjusted for what he knows of his condition. Indeed, those who will die soon will be unduly optimistic; but those who will recover will be unduly pessimistic. Hence, withholding information will make some feel better off only by making others feel worse off.

Suppose, then, we inform those who will recover of their good fortune but withhold the bad news from the others. If this policy is known, it will be futile; those who receive no information can deduce from that lack that they are not among those who will recover, so in fact there is

*Information from an unpublished manuscript.

no concealment. To make the withholding of unfavorable information effective, it would be necessary to conceal the policy as a whole. We are getting far down the line of general social manipulation.

(I will not deny that the psychology of individual self-protection is being slighted here. Clearly, many individuals do not wish to know of their imminent death. In accordance with the general libertarian position, I see no reason to impose this knowledge on them. But I do not see the argument for removing the choice from individual patients to individual physicians or to the medical system.)

I have apparently wandered far from my assigned topic—from the value ascribable to human life in governmental calculations to the virtues of truth in regard to life and death. But I think this wandering path leads to a perspective on one of the clearest-cut issues involving the preciousness of human life—that of euthanasia and suicide. In its simplest form, the libertarian case for suicide and for voluntary euthanasia is overwhelming. The case indeed is in some ways stronger than that for abortion: One might at least raise the possibility that the fetus has some rights as against the mother, but it is hard to see who else has any rights in the case of voluntary death. (There may be family or other social obligations, in individual circumstances, but it is hard to see that they are matters for governmental intervention; rather, they are legitimate social obligations only to the extent that they are voluntarily accepted.)

This is not to say that there are no problems with regard to euthanasia. Rather, the problems are to be found precisely in the inequality of information between physician and patient and in the ethical and practical decision problems that we have already explored. Should a physician give an unfavorable prognosis that he realizes will very likely lead to a voluntary choice of death? If the prognosis is so complicated that the patient finds difficulty in understanding it, should the physician simplify by giving advice for euthanasia? If—contrary to the general views I have expressed earlier—it is considered appropriate for the physician to choose a dangerous course of treatment after weighing the alternatives, should he be allowed to choose euthanasia for the patient?

The danger arises, so it would appear, from the difficulties in enforcing meaningful and accurate flows of information; they may be deficient either because of the motivation of the physicians or because it is so difficult to convey a true assessment of the situation accurately under conditions of uncertainty.

I would summarize my views as follows: The basic aim should be to give the dying individual as free and well-informed a choice as possible. To do this meaningfully, it is necessary to create a code of conduct that will guide the physician in the supplying of information and advice, that will create appropriate expectations for diligence and legitimacy. A code will be a natural extension of present codes of medical ethics and will serve the same functions: i.e., creating definite but limited obligations on the part of physicians so as to provide some sort of guarantees for the information exchanged. Clearly, in this day and age, the ultimate sanction for such codes will have to be the government.

II

My original intention was to consider how life should be valued as part of the benefit–cost analyses underlying various possible government programs. That is, on the assumption that a human life is worth a finite amount of resources (possibly varying with the particular life in question, old, or young, high-wage or low-wage, or whatever), a program designed to save lives or having lifesaving among its incidental implications (or indeed lifelosing), should be evaluated by a calculation of benefits and costs that include the value of human lives. The programs involved cover a wide range: safety on the highway, in products, in the factory; increasing the supply of medical services through more medical education, increased use of paraprofessionals, more hospital facilities, or changing the methods of financing medical care; or support of biomedical research. We also have the issues of the government's role in increasing personal safety, of forcing or inducing individuals to improve their protection against illness or accident; the regulation of cigarette smoking, alcohol, or narcotics, safety belts in automobiles, swimming in unsafe waters, or rescue and protection of mountain climbers.

The first group of issues seem like standard resource-allocation problems. The straightforward answer is to value life as the individual himself does: What he would pay for it if it were available on the market. The measurement problem is complicated, as it always is when we seek to put a value on something not traded on the market.[1] But the second set already moves us toward problems of the kind raised above. Obviously, there are grounds for informing individuals of risks they might not otherwise be aware of. That there is a demonstrable statistical relation between smoking and lung cancer and other diseases, that safety belts can prevent injuries in automobile crashes, or that a given body of water has an undesirably high level of germs are clearly pieces of information that should improve the individual's decision making. But should we go further in the direction of compulsion? Clearly, this issue is thoroughly analogous to that with which we have been mostly concerned; however, it is no longer the special role of the medical profession but the general role of the expert that is in question.

The government may be in a position to know a good deal more
about the effects of, say, drugs on a human being than is the individual.
The acquisition of such knowledge is a specialized activity. This is especially true, since for the most part we are talking about statistical
risks. No individual from his own experience can learn much, partly because he is in any case a sample of one, partly because in most instances
the effects are irreversible, so that experimental behavior on the individual's part is highly risky. Does the government then proceed by making
the decisions for the individual? One can raise the same set of questions
as we did before for the physician–patient relation. Before that, one
difference in the two situations must be noted.

The relation between the government and the individual is essentially
statistical and impersonal. A government regulation is applicable to a
wide variety of individuals and cannot differentiate sharply among individual cases. It can, to be sure, create categories and treat different
categories differently. But the very equity and impersonality that essentially characterizes a government, particularly a democratic government, "the rule of laws not men," mean that differing personal situations must be treated as identical. The government has superior general
information, but it does not and cannot take account of individually
varying facts. The individual knows many things about himself (his
technology, his tastes, even some aspects of the conditions for his
health) better than the government possibly can. The physician's role
lies somewhere in between. He can know more about the individual
case than the government, though, as I have suggested before, he too
should perhaps be modest in the face of those individual preferences
that the patient should be presumed to know best.

Hence, I would conclude that there is even more reason for the government to adopt a laissez-faire mode in its safety-regulating behavior
than for the physician. That is, with regard to the second class of government interventions discussed above, those not involving major re-
allocations of resources (e.g., policy toward cigarette smoking), my personal preference would be that government's role should be confined
to the supply of information. Effective supply of information may still
involve considerable interference with classical notions of laissez-faire—
tax-financed expenditures for publicity, even compulsion on private economic agents to dispense reliable information along with their possibly
offending products (as with cigarettes and pharmaceuticals). But going
further, prohibition of cigarettes or, to take a famous instance, alcohol
exceeds the boundaries of the libertarian principle. It can only be justified on the basis of a thoroughgoing paternalism, a firm assertion that a
significant fraction of the people are judged by their peers to be in-

competent to handle their own affairs, to understand themselves so poorly that the necessarily imperfect and impersonal knowledge that remote experts have of them is better control than they can have over themselves.

Clearly, if the fraction who need this control is very large, the position I have just sketched is contradictory to the principles of a democratic state. If many individuals, given proper information, refuse to fasten their seat belts or insist on smoking themselves into lung cancer or drinking themselves into incompetence, there is no reason to suppose they will be any more sensible in their capacity as democratic voters. It is no answer to say that the government has the advantage of expert advice; the same advice can be made available to individuals in their private decision making. Only when the advice becomes highly technical, as in safety regulations for chemicals or nuclear power plants, does the delegation of responsibility to the government become reasonable.

The case of heroin and other similar narcotics poses a great dilemma for my libertarian position. My own view is that those individuals who are willing to eliminate themselves from a normal life after all the warnings they have been given should be allowed to do so. It could be argued that the fact that they have made this tragic choice is evidence of their incompetence, and the others, who in this case are still a large majority, have the right to protect them. But, as may be surmised, I am reluctant to substitute my judgment for that of an individual, even when the decent majority agrees with me.

Finally, let me turn to what might be regarded as the most obvious cases of the governmental role in the determination of life span, those involving the allocation of resources to what the economist would call "public" or "collective" goods, that is, life-enhancing measures that are clearly best undertaken by the collectivity. The improvement of safety in public transportation facilities (highways, aircraft) is an obvious example; so would medical research be if its health implications were not so uncertain. In my view, the criteria for choice among alternative forms of medical insurance include improvement of life chances only marginally. Basically, medical insurance is insurance against financial troubles; only for extremely costly cases is the effect on lives saved likely to be consequential.

As I have said earlier, the libertarian-economic way of dealing with the effects on human lives is to price them, essentially at the value a human being is willing to put on it. For any given project, the benefits so computed should be compared with the costs. There are two difficulties with this cursorily described procedure: (1) It is difficult to find the benefits so computed; (2) a poor man's life is valued less than that of a rich man, simply because the poorer man cannot afford to pay as much.

The value of a marketable good can be derived by observation on the market. But the provision of collective goods becomes efficient precisely when markets fail; therefore, in all cases of collective goods (e.g., defense, police) there is an intrinsic difficulty in observing the values that individuals place on the goods. Collective policies to improve life chances have the same problems in measuring benefits as any other collective policies. In addition just because the choice of life is rarely possible to an individual—and when it is possible, it is frequently delegated to others—the measurement of benefits from prolonged life becomes even more difficult.

Also it is not so clear, from introspection or from the judgments expressed in the great literature of the world, that sheer length of life is such a great value as compared with its quality: "Men must endure / Their going hence, even as their coming hither: / Ripeness is all" (Shakespeare, *King Lear*).

The conventional though often-challenged view of economists is to accept the sum of individual benefits as a criterion for social action, even though they are influenced by income. The usual argument is that if it is the income distribution that is undesirable, it is that distribution that should be changed and not the distribution of a particular good, even life. Suppose in deciding on a safety program, we compute life-increasing benefits for some individuals in excess of what they are willing to pay for them. Then it can be seen that the individual would be better off if he were given the same amount of money to be spent as he chooses; for what is meant by saying that he would be unwilling to pay so much for an increase in length of life is precisely that he values other goods of the same cost more. (I skate over a technical question here; once money is paid out, the individual is richer and might be willing to pay more for life extension. But for amounts of resources that are small per capita, the argument is sound.) In the absence of a paternalistic counterargument, that individuals underappreciate life extension, the argument for using individuals' own evaluation of improved life span seems valid.

Some of the arguments just advanced are less important in practice than in theory. They do show that no perfectly satisfactory solution is possible. But if health and safety measures affect individuals more or less independently of income, then the second difficulty becomes unimportant. For the first, it may suffice to use a conventional, but reasonable, figure for each additional year of one's life.

I wish it had been possible to provide more direct guidance than is contained in this paper. But, despite a basically libertarian bias, I cannot deny the claims of paternalism completely when the unequal distribution of information between the general public, on the one hand, and the physicians and experts, on the other, is considered.

REFERENCE AND NOTE

1. For two excellent studies, see Schelling, T C: The life you save may be your own. Edited by SB Chase. *Problems in Public Expenditure Analysis.* Washington, D.C., The Brookings Institution, 1968, pp 127–162; Fromm G: Aviation safety. Law Contemp Prob 33:590–618, 1968.

GUIDO CALABRESI
Professor of Law, Yale University

Commentary

I

One should realize that when Professor Arrow talked about maximizing
welfare or efficiency, as he did when he suggested that maximization
of patient welfare might require a move away from laissez-faire, he talked
about efficiency in a very different sense from the way it is often talked
about by economists. The moment one talks, as he did, about any kind
of governmental or other intervention, one is not talking about a Pareto
optimal definition of efficiency. One is not talking about a situation in
which those who gain as a result of a change actually compensate those
who lose. Instead, one is talking about something that is better called
potential Pareto optimality, a situation in which the winners do not
compensate the losers but in which there is some kind of collective judgment that the winners could, in theory, compensate the losers and still
come out ahead. Sometimes the winners may actually try to compensate
the losers according to some collective determination of what adequate
compensation is. But since the losers did not agree to the change and to
the compensation, it is impossible to be sure that the compensation
was sufficient to make the losers as well off as they had been originally.
As a result, this kind of decision necessarily involves interpersonal comparisons of utility. It necessarily involves saying that somehow it was
more important to have this more efficient way (to have the winners

48

win) than it was to take care of those who lost as a result of the intervention. The moment one recognizes that such a result is implicit in any intervention, one must also recognize that failure to intervene in a situation where intervention would in this sense be efficient also involves interpersonal comparisons of utility. That is, failure to intervene implies failing to better the lot of some people who could be made better off through collective action and not compensating these people for that failure. Thus, their utility loss is counted for less than that of those who would lose as a result of intervention. In short, there is always a trade-off of people once one moves away from a society in which transactions are costless and compensation of losers is, therefore, always feasible.

It is crucial to realize this because, if we think of our society as one in which full compensation can occur, as one in which a unanimity principle like Pareto optimality is feasible, then—even if it is not true that everybody always gets everything in a scarce world—it is at least true that everybody always gets the best that he can, given his starting point. Instead, once one moves from that to what implicitly Arrow advocates, to trying to maximize total gains even if losers are not compensated, then one has a much more complex ethical situation. It is not just the starting point that is suspect; any intervention, or any failure to intervene, implies a choice that some people are more important than others and hence is suspect. It is in this complex ethical context and not in the simplified classical context of economists that Professor Arrow discusses the problem of information.

II

The problem he poses is what ought one do to maximize welfare in a patient–doctor situation where one of the parties has more information than the other. I'd suggest that this problem, far from being unique to the doctor–patient relationship, exists very commonly. It exists, for instance, in almost all accident law cases. The answer some writers, like me, have given in this last context is to put the burden, the costs that result from a decision either way, on the party who has the access to the best information, to the most information. This is sometimes called— unfortunately, I think—the strict liability approach. Its aim is to create an incentive for the party who has access to information to choose correctly, to make the best cost–benefit analysis. It is an appropriate approach, regardless of the reasons why a transfer of information is impossible between the party with knowledge and the party with less knowledge.

In the doctor–patient context, Arrow assumes that a transfer of information is often undesirable or impossible either because it is too expensive to inform the patient, or because it is psychologically difficult to get the facts across to the patient, or finally because it creates a new harm, "anxiety," to inform the patient. In other contexts, the transfer of information may be difficult simply because one cannot get the parties together to negotiate.

I do not know all the people whom I may hit with my car; hence I cannot inform them of the danger they incur by letting me drive and then buy from them the right to drive. To require this would cost too much. To say that a driver must inform the potential victim and buy from him the right to subject him to risk is, in practice, to say that there will be no driving, and we're not prepared to do that. That would be inefficient in the potential Pareto optimality sense we have been using. We require compensation at a collectively determine level to guarantee that the party with knowledge will take the risks he imposes on the other into account. This is needed to make the result "potentially" Pareto optimal. Such *ex post* collectively determined compensation is not as *good* as a true negotiation (between victim and injurer) of the right to cause a risk of injury. But since *that* is impossible, the incentive created (by putting the burden of compensating, at the collectively determined level, on the party with the greater knowledge) is the best we can do.

What is fascinating to me about Arrow's discussion is that when it comes to putting a burden, or an incentive, on a doctor (the party he assumes has greater knowledge), he automatically suggests an internalized code of ethics. He mentions malpractice but only in passing and perhaps with the slap on the face that it deserves. Basically, he says, we want the physician to maximize the welfare of the patient, as the patient would see it, but we need a code of ethics to make the physician do this. A code of ethics, however, is very different from what we normally rely on to cause analogous behavior in the party with the informational advantage. In most other contexts, instead of relying on ethics, we place a cost burden on the party with the most information. He bears the burden regardless of the choices he makes, and this gives him an incentive to reduce the burden by choosing that which harms least.

It may be that this approach is impossible in a medical situation. It is often said that it is not feasible because it is virtually impossible to define the cost to the patient of a medical adverse reaction. How can one tell if the patient is made better off by one treatment than he would have been by another? This obviously is a tremendously difficult problem. But it is a problem that we do not avoid by relying on a code of

ethics rather than on allocation of costs to induce proper physician behavior. If the job of the physician, enforced through the code of ethics,
is to maximize the patient's welfare, then that maximization must involve the analogous valuation on his part of the costs to the patient of
the alternative possible treatments. The physician is required by the
code of ethics to balance the very same costs we have said were so hard
to measure. We have not done away with the cost–benefit analysis for
the costs and benefits are still the same; we only act as if they are not
there by requiring the physician, through a code of ethics, to divine
them. If he can't divine them adequately, then the code of ethics cannot work.

There are, in fact, three generalized approaches to such cost–benefit
choice situations. Each of them must resolve the same basic cost valuation problem, but each of them does it in a slightly different way. (1)
We can set up a code, governmental, peer group, or what have you, that
determines which choices are proper and which are not and enforce
this collective decision through whatever pains or penalties seem appropriate. We can have any amount of decentralization in the application
of the code. Thus, Arrow would suggest application of a code of ethics
by physicians. But he would also have some guidelines decided centrally
as to what ought to be done and what ought not to be done. (2) We
can instead do what the fault system does. The fault approach looks
retrospectively and says, if after the act we can collectively say that the
physician ought to have known before the choice that he ought not to
have chosen as he did, then and only then will he pay for the bad effects of his choice. But even then he will be allowed to ensure against
having to make such payments. This is a very peculiar way of doing
things, which we don't use in most other incentive creating situations.
(3) Finally, we can simply try to evaluate the costs that result from
either choice as best we can, put them on the party who has the best
knowledge as to possible harms, and let him make the choice.

In the context of medicine, this last approach presents more problems than the ubiquitous valuation problem. We are often not at all
clear on whether the physician is in the best position to choose and
therefore is the one who ought to bear the costs. It is very difficult to
define the cases in which we want the choice put on the physician. But,
it is not impossible. Professor Clark Havighurst of Duke and Dr. Laurence
Tancredi have in certain areas attempted to do precisely this. They have
shown that, where the choice is between various types of anesthesia, for
instance, a system of incentives that is based neither on fault nor on an
outside code of ethics can be established.

All of this still leaves the problem, as Arrow has recognized, of the patient who does know more than most people or who wants to be treated differently from most other patients. Such a patient poses a difficult problem, but again one that is in no way unique to the medical context. Again, since we are in a world of potential Pareto optimality, and not true Pareto optimality, such a patient is going to lose because to fashion a rule for his benefit would cause others to lose more. Sometimes his burden can be eased by allowing an exception to the normal cost allocation rule if he successfully informs the physician that he *is* the unusual man, if he lets the physician know that he is in a different situation from most. But such individualized exceptions are, in practice, fairly hard to work out. It is simply not worth the administrative costs of making exceptions to general liability rules to take care of a really unusual patient or doctor.

III

Arrow's discussion essentially ends at this point with an examination of those cases in which the patient, as a rule, will have more knowledge as against those in which the doctor has the informational advantage. In effect he ends the discussion just where the most interesting problems begin, where the question becomes not who has better access to information, patient or doctor, but rather what is involved in valuing a life for either of them. And that is where the discussion must turn next.

I'd like to know, for instance, if any individual does value his own life in a way that can meaningfully be used in choosing between life and death risks. If each of us were paid to take a one in a million chance to lose our life, realistically, how much would we ask? How much more would we ask if the chance of death were one in one thousand? Or one in two? I would suggest that the value that most of us would give to our lives would not be the same value in the three cases, after discounting by mathematical risk. In other words, the value we as individuals put on our life is not independent of the gamble we are taking. This fact makes it very, very difficult as a practical matter to define any value as the appropriate one in creating incentives for safety.

Beyond this problem is the further difficulty that human life does not have value only to the person who loses it. That is, the problem of external costs and benefits seems to me to be fundamental when one is dealing with value of life. There are two aspects to this problem. First and most obvious, society may value a person's life more than he does. A saint may be perfectly ready to die, while society may need him alive. Yet, any *explicit* recognition that the saint's life is worth more than a scoundrel's is, and should be, exceedingly costly in an egalitarian society.

The second aspect goes less to the fact that there are external costs and benefits that attach to most individuals' lives. It is concerned, instead, with the external costs involved in the manner, the process, through which a life is valued or taken. Let me suggest one example of this. When the Pentagon Papers case was being tried, Justice Stewart asked my colleague, Alexander Bickel, who was counsel in the case, what he would do in a case in which it was known that if the papers were published a hundred lives would be lost. He added, "Would not permitting publication amount to a judicial sentencing to death of a hundred people?" Implicit in his question was the belief that such a judicial sentencing to death would be catastrophic, would be horrible. Professor Bickel answered properly that the case before the Court involved no such catastrophes and the Court should not worry about such a future case until and unless it came up. Justice Stewart didn't worry about it and decided the Pentagon Papers case in favor of publication.

A deeper answer than that which Professor Bickel gave did exist, however (though it is an answer that was probably less appropriate to counsel in the specific case). It is the answer that I imagine Justice Black, had he been a little younger, would have given. His answer would have been precisely that judicially sentencing a hundred people to death is a terrible thing to do and must be avoided, but that sacrificing a hundred lives, in exchange for freedom of speech, is nothing! We sacrifice many times a hundred lives in exchange for things that are far less important. The whole object, therefore, is to create institutions that avoid a "judicial sentencing to death" in this context. Black might have said, "Don't let a case like that even get to court." We must create structures such that the lives are taken before a judicial sentencing to death can occur.

Whether one likes the result I hypothesize or not, the suggestion implicit in the discussion before the Supreme Court has to be that there are external costs, that there are harms, that depend on the process used to decide terribly important issues like life or death. There are also benefits. Thus a dramatic decision to spend millions of dollars to save a fool who has chosen to row across the Atlantic has external benefits, which spending much less money to make a highway safer—with far greater lifesaving effect—apparently does not. It's when we discuss such situations that I think we come face to face with the fundamental issues involved in the topic "the preciousness of life and governmental decisions."

IV

I have been playing around with analogous problems recently in the context of what I call tragic choices. Tragic choices for me are situations where there is no right decision. Assuming that a society has made some kind of a decision as to how many kidney machines it will produce, how many soldiers it will need for a limited war, or how many births it can tolerate, how does it decide, explicitly or implicitly, who gets the kidney machines, who gets picked to serve in that limited war, who gets to have children. [And don't think for a moment that we do not have a system of implicit incentives and suasions that decides today who gets to have the children. It's just that that system is not as knowingly chosen as the systems we have used (unsuccessfully on the whole) to choose recipients of kidney machines or soldiers for limited wars.]

In fact, virtually every system of choosing in these situations has tremendous costs associated with it. This is so if the choice is made by a market system, which would place a value on the resources and let people bid for them. It is so if it is made by a market system corrected for wealth differences. It is so if it is a system of political choices, a deferment system. (Consider, for instance, a deferment system in the context of the right to have children. Consider a system that says that a certain group can have more children than another because its children are in some sense more valuable to society than those of the other group.) It is so whether the choice is made by a lottery or by a topsy system, a system like the one we are using to allocate children today—a system, that is, which we can claim has never been chosen, because it "just kind of grew."

The external costs are different for each one of these possible choice mechanisms, and they do not always apply equally to all possible choices in each of the three paradigmatic "tragic situations" I have mentioned. For instance, we may not be bothered by excluding people under 18 from the army because they don't make good soldiers. That's all right. Indeed, we can exclude them even if they want to serve. Yet we are likely to be very troubled by a rule that exempts college students from the army because *they* don't make good soldiers. And this would be so even if it were clear that college students are every bit as bad as soldiers as are 16 year olds. All this suggests that we may be able, without undue external costs, to make one decision through political choices in a tragic choice area, but not able to make others. It seems to me, therefore, that when one is talking about governmental decision making and the preciousness of life, one has to concentrate on external effects and on different procedures that, while they don't avoid, at least minimize the external effects.

I don't have time in these comments to go into adequate detail on what is involved in choosing among possible choice mechanisms where life is at stake. I gave a series of lectures at Pennsylvania last year, which

I haven't published yet, that dealt with this topic—still inadequately but at least more fully. My conclusion in those lectures was that none of the choice mechanisms available will work ultimately and that perhaps the way in which one can minimize the external cost of choosing is to shift from system to system. This conclusion follows from my belief that in our society there is, and probably should be, a basic inconsistency in fundamental values. So long as we have an inconsistent series of values, the only way we can attempt to uphold all of them is to ignore some of them for a period of time and then reassert them with great fanfare (as we've done in every change in the selective service system from the Civil War to the present). The fanfare is designed to call attention to the fact that we are now re-establishing a value that is fundamental and previously had been ignored. But at the same time that we re-establish one value with great fanfare, we tend to hide the fact that we are now ignoring another value that is equally important and that we will have to re-establish later. Such an approach is hardly a happy one. But it may be the best we can do when we deal with a problem as knotty as that of human life and governmental decisions.

V

In summary, the problem of governmental decisions and human life is a terribly hard one because it involves at least four fundamental problems, any one of which is enough to warrant a lifetime's study. The first is what happens when one moves from a system of choices in which everyone consents to a system that necessarily involves intervention or the intentional failure to intervene and, hence, implicitly involves comparing the value of different human beings. The second is how should a society deal with situations where harms are likely and where there is an uneven division of knowledge between different parties as to the likelihood and severity of the harms, as well as to the likelihood and severity of what must be borne to avoid the harms. The third is that a human being's own valuation of the worth of his life, even if possible, is an inadequate gauge of the value of that life to society. And the fourth is that any process or system for choosing among lives has external costs associated with the use of that process in making such, literally, vital decisions. All four of these problems are enormously difficult to deal with, and yet all must be examined together if we are to deal at all humanely with the relationship between human life and governmental decisions.

EDMUND D. PELLEGRINO, M.D.
Professor of Medicine and Humanities in Medicine,
The University of Tennessee College of Medicine

Commentary

Professor Arrow has provided a disquisition on the economics of medical decision making based on libertarian principles. He recognizes the complexities of assessing the value of life and health without benefit of the classical market determinants that operate for most consumer goods. His leitmotiv is freedom for each individual to set his own value on his life and to do so with a maximum of information possible about the nature and consequences of each alternative.

Arrow's line of argument starts with the assertion of the libertarian principle as the primary value and laissez-faire as the preferred policy. His ordering principle is information since the individual is most free when he is best informed. When the individual is well informed, Arrow grants him the right to make decisions harmful to himself and to reject technical and professional advice. Thus each man sets his own price on his life rather than having it set by government or some other external agency.

Arrow takes a very reserved view of government's role. Its major function should be to improve the quality of information available to the individual and thereby to close the gap between the professional and the patient. He admits a role for government in such instances as setting safety regulations for nuclear power plants, and he is uneasy about the application of his principle in the case of heroin usage. But, he finally opts for the individual's right to make even the "tragic choices."

Professor Arrow fears paternalism of any kind. He rejects any but the most necessary intrusions on individual liberty even when it comes to the equity of distribution of goods and services in the economics of health care. He admits that the libertarian criterion may not necessarily imply a laissez-faire policy, though for most of his argument the two are so closely aligned as to be indistinguishable.

I hope this is a fair unraveling of the major thrust of Arrow's reasoning. I have chosen four features of this line of thought for comment: (1) the inherent limitations of the libertarian criterion; (2) the emphasis on information in the physician–patient transaction; (3) the guarantee of freedom and consent; and (4) the relationships of law and ethics in this guarantee.

THE LIBERTARIAN AXIOM: SOME LIMITATIONS

Professor Arrow is, of course, aware of the dilemmas in any absolute application of the concept of individual freedom of choice in matters medical and otherwise. If each of us were isolated, individual units, each of whose actions could be encapsulated and separated from the actions of others, the libertarian principle might apply absolutely. But we are also, and necessarily, social beings. As such, the freedoms we enjoy are licit only when they do not limit similar free choices by others. The libertarian ethic is built therefore on a contingency that makes its absolute application self-defeating.

We cannot be left free to make certain choices—to run red lights, drive while drunk, to pollute, to deforest, to spread nuclear waste. Even a predominantly self-noxious action like smoking, when done in a public place, limits the rights of nonsmokers to be free of this noisome habit in their vicinity. The absolute right to self-determination even in the smallest things is a mirage, since to grant this right to anyone for one thing is to limit it for someone else in other things.

In matters medical, Arrow argues that the individual should be free to reject knowledge of what is harmful to health and to make his own choice as to whether he shall smoke, wear seat belts, drink excessively, or use heroin. But he overlooks the social burden placed upon all of us by the costs in money, facilities, and personnel required to treat the victims of self-abuse. The individual may indeed place a low price on his health and his life. Society has, however, placed a higher value on that individual's life and comfort. We do not let the person who opts for a "tragic choice" and, in Arrow's words "eliminates himself from a normal life," perish in isolation without medical assistance. We do not suffer him to lie where he has fallen, so to speak. We build hospitals, train physicians, and employ researchers to help the victim of lung cancer, emphysema, or cirrhosis of the liver, or the victim of a motorcycle accident.

Manifestly, the individual's free choice, even if based on the most complete information, has social implications that make the application of the libertarian principle more than dubious for other individuals. I am not suggesting that we abandon those who have made the "tragic choices" or coerce them into healthy living. But we must weigh the social consequences of individual decisions however free they may be. When resources are limited, to what extent can we permit individual decisions that predetermine priorities and distribution of public resources in favor of one category of needs as opposed to others?

Fortunately, we live in a society that provides for its members who may become a burden to themselves and others by their self-destructive behavior. This is a civilized act of indulgence, an acceptance of the human condition. It does not derive as a right, however, from the libertarian ethic.

We touch here on the still largely unexplored tension between an ethics of individual good and an ethics of social and communal good. One of the challenges in a free society is how to strike a reasonable balance between these polarities. Neither individual nor social good can be absolute in health care decisions or in any other realm.

In the microcosm of the choice of a mode of treatment in the individual physician–patient relationship, the libertarian principle has more substantial validity. In general I would concur with Arrow's analysis of the varying degrees to which the physician might intrude; I too would opt for the freedom of the patient to make the choice himself wherever he is intellectually, emotionally, and physically capable of doing so.

In the circumstances of curative medicine we deal with the fait accompli, with the end result of illnesses, some of them preventable, others not. Let us hope that we never have to face the situation in which resources are so limited that even these decisions come into conflict with other social needs—e.g., better nutrition, housing, public safety.

The libertarian principle, even though limited, is desirable for the individual isolated from the group and pursuing his own ends and values. As an absolute criterion in decisions about health in a democratic society, it has significant limitations.

BEYOND THE INFORMATION GAP

The second aspect of Arrow's paper that elicits comment is his emphasis on the information gap that separates physician and patient. This

gap, he is right in saying, limits the freedom of the patient's freedom of
choice and thus of the libertarian principle. Arrow implies that if only
this difference in knowledge could be eliminated, the patient could
make truly free choices. This is a simplistic view of the complicated
phenomenology of the physician–patient transaction, especially of the
process of consent that is so central in decision making.

What is really at issue is the process of consent, by which one person
(the patient) seeking assistance from another (the physician) agrees to
follow one of several courses that presumably maximize benefits and
minimize hazards, costs, and discomfort. Information transfer is only
one part of this transaction. Even if it were the only factor, we would
have to ask if a patient's consent can ever be fully informed—that is to
say so clear that a rational choice could be made on the basis of the
facts known about the courses of action presented as alternatives. Manifestly, we deal in the majority of instances with limited knowledge no
matter how diligently the physician may try to disclose "all" the facts.
The sorting of these facts, putting them in a priority order, giving each
its proper weight, and then relating them to the context of a particular
patient are matters that the patient can address with limited competence
and then only with the physician's guidance.

But, granting that the physician tries consciously to close the deficiency
in knowledge between himself and the patient, is the patient ever totally
free to act on that information? He is after all seeking help; he is anxious, perhaps in pain, or otherwise discomfited. He sees his life style
threatened, his own values put awry, and his person subjected to the in-
dignity of petitioning another for help. The patient's capacity to deal
with the information is modulated by a dozen factors that make his
transaction with the physician an unequal one. If the patient is a child,
or elderly or emotionally distraught, there will be psychologic and physical barriers to the reception of information. Socioeconomic, ethnic,
and cultural inequalities compound the difficulties. The mere transfer
of available knowledge will not suffice for most cases; thus, the libertarian principle, even if it were a valid a priori principle, would be difficult to apply to most of the decisions clinicians and patients must make
daily.

Perhaps the most subtle influence that limits the freedom of the physician as well as the patient is the intersection of their value systems
that each transaction involves. The disproportion between these value
systems may be as great as the disproportion in information. What each
thinks of the meaning of life, pain, disability, the value or nonvalue of
suffering, the existence or nonexistence of God, and a hundred other
like issues will all color *how* the information is delivered by the physi-

cians and received by the patient. The same information can be delivered by two surgeons on the benefits and dangers of elective gall bladder surgery or the treatment of breast or cervical cancer between radical surgery or radiation. Each surgeon will unconsciously place certain emphases that can weigh the decision in the direction that more closely fits his own value system. Two patients, of different social or cultural background, will "hear" different things, though the facts presented might be the same.

It is as important to maintain the integrity of the patient's own values as it is to maintain the integrity of his body. The physician is impelled morally not only to disclose the information requisite to a free decision but to do so in a way that assures the patient's values are safeguarded. The decision, or in Arrow's terms, the value placed by the patient on his life and health, cannot be self-determined without recognition of many nuances that often supersede the mere transfer of information.

The point is further illustrated by Arrow's assertion that, even if the information produces anxiety and if that anxiety may be detrimental to the patient's welfare, he favors telling the truth. It is just such axioms that underlie the physician's advice and the patient's decisions. Others may well not wish to know, and they have a right to be "protected" from such information. The ticklish question is how the physician can discern this desire in his patient and allow the patient to make the choice of how much he wants to know, especially if the case is hopeless.

Arrow is especially emphatic in the case of euthanasia. He sets forth his own value-laden axiom—here the libertarian case, he says, is "overwhelming." But once again, the limitations on the certitude of the data and the modulations in communicating those data are significant enough to place qualifications on the absolute application of the libertarian ethic.

Another serious limitation on the transfer of information is the lack of certitude about what in fact is the "correct" decision. The probabilities we assign to any choice in a decision matrix vary from one authority to another or, are based on samples of varying validity. Professor Arrow assumes that we can simply fill in the probabilities of this or that outcome and make the decision on the basis of a rather simple summing of the probabilities pro and con. The more mature a clinician becomes, the more critical will he be of the seeming certitudes upon which he bases his actions. The critical factual data needed to make these decisions are still seriously lacking in clinical medicine today. One needs only to recall the still dubious character of the data relating to the use or nonuse of anticoagulants in myocardial infarction, during the acute episode or in prophylaxsis.[1]

Of equal importance with information transfer is the "quality" of consent. Consent has the highest quality, in human terms, when the patient feels he has truly participated, that the decision is his own and made in his own terms. Freedom, then, manifestly includes much more than information transfer. It is found only when the complex conditions surrounding consent permit a decision appropriate to the patient's existential situation—the one that best fits the particular life context within which the patient resides at the moment of decision.

The physician has therefore a fiduciary responsibility[2] that transcends closing the information gap. He must assure as much freedom as the complicated web of circumstances and values will allow. He must attend to all the nuances that modulate information transfer. Mere information, however complete or accurate, can be dehumanizing. In sum, then, we agree with Arrow's desire for maximal freedom, but the conditions for that freedom are far more intricate than his essay suggests.

WHO SHALL GUARANTEE THE PATIENT'S FREEDOM AND HOW?

If the libertarian principle has practical as well as ethical limitations, how shall we assure that freedom of choice is guaranteed? A democratic society requires freedom in decision making, on the one hand, and participation by the group, on the other. Some form of social sanction appears to be necessary. Public sensitivity on this issue is evident in the current discussions about a patient's "bill of rights" and in the recurrent themes of "accountability" and "quality assurance" in present-day legislation.

In the realm of individual decisions, Professor Arrow feels the role of government should be limited largely to assuring that information is complete and accurate. In certain instances, he reluctantly agrees that some combination of government regulation together with an upgrading of professional ethical codes and public participation will be essential. We must take very seriously Arrow's concern about the dangers of societal and governmental intrusions into the individual's decisions about his own life and health. Governmental regulation of necessity will tend to the impersonal and will be based on far less intimate knowledge than the patient and his physician possess.

Yet, having said this, we must also seek other options that will permit some attention to the remote effects of personal choices. We must strive consciously for some means of setting some of these values by the community. We do this now only implicitly. The capabilities of modern medicine, the costs of its wide application, and the right of each citizen to a healthful existence now require that we set some of these values explicitly. The statement of value will not be in terms of dollars but in terms of the restrictions each of us is willing to accept on our absolute freedom to gain a more healthy existence for all.

In the broader realm of decisions on how to allocate our national resources, or where technical expertise is beyond the ordinary citizen's ability to grasp (safety measures for nuclear power plants), Arrow is readier to admit government regulation. Every conceivable mechanism of practical value should be examined to ensure social sanction for even these decisions. Regulation cannot be left to government alone. Rather, a balance between government regulation and public surveillance of government must be achieved. Some modification of the public utility concept would probably be most apt, provided it can be designed to meet regional as well as national interests.

To enjoy the benefits of a democratic society, the individual yields some of his absolute freedoms in many civil matters. This is also true in matters of health. What is yielded and under what circumstances are the crucial issues, not preserving the libertarian ideal as an absolute. We have yet as a nation to define what values we deem inviolate and which ones can be compromised to maximize social benefit and minimize restraints on the individual. This may well be the focal social and political issue of our times. Our discussion of the government rule in setting the value and quality of human life is a subset of this larger human problem, albeit an exceedingly important one.

Professor Arrow examines only the extremes of the regulation of decision making—the absolute right of the individual, on the one hand, and government intervention, on the other. He does not discuss at all the role of health care institutions in guaranteeing the freedom of the patient's decision. The locus for these decisions is often in the hospital or other health care institutions. Few of these institutions have assumed their responsibility for assuring disclosure of the information necessary if the patient's consent is to be as informed and free as possible.

Institutional mechanisms have in recent years been established when consent is sought for experimental procedures. I believe that the same guarantees and the same degree of disclosure will be required for ordinary therapeutic and diagnostic procedures, especially when they carry risks, are expensive, or can be conducted in alternate ways. Legal opinion is already moving in this direction. We can expect the hospital more frequently to be held to account if its staff does not assure consent that satisfies both legal and moral criteria. Many levels of institutional regulation will be required. This will in turn force a transformation in the physician–patient relationship, opening it up to wider scrutiny. Properly

conducted, this scrutiny should afford greater safety and better participation by patients in the decisions that affect their lives. The patient's
right to set the value of his own life himself will become part of his "bill
of rights." Some of these possible mechanisms have been examined elsewhere.[3]

RELATIONSHIPS OF LAW AND ETHICS

Legal mechanisms will multiply to meet growing public demand for
more regulation and accountability in the provision of health care.
There will still remain a significant realm for the operation of professional ethics. To be effective, however, professional ethical codes will
need to be expanded to include new realms of responsibility. Existing
ethical codes in medicine, except those that apply specifically to medical experimentation, are silent on these matters or leave them entirely
to the judgment of the physician.[4] The synergistic interplay of new legal
means and an expanded professional ethic promise to avoid the imper-
sonalization, standardization, and bureaucratic obfuscations that government interventions have inevitably brought with them in the past.

Law can guarantee the validity of consent by providing that certain
procedures be followed and recorded for later examination. It can penal-
ize the professional who fails to meet statutory requirements for valid
consent. It is a far more difficult thing to assure that the patient's decision and his consent to a given course of action are of high "quality" as
a human action; that is, they take the full dimensions of the medical encounter into account. Here, we are more dependent on the ethical behavior of the physician. It becomes urgent for ethical codes to be more
explicit about the physician's responsibility to make the patient's bill of
rights a reality, not a mere formal adherence to a set of procedures.

In a sense, the law is the coarse adjustment that guards against the
grosser violations of human rights; ethics is the fine adjustment that sets
a higher ideal than law can guarantee. Government must not become the
sanction for a code of ethics but only a substitute that recognizes the
human frailties of professionals. What is legal is not always ethical. Ethics
is the realm in which professional conscience transcends law, strives for
equity in its application, and anticipates the higher dimensions of assurance that human decisions shall be as truly human, i.e., as informed
and free as it is possible to make them.

Professional ethical codes have adapted too slowly to the new responsibilities that medicine in the modern world demands. They need constant refurbishing. They should be ahead of the law in divining what
duties should be required of professionals. Indeed, the separation of

ethics and law is essential in a free society to prevent an unjust government from identifying the law with what is ethical. If government sanctions ethics, then an infraction of the ethical code is a crime against the state. The twentieth century has already seen too much of this abomination.

SUMMARY

Professor Arrow is a man of the Enlightenment and all of us who respect and have high hopes for human reason and freedom want the kind of liberties he argues for so cogently, whether in the realm of medical decisions or in other aspects of our lives. What I have tried to show are some of the limitations of libertarian absolutism and a laissez-faire policy in decisions affecting the health of individuals and society. These modulations of the libertarian principle are central to any genuine balancing of the rights of individuals and of society. To achieve this balance requires a creative interaction between the patient, the physician, and society, each operating orthogonally with safeguards guaranteed by the interplay of law, ethics, government, and institutional regulation. The resultant matrix is a complex one, and the job of defining each box in that matrix is sure to be lengthy, tedious, and vexing. There is no alternative to beginning that examination immediately before the capabilities of medicine and its technology obscure the human purposes they presumably were meant to serve.

REFERENCES

1. Pellegrino ED: Myocardial infarction, during the acute episode or in prophylaxsis. Med Lett 16, No 4, 1974.
2. Pellegrino ED: Humanism in human experimentation: some notes on the investigator's fiduciary role. Tex Rep Biol Med 32: 106–111, 1974.
3. Pellegrino ED: The changing matrix of clinical decision making in the hospital. Edited by BS Georgopoulis. Organization Research on Health Institutions. Ann Arbor, The University of Michigan, 1972, pp 212–219.
4. Pellegrino ED: Toward an expanded medical ethics: the Hippocratic ethic revisited. Edited by RJ. Bulger. Hippocrates Revisited. Medcom Press, New York, 1973, pp 133–147.

III

Consumer Evaluation of Health Care

A strong consumer movement in health care has developed over the past few years. The expectations of the health system are different for the consumer than for the provider, and the values of these two groups are often at odds. This topic looks at the overall social ends that are to be achieved in the health care system and examines from that perspective how the values of the consumer and those of the provider are shaped—the mass media is particularly influential—and how they affect the health care system.

DAVID MECHANIC, Ph.D.
Professor of Sociology, University of Wisconsin

Patient Behavior and the Organization of Medical Care

Throughout most of the history of medicine, physicians could do little to prevent disease or to intervene effectively in its progress. But people sought the assistance of physicians, healers, and shamans to relieve their sense of subjective distress and uncertainty. Seeking care was in part a symbol of continuing hope, in part an expression of a desire to alleviate pain and restore functional capacity. These basic human needs persist today as well, perhaps overshadowed by the scientific development and technical elaboration of medical activities, but have a profound effect on the perception and response to medical services.

It is trite to observe that persons live in families and communities and that these social contexts shape their perceptions and behavior. Nevertheless it is true that how people come to identify problems, why they become concerned about them, and how and when they seek assistance are influenced by their social context as much as they are by objective symptoms or the character of the medical care system; and their reactions to treatment, their willingness to return to the physician, and cooperation in following medical advice are all affected by the extent to which the medical context conforms or clashes with social and cultural expectations.

The medical practitioner, by virtue of his activities, is in a position from which it is difficult to obtain an unbiased view of the social behavior systems affecting the occurrence of illness and the responses to it. The persons he ordinarily sees are those who have selected themselves for care, and the practitioner has little basis for an accurate construction of the populations from which the patients were selected, or how they are different from those who did not seek care. Even a cursory examination of the potential population at risk demonstrates considerable overlap in presenting symptoms between patients who seek care and symptoms reported by others in the population who do not choose to consult a physician.

Using relatively conservative estimates of the occurrence of physical symptoms in the population—that is, symptom reports based on an action criterion such as taking bed rest or medication—it is apparent that a large proportion of the population, approximately three quarters, have symptoms in any given month comparable to those that physicians see every day.[1] Approximately only one in three of these patients will seek a consultation with a physician. These estimates are based largely on acute and chronic physical illness and do not consider the wide range of psychiatric morbidity in the population. Estimates of such morbidity are difficult to provide since they vary so substantially from one study to another depending on the criterion used.[2] Obviously, if the criterion is too loose, the category becomes too inclusive. Various studies suggest that an estimate that from 5 to 10 percent of the population have serious psychiatric problems requiring care—such as depression, alcoholism, and the like—would be conservative.[3] Some epidemiological studies have reported that as many as 60 percent of the population suffer from psychiatric impairment.

To understand the process of medical care, it is essential to understand why some patients decide to seek care and others do not, why care seeking is initiated at particular points in time, and how the needs of patients and their motivations for medical care interact with the organization of the delivery system.

Differences in response to symptoms are dependent on the manner in which problems become manifest and their severity, on the social and cultural background and experience of the persons involved, and on the immediate contingencies of patients' life situations.[4] But before elaborating on each of these points, it is useful to examine what people mean by health, and how it relates to medical conceptions.

Although persons in Western nations have a fairly sophisticated view of health and illness, it is quite different from the professional viewpoint of physicians. Medicine as a science has developed by making abstract distinctions and classifications that have been incorporated in the way in which physicians define and treat patients. Patients react to illness more experientially and in a fashion that does not distinguish between feeling states and specific symptoms. Health is a state of perception and experience, and not the absence of one or another disease entity. Thus, when the correlates of persons' perceptions of their physical health are examined, psychological distress is a major predictor of how they see themselves.

Since reactions to illness are largely experiential, it is not surprising that persons who have symptoms are more likely to define them as worthy of care when such symptoms disrupt their ability to function and interfere in some fashion with their life activities. Investigators have consistently observed that illness is most salient when it is disruptive to usual functions, activities, and routines.[5] However, the seriousness of symptoms from a medical perspective may or may not be related to their salience or disruptiveness. Patients are also more likely to define symptoms as worthy of care when bodily indications are unfamiliar and frightening and when the person lacks an interpretation that allows "normalization" of the symptom. Some symptoms are much more easily normalized than others; chest pains might be attributed to indigestion, muscle ache to physical activity, or headaches to tension and stress.

How people react to symptoms is also related to their prior learning and experience and to the cultural and social definitions of the groups within which they live. Some years ago I characterized this concern as the study of illness behavior, and a fair amount of information on such reactions has accumulated in the last decade. Individuals as part of their social development acquire various attitudes and behaviors that are in part characteristic of their social contexts. Some groups encourage the expression of distress, while others expect stoicism and denial. Some cultural contexts provide a detailed psychological vocabulary to conceptualize and describe personal problems, while others communicate disapproval of any such suggestions.[6] These norms differ not only among social and ethnic groups but also may vary for men and women, children and adults. Such norms—and experience in reference to them—come to have an important effect on how persons define their difficulties in functioning and how they adapt to life problems.

Going to a doctor is only one of many possible responses for persons suffering pain and distress or disruption in life activities. In some of our studies we have attempted to measure in a rather crude way the varying propensity of persons to go to a doctor when they face illness. In some subgroups persons learn to seek out physicians readily when they have a problem, to have faith in doctors, and to have little skepticism about the value of medical care. In other contexts, learning experiences lead to delay in seeking medical care, denial of symptoms, and little trust in doctors. These propensities are not unfixed or unchanging, but frequently interact with the organization and typical response of the health care system and other factors in the individual's environment.

Various studies indicate that life difficulties and psychological distress are frequently present among persons seeking medical care.[7] Such stressful life situations have been alleged to contribute to the occurrence of illness, and this indeed may be the case.[8] But as Balint[9] has maintained, life difficulties and psychological distress frequently trigger the use of physician services, although some physical symptom might be presented as a justification for coming to see the doctor. Thus the high rate of psychological distress among patients seen may result either because such distress contributes to symptoms and illness, contributes to illness behavior and help seeking, or both. Our research suggests that psychological distress appears to have a larger influence among patients with high readiness to use physician services. Among patients with less readiness and greater skepticism of medical care, psychological distress may result in other forms of coping.

There are limits within which discretion in help seeking operates. When symptoms are sufficiently acute and severe, the impact of definitional processes is limited. But when symptoms occur less dramatically, in a milder form, and have limited impact on functioning, such social processes may be crucial. Much of ambulatory care falls within this latter categorization, and thus social definitions and response have an important impact on the content and process of primary care.

In part, patients who seek medical care as a result of life difficulties and high readiness to depend on physicians may present their problems in a variety of ways, and underlying problems are frequently identified only with difficulty. Some patients, of course, have a highly developed psychosocial vocabulary and present their problems to the doctor in psychosomatic and psychosocial frames of reference. They may complain of family conflict, depression, difficulties on the job, or whatever. Studies indicate that patients with such constructions of their complaints tend to be more urban, more educated, and tend to come from backgrounds encouraging a psychological vocabulary—such as among Jewish populations. A second type of patient, however, chronically complains of diffuse physical symptoms that are characteristic of both psychological and physical disorder: loss of appetite, difficulty sleeping, fatigue, aches and pains, and so on. Such patients are more likely to be of rural origins, to have less education, and to come from cultural backgrounds that discourage the open expression of emotions and complaints. Various data suggest that these patients subject themselves to considerable diagnostic work and to a high prevalence of surgical procedures. Other types of presentations fall between these two extreme types. A common complaint by patients is "nerves," a category between a physical and psychological presentation. Patients describing their problem as one of "nerves" frequently resist any interpretation that directly implicates factors in their immediate life situations, but seem to recognize their problems as somewhat different than more conventional physical disorders. Finally, many patients presenting self-limited acute complaints of mild or moderate severity may have come to the doctor as much because of life difficulties as of the symptom presented. But, then again, the physician does not really know, and that contributes enormously to the difficulty of his task. Let us now consider how this all appears from the physician's perspective.

PHYSICIAN RESPONSES TO PATIENT COMPLAINTS

The capacity of the doctor to cope effectively with the types of problems characteristic of primary medical care depends not only on his personality, attitudinal orientations, and prior preparation but also on the practice pressures and incentives he faces and the manner in which care is organized. The physician must manage not only his patients but also his time so as to complete the day's work and be reasonably responsive to his patients in the aggregate. How he does this will depend on both the organization of his practice and incentives implicit in how he is paid.

The discussion that follows must be somewhat exploratory since there is very limited research on how practice structures affect the physician's behavior. I, therefore, must depend substantially on my own inquiries that have certain limitations. Most serious of these limitations is that the studies that I will report are cross-sectional and nonexperimental in character and depend exclusively on what the physician reports about himself and his practice. When one observes an association in nonexperimental, cross-sectional studies between a mode of practice and other behavior, it is impossible to precisely determine to what extent the outcome is attributable to organizational effects from the degree to which certain persons with particular behavioral orientations select certain modes of practice. Also, without independent observations, self-reports of physicians concerning their own work must be viewed with a certain skepticism. Wherever possible, I seek data from other studies that either strengthen or contradict my conclusions, but I emphasize that the types of investigations I discuss cannot prove the contentions I will put forth.

When I first became interested in general medical practice in England

and Wales in the early 1960s, I was impressed by the frequency with which practitioners complained of the triviality and inappropriateness of medical consultations. As I inquired into the issue I became more puzzled because the usual interpretations of the reasons for such complaints appeared to be inconsistent with existing information. Although there was a tendency to explain such attributions of triviality by the fact that the National Health Service was free—and thus the argument that the absence of economic barriers led to exploitation of the doctor the available data on practitioner utilization could not sustain this contention. Average medical utilization was not substantially higher in England than in the United States, nor was it likely that differences in utilization or patients' behavior from one practitioner to another could account for their widely varying attributions of triviality. Also, it appeared that doctors with larger panels complained more vigorously of trivial patients; yet existing data suggested that the patients of such doctors had lower average per capita utilization of medical services than patients of doctors with smaller panels. I came to the same conclusion as Ann Cartwright,[10] who was also working on similar issues at the time, that the attributions of triviality told us more about the doctor and his practice than about the objective characteristics of his patients or the nature of their problems.

When we examine the reports of official bodies—such as the Gillie Committee[11] or the Royal Commission on Medical Education[12]—we find that the dissatisfaction of physicians and their frustrations are explained by such factors as a lack of hospital attachment, the absence of group practice or adequate ancillary help, or the unsatisfactory educational preparation of the general practitioner. When we studied a national sample of general practitioners in 1965–1966, we could find little evidence in support of any of these arguments except that doctors with training in psychiatry and behavioral science seemed somewhat more content.[13] We cannot determine whether this is attributable to the training or to the types of people who select to have such training. I should emphasize that our sample of 800 general practitioners did not provide many who were working in modern practice structures, containing the advantages usually attributed to group or health center practice or to the effective use of paraprofessional manpower. Thus, it is conceivable that the implementation of the suggestions of these official committees could have a real effect. But within the prevalent variations then existing—and still existing—I am frankly skeptical.

In the study of English general practitioners a large number of variables was examined. Most variables describing the doctor's background or modes of practice had little effect on how he viewed his patients or his own satisfactions and dissatisfactions. Only one type of factor appeared to matter very much—patient demand. The more patients the doctor saw, the more likely he was to describe them as trivial and inappropriate. The influence of patient demand was pronounced even when controlling many other variables simultaneously.

Such an association is, of course, open to a variety of interpretations. We were able to exclude some of these since we had collected a great deal of data on various facets of the doctor's practice. One could not account for the differences on the basis of geographic area or the doctors' descriptions of the social class characteristics of their patients. Nor is it likely that the different perceptions of triviality reflect real differences in the distribution of morbidity or help seeking in varying doctors' panels, although this issue deserves more study. I, thus, came to the following *post hoc* interpretation of these findings.

English general practitioners, paid on a weighted capitation basis, develop some concept of how much time they ought to devote to their practices. Although they may adjust to varying patient demands in their practice, they do this within some concept of what constitutes a reasonable workweek. They then establish fixed surgery hours within which they accommodate the patients who wish to see them. Doctors who have larger panels and who schedule more limited surgery hours relative to patient demand must practice an assembly-line medicine that basically involves symptomatic treatment. As patient demand grows, the doctor must practice in a more hurried way to get through the daily queue. The doctor, of course, can cope by increasing his surgery hours substantially, but a capitation system of payment provides no incentive for him doing so. Obviously, some do so because of their own compulsiveness or sense of obligation, but our concern here is with the average tendencies and not the exceptions.

The general practitioner sees many patients with psychosocial problems who suffer from significant psychological distress, and this has been well documented by the studies of general practice carried out by Michael Shepherd and his group.[14] Such patients may present common physical complaints to justify their consultations, but such visits may be motivated by underlying distress. These patients are difficult to care for under the best of circumstances, but under conditions that prevail in the busiest surgeries the doctor has little time to talk with the patient and explore in any detail the nature of his concerns.

The doctor, in treating the patient symptomatically, is aware of his failures to explore the patient's problem and feels frustrated by his manner of practice. The attribution of triviality is probably a reflection of this feeling, and, indeed, we find that doctors who report that a large proportion of their patients are trivial also report that they frequently do not have time to do an adequate examination and to do what is necessary for the patient. They also report more frequently than other doctors that they more commonly issue prescriptions without seeing the patient and give patients certificates although unconvinced that the patient is too sick for work.[15] In short, I am suggesting that British general practitioners define patients as trivial because the nature of their practice induces them to treat patient complaints as if they are trivial.

We anticipated that fee-for-service arrangements would create different incentives for the doctor's behavior; thus, we carried out a similar investigation of a national sample of 1,500 American general practitioners, internists, pediatricians, and obstetricians.[16] Although perceptions of triviality are not uncommon in the American context, such reports are much less frequent than in British practice. In general, American doctors see far fewer patients, and expectations require that they give the patient more time than in typical British practice. We anticipated that, in fee-for-service practice, doctors would be subject to a larger extent to what Freidson has called "client control" and, thus, would anticipate that their patients expect the doctor to spend a reasonable amount of time with them. Because of the fee-for-service incentive, we anticipated that doctors would be more likely to respond to such patient expectations by increasing office hours in order to see patients. Indeed, this is what we and others find. Doctors in fee-for-service practice, who face large patient demand, work very long hours.[17] Unlike the British practitioner, the doctor is rewarded for every additional patient he sees. Consistent with this is the finding that when physicians move from a fee-for-service to a salaried structure, as occurred in Canada, they report a decrease in hours worked.[18]

In the American context, we anticipated that prepaid physicians in large prepaid group practices would be exposed to incentives very much like those characteristic of English general practice. Although our sample of doctors in prepaid groups was very limited within the context of our national sample, our fragmentary data suggested that they responded very much like the English general practitioners and that they were much more likely to attribute triviality or inappropriateness to the patients they see.[19]

This finding was sufficiently provocative so that we selected still another national sample of physicians who practiced in prepaid groups. For reasons that I would not go into here, this sample includes only general practitioners and pediatricians. The analysis of these data is still incomplete, but they suggest a complex and differentiated response depending on the practice conditions prevailing. Consistent with our pre-

vious survey of American physicians, general practitioners and pediatricians in prepaid group practice are more than three times as likely as nongroup fee-for-service practitioners to indicate that 50 percent or more of
their patients are trivial or inappropriate (Table 1). While only 9 percent
of nongroup general practitioners report this many patients as trivial, 32
percent of general practitioners in prepaid practice give such a report.
The comparable figures for pediatricians are 9 percent and 29 percent. I
should note that the proportion of American general practitioners and
pediatricians in prepaid practice reporting 50 percent or more of their
patients as trivial is higher than the 24 percent of British general practitioners who give such reports.

One possibility, of course, is that prepaid patients exploit medical
care in the absence of economic barriers, and perceptions of triviality reflect such abuse. We have carefully examined existing data involving
studies of prepaid practice and utilization data reported by the large pre-
paids, such as Health Insurance Plan and Kaiser–Portland. In some cases,
average utilization in prepaid practice is a little higher than in other
forms of practice; in some cases, there are no clear differences; and in

TABLE 1   Reports Concerning Trivial Consultations in Varying Practice Settings

	Percent Reporting 50% or More Patients Are Trivial	Percent Reporting 10% or Less Patients Are Trivial
British general practitioners (N = 772)	24	12
All nongroup American primary care physicians[a] (N = 1148)	7	36
All group American primary care physicians[a] (N = 310)	10	36
Nongroup American general practitioners (N = 604)	9	33
Group American general practitioners (N = 113)	13	27
Nongroup American pediatricians (N = 136)	9	31
Group American pediatricians (N = 43)	9	33
Prepaid American general practitioners[b] (N = 108)	32	7
Prepaid American pediatricians[b] (N = 154)	29	14

[a] Includes general practitioners, pediatricians, internists, and obstetricians.
[b] Includes physicians in practices involving 50 percent or more prepaid practice activity.

still other cases there is even evidence of lower rates of utilization than in the population at large.[20] This should not be surprising in that we know that there are many noneconomic barriers that control rates of utilization: the resources made available, distance to the outpatient facility, difficulty in making an appointment, waiting time, and the responsiveness of care once one arrives.

On the basis of our two earlier surveys, we suspected that physicians in prepaid contexts viewed themselves as working on a contractual basis. They receive a fixed salary for a defined period of work, and unlike fee-for-service physicians, there are few existing incentives to substantially increase the amount of time they spend seeing patients. Thus we suspected that when prepaid practices faced large patient demands, they scheduled extra patients within the physicians' defined hours of work rather than have the physicians work longer hours. This would result in a more assembly-line practice, one that is less responsive to the patient as a person. Studies of consumers of prepaid practice also report that they are more likely than in fee-for-service practice to feel that practitioners are less responsive to their needs and seem less interested in them,[21,22] and this is consistent with the overall argument.

When we more closely examined the specific components of the physicians' satisfactions and dissatisfactions in our large American sample, we found support for this interpretation. Fee-for-service physicians have longer workweeks than prepaid physicians and complain the most of their long hours of work and lack of leisure time. In contrast, prepaid group practitioners are more satisfied with their overall workweek, but they are more dissatisfied with the amount of time for each patient.

Our sample of general practitioners and pediatricians in prepaid group practice provided a further opportunity to examine factors affecting the perceptions and attributions of physicians working on other than fee-for-service arrangements. As we anticipated, physicians in prepaid practice are much more likely to have a shorter workweek, although they spend more of their total working time in direct patient care. Doctors in prepaid practice, in contrast to both other group and nongroup practitioners, are more satisfied with the total time their medical practice requires and with the leisure time available to them. Although prepaid group general practitioners were most likely to be dissatisfied with the time available for each patient, this expected relationship was not obtained for the prepaid group pediatricians. Unexpectedly, we found the opposite to be the case: The nongroup pediatricians were most dissatisfied with having adequate time for each patient. This finding required a more detailed examination of the practice characteristics of nongroup and prepaid group pediatricians.

Our data conform with the typical picture of the highly harassed nongroup pediatrician. In comparison to the prepaid group pediatricians, nongroup pediatricians saw many more patients, worked many more hours, and took on a wider range of functions and responsibilities. For example, on the previous day, 43 percent of nongroup pediatricians saw 33 or more patients in contrast to 18 percent of prepaid group pediatricians who saw this many. More than half of the nongroup pediatricians reported seeing this many patients on a typical busy day, but only 34 percent of prepaid group pediatricians gave a comparable report. While 31 percent of nongroup pediatricians reported that they saw more patients than reasonable, only 13 percent of group prepaid pediatricians gave a similar report. Furthermore, nongroup pediatricians reported spending more time on the phone, on hospital rounds, on administrative work, and the like. They made more house calls and spent more time managing their practice. In contrast, although prepaid group general practitioners had a much shorter workweek than nongroup practitioners, they saw a large number of patients when they worked. Two fifths of the prepaid group general practitioners saw 33 or more patients on the previous day, and 37 percent reported that they had responsibility for more patients than was reasonable.

Because of the different practice demands faced by prepaid group general practitioners and pediatricians, we pursued the analysis separately for each group. While such reports as having responsibility for too many patients were associated with reported trivial consultations among prepaid general practitioners, they were not very useful as predictors among prepaid group pediatricians who faced a much smaller patient load. We thus examined all of our samples of physicians to establish those findings that were consistently associated with attributions of triviality across all samples. As a consequence, we ignored many strong findings that appeared in some samples but not in others. For example, among prepaid group general practitioners, the correlation between the doctors' disagreement that they have a "responsibility to advise and care for the psychological problems of patients" and the proportion of patients perceived as trivial is 0.34; among prepaid group pediatricians it is 0.14; and in the overall sample of American primary care physicians it is only 0.07. By the criterion stated above, the association between these two variables would not be regarded as stable, but it is probably suggestive of the true complexity of the phenomenon at issue. I suspect that the relationship between perceived responsibility for psychological problems and attributions of triviality is only strong when the physician is paid on a capitation basis and when he has more patients than he can reasonably cope with. At present we are pursuing these ideas in a multivariate analysis.

In examining those correlations consistent throughout all samples, we find that attributions of triviality are associated with concern about people bringing less serious disorders to doctors and more readily seeking help for problems in their family lives and with less overall satisfaction. We also find that attributions of triviality are consistently higher among physicians who report that they are dissatisfied with the amount of time they have for each patient and among those who report seeing more patients on a busy day. We suspect that attributions of triviality reflect the reactions of a technically inclined physician burdened by a heavy patient load and with few incentives to be responsive to the psychological and social concerns that are associated with many patient consultations.

These findings reinforce our understanding that each type of practice organization has its own distinctive advantages and disadvantages. There is a great deal of data suggesting that a fee-for-service system, in the absence of other controls, promotes incentives for unnecessary and perhaps dangerous work and increases the rate of discretionary surgery.[23] Physicians in this type of practice frequently work themselves to exhaustion, taking insufficient time for continuing education and leisure. The direct dependence on the patient's satisfaction, however, may produce a more responsive attitude and one that communicates greater interest in and concern for the patient. This may be reflected in a greater willingness on the part of the physician to answer the patient's inquiries, to talk with him, and to have an interest in his viewpoint.

In prepaid group practice the physician is less attuned to his patient, and as Freidson[24] has suggested, colleague control is more prevalent. This may be conducive to a high quality of technical medical care and an avoidance of unnecessary treatment, but it also may be conducive to a certain inflexibility and lack of responsiveness that may not be consistent with a high level of primary care. The point is not to engage in mindless polemics about the value of one or another system of organization, but to seek models of care that maximize the advantages and minimize the costs of each. In talking about new models of primary medical care, we must be continually aware of the human problems of medical care and the factors that bring patients to physicians in the first place.[25]

A certain level of morale is necessary for decent performance, and we should bolster physician morale as much as possible to the extent that it does not undermine other functions. I believe that we must combine the advantages of prepaid group practice with new incentives for physicians who work within such practice contexts. The most important goal of such incentives would be to make the physician more responsive and interested in the types of problems typical of ambulatory care. Since such responsiveness is closely associated with the number of patients the physician is responsible for and the types of problems they have, we cannot neglect the issue of the amount and types of patient demand, the effective use of ancillary assistance, and the implementation of new paraprofessionals as a way of dealing more effectively with some of the problems discussed.

CONSIDERATION OF ALTERNATIVE INNOVATIONS IN PRIMARY MEDICAL CARE

In discussing patient motivation in seeking medical care, I maintained that psychological concerns were of great importance. From a practical point of view we might distinguish services for such patients in terms of the complexity of their needs. Conservative estimates suggest that approximately 5 to 10 percent of patients populations have formal psychiatric difficulties and that of these approximately 5 percent are acutely psychotic. Some proportion of this group is clearly beyond the capabilities and experience of the typical primary care physician and requires referral. The remainder of this group is probably manageable within primary medical care with supportive specialty assistance for the primary physician. Beyond this group of formal disorders are others that require time and attention but no complicated regimen. Then there are many chronic patients with considerable psychological and psychosocial problems who could be served quite effectively on a continuing basis by nurse-practitioners supported by the primary care physician.[26]

There is now increasing evidence that providing psychiatric assistance to chronically complaining patients is related to an overall reduction in medical and hospital utilization.[27] However, since these studies tend to be nonexperimental, it is difficult to project whether the same outcomes can be achieved among chronic complainers who now resist psychiatric care or a psychiatric interpretation of their problem.[28] Such patients are probably better managed by the primary care physician. It is important to also note that the utilization reduction reported in these studies mainly characterizes patients with mild and moderate disorders. The seriously disturbed psychiatric patients do not appear to reduce overall medical utilization despite the provision of psychiatric care.

Primary care physicians treat the vast majority of patients with psychiatric disorders. Only a relatively small proportion is referred, or refer themselves, to psychiatric facilities. This process of pathways into psychiatric care has been extensively studied, and for the less extreme disorders it is clear that social and cultural characteristics are important in determining the use of psychiatric referral.[29] Patients more willing to accept psychiatric referral are better educated, more cosmopolitan, and are more likely to associate with others who have used or are receptive to psychiatric services. Also, such receptivity is more common in urban areas, among particular ethnic groups such as Jews, and among persons with lower religiosity.

No matter how good psychiatric services are—and they are far from optimal—much of the responsibility will continue to reside with the primary care physician. Many primary care physicians have negative attitudes toward both psychiatry and psychiatric patients, and rates of recognition and referral of psychiatric patients fluctuate widely from one practitioner to another.[30] But regardless of the attitude of physicians, the management of patients with psychiatric and psychosocial difficulties can be exceedingly difficult. Some probably need no more than a professional who expresses an interest in their problems and who is willing to listen to them, but the patient with diffuse physical complaints who may indeed have a serious physical condition poses a much more difficult problem.

Physicians, of course, have an obligation to satisfy themselves that the complaints have no basis in detectable organic disease, but if they are not to exaggerate such physical detection processes, they must also be attentive to patients' psychological states and provide opportunities for relevant psychological and social information to become salient. Many complaining patients are significantly depressed and anxious, but do not feel free to discuss these feelings unless the physician provides an appropriate opening.

There is growing evidence that indicates that dealing with many psychosocial problems requires more than social support and encouragement that contributes to the reduction of feelings of anxiety and distress.[31] In many circumstances patients require specific instructions that assist them in dealing with their life circumstances. To be effective, such instructions must be relevant to their problem and consistent with the patient's experiences, and they also must be psychologically and culturally credible. The growing utility of behavior modification approaches offers some promise for the practitioner dealing with problems of child care, obesity, alcohol abuse, and the like. In many areas of behavior, it is not clear what directions for behavior change are credible, but it is valuable for the practitioner to keep in mind not only the needs of the patient to maintain greater psychological comfort but also the necessary instructions and skills required for the patient to cope with his or her life situation.

I emphasize the dimension of credibility since every practitioner knows that there is a substantial difference between recognizing a patient's level of psychological distress and obtaining the acceptance of the patient that this is part of the problem. I also noted that there are many persons who resist psychological attributions to their distress because of prior cultural upbringing and existing social norms in their important primary groups. The physician who forces a definition on a patient that the patient is unprepared to accept achieves little and may undermine whatever source of help he can be. He must work patiently and subtly within the patient's frame of reference if he is to achieve desired results.

If, indeed, this is part of the responsibility of primary care physicians, it is not difficult to understand why a technically efficient and operationally hurried practice may not be conducive to its fulfillment. The realities of care require certain trade-offs between optimally responsive care and the need to meet demands for access to the physician, but we would do well to recognize what it is that is sacrificed and attempt to develop appropriate models of care that are better attuned to the forces that create concern in the population and that bring patients into medical care.

IMPLICATIONS FOR THE RESOLUTION OF CONFLICTS

The problem in meeting patient expectations is inherent in the different conceptions of physician and patient and in the conflict between giving patients more comprehensive care in contrast to seeing more patients. To the extent that physicians take a broad view of their responsibilities, and devote time to exploring life situations and providing support and advice, curtailment of patient load becomes mandatory. When resources are limited, however, those without adequate access to care might not experience such modifications as beneficial.

It should be apparent that patients have diverse needs and orientations, and no simple uniform assumptions will allow physicians to proceed effectively. If the physician is to respond to the patient as an individual, he must have some acquaintance with him and be sensitive to changing needs, and this requires time and continuity. Physicians, of course, complain that they lack the time and, in any case, it is not clear to them that such investments yield much in the way of tangible benefits. Thus physicians focus on identifying and treating recognizable disease states that are relatively clear-cut, subject to routinization, and are consistent with the models of behavior with which the physician has learned to feel comfortable.

The more specialized approach to the patient has other consequences as well. In focusing on the search for disease, which is largely a technical activity, the physician can proceed in a manner less dependent on the patient or on his cooperation and involvement. Thus, the physician can deal with the patient as an object with little attention to the patient's wishes or consent. He proceeds independently, making decisions on the tests to order, the procedures to use, and the expenses involved. Even with such major decisions as hospitalization, length of stay, and the use of discretionary procedures, the involvement of the patient is usually limited to providing nominal or legal consent. The organization of medical activity generally is one that leaves the patient with the impression of being worked on and is hardly conducive to maximize the play of the patient's values and choices against those characterizing the predominant medical approach.

While in ambulatory settings the pressures of time and the limited scope of the physician's approach result in constraints on patient expression and choice, such constraints are greatly exacerbated by the elaboration of conflicting interests in multipurpose institutions such as teaching hospitals and medical centers.[32] In such contexts there is an elaboration of potential conflicts of interest between patients' wishes and the constellation of pressures on the physician from patient load, service needs, research, and teaching. As these institutional forms have grown and as new programs have emerged, such conflicts are actually built in as a way of coping with particular problems. Thus, a health maintenance organization (HMO) may provide economic incentives for the physician to cut down patient utilization of services, a teaching hospital may give awards to the house officers who achieve the greatest participation of patients in research work[33] or who get the most autopsy permissions,[34] and patients may be kept in the hospital to protect and enhance the vitality of a developing unit that requires a minimum patient load to ensure its continued financing.

The existing pressures toward the specialization and institutionalization of medical work—and the emphasis on efficiency and productivity— make it difficult to reorder priorities in a way that ensures patient care that is responsive to them as persons rather than as objects, that maximizes opportunities for expression and choice, and that provides occasions for participation and instruction in relationships with professionals. But if one measures the success of medical care by its effective implementation rather than by the number of consultations and number of procedures performed, then what now appears inefficient and wasteful may turn out not to be as costly as alleged. Current medical practice is characterized by frequent disruptions in communication and in mutual expectations of patients and physicians and in frequent failure to conform with medical advice.[35] Care that is responsive to patient perceptions and expectations, that provides the patient an opportunity to be heard, and that instructs the patient in a fashion consistent with knowledge of life situations and problems may result in greater cooperation and implementation of medical care.

In conclusion, I do not want to exaggerate what we know about managing human problems in the context of medical care. Serious research in this relatively neglected area is of high priority. From the perspective of human values, however, medicine has a social role that far transcends the technical procedures that doctors perform. To deny these needs and motivations is to debase the practice of medicine and its traditions. In social life symbols are of immense importance, and the character of medical activities and their scope help define those aspects of man that we value.

I also would not want to minimize the practical issues. The implementation of comprehensive medicine depends on a more adequate distribution of medical manpower, better models for organizing health care tasks between physicians and among health workers generally, and the development of new educational settings in which the larger problems of medical practice are given attention as a major priority in the work of faculty and the training of students. This is not possible without fundamental changes in medical education and medical practice, and in the reward structures that determine not what people say but how they behave.

ACKNOWLEDGMENTS

The work reported here was supported in part by the Robert Wood Johnson Foundation Project on Ambulatory Health Care and the National Center for Health Services Research (grants HS00253 and HS00091).

REFERENCES

1. White KL, Williams TF, Greenberg BG: The ecology of medical care. N Engl J Med 265:885–892, 1961.
2. Dohrenwend B, Dohrenwend B: Social Status and Psychological Disorder. New York, Wiley Interscience, 1969.
3. Gardner E: Emotional disorders in medical practice. Ann Intern Med 73:651–652, 1970.
4. Mechanic D: Public Expectations and Health Care. New York, Wiley Interscience, 1972, pp 203–222.
5. Mechanic D: Medical Sociology. New York, Free Press, 1968, pp 145–146.
6. Mechanic D: Social psychologic factors affecting the presentation of bodily complaints. N Engl J Med 286:1132–1139, 1972.
7. Shepherd M: Psychiatric Illness in General Practice. London, Oxford University Press, 1966.
8. Hinkle LE, Jr: The effect of exposure to culture change, social change, and

changes in interpersonal relationships upon health. Presented at the Conference on Stressful Life Events, University Center of the City of New York, June 1973.

9. Balint M: The Doctor, His Patient and the Illness. New York, International Universities Press, 1957.

10. Cartwright A: Patients and Their Doctors: A Study of General Practice. London, Routledge, 1967.

11. Great Britain Ministry of Health: The Field of Work of the Family Doctor. London, Her Majesty's Stationery Office, 1963.

12. Royal Commission on Medical Education, 1965–68 Report. London, Her Majesty's Stationery Office, 1968 (Cmnd 3569).

13. Mechanic D: Correlates of frustration among British general practitioners. J Health Soc Behav 11:87–104, 1970.

14. Shepherd M: *op. cit.*

15. Mechanic D: Correlates of frustration among British general practitioners. *op. cit.*

16. Mechanic D: General medical practice: some comparisons between the work of primary care physicians in the United States and England and Wales. Med Care 10:402–420, 1972.

17. *Ibid.*

18. Enterline PE, et al: Effect of "free" medical care on medical practice—the Quebec experience. N Engl J Med 288:1152–1155, 1973.

19. Mechanic D: Physician satisfaction in varying settings. Paper presented at the NCHSRD Manpower Conference, Chicago, Illinois, 1971.

20. Health Insurance Plan of New York: H.I.P. Statistical Report: 1968–1969. New York, Division of Research and Statistics, 1970; Saward E, et al.: Documentation of twenty years of operation and growth of a prepaid group practice plan. Med Care 6:239–244, 1968; Columbia School of Public Health and Administrative Medicine: Family Medical Care under Three Types of Health Insurance. New York, Foundation on Employee Health, Medical Care and Welfare, Inc., 1962; Committee for the Special Research Project in the Health Insurance Plan of New York: Health and Medical Care in New York City. Cambridge, Harvard University Press, 1957; Darsky BJ, et al: Comprehensive Medical Services under Voluntary Health Insurance. Cambridge, Harvard University Press, 1958; Anderson OW, Sheatsley PB: Comprehensive Medical Insurance: A Study of Costs, Use and Attitudes under Two Plans. New York, Health Information Foundation Research Ser No 9, 1959.

21. Freidson E: Patients' Views of Medical Practice. New York, Russell Sage Foundation, 1961.

22. Donabedian A: A review of some experiences with prepaid group practice. Bureau of Public Health Economics Research Ser No 12. Ann Arbor, School of Public Health, University of Michigan, 1965.

23. Roemer MI: On paying the doctor and the implications of different methods. J Health Human Behav 3:4–14, 1962; U.S. Department of Health, Education, and Welfare: Toward a Comprehensive Health Policy for the 1970s: A White Paper. Washington, D.C., Government Printing Office, 1971.

24. Freidson E: Profession of Medicine. New York, Dodd, Mead, 1970.

25. Mechanic D: Public Expectations and Health Care. *op. cit.*, pp 67–79.

26. Lewis CE, Resnik BA: Nurse clinics and progressive ambulatory patient care. N Engl J Med 277:1236–1241, 1967.

27. Follette W, Cummings NA: Psychiatric services and medical utilization in a

prepaid health plan setting. Med Care 5:25–35, 1967; Goldberg ID, et al: Effect of a short-term outpatient psychiatric therapy benefit on the utilization of medical services in a prepaid group practice medical program. Med Care 8:419–428, 1970.

28. Follette W, Cummings NA: Psychiatric services and medical utilization in a prepaid health care setting. Part II. Med Care 6:31–41, 1968.

29. Kadushin C: Why People Go to Psychiatrists. New York, Atherton, 1969.

30. Shepherd M: *op. cit.*

31. Leventhal H: Findings and theory in the study of fear communications. Adv Exp Soc Psychol 5:119–186, 1970; Egbert LD, et al.: Reduction of postoperative pain by encouragement and instruction of patients: a study of doctor-patient rapport. N Engl J Med 270:825–827, 1964.

32. Duff RS, Hollingshead AB: Sickness and Society. New York, Harpers, 1968; Cartwright A: Human Relations and Hospital Care. Boston, Routledge and Kegan Paul, 1964.

33. Miller S: Prescription for Leadership: Training for the Medical Elite. Chicago, Aldine, 1970.

34. Duff RS, Hollingshead AB: *op. cit.*

35. Ley P, Spelman MS: Communicating with the Patient. London, Trinity Press, 1967.

RICHARD ZECKHAUSER, PH.D.

Professor of Political Economy, Harvard University

Commentary

In the health care sector, modes of delivery and value norms are closely entwined. They evolve together. To explore this theme, we must understand the way alternative medical care settings mold consumer (patient) and producer (physician) attitudes and shape their behaviors. Professor Mechanic addresses these issues, paying particular attention to fee-for-service and prepaid capitation practices. His analysis provides insights on such questions as, "Why do patients seek medical care?" "What aspects of medical care delivery systems are most influential in determining attitudes of physicians toward their patients?" Having identified significant advantages for two competing delivery modes, Professor Mechanic, quite appropriately, is loath to recommend one system over the other. Still, he might have given us some thoughts on procedures for financing medical care that can be expected to promote efficiency in either delivery mode.

Professor Mechanic concludes with a plea that all can applaud. We should improve our performance in managing the human problems in the context of medical care. In particular, we should ensure that physicians respond to each patient as an individual.

WHY ETHICS ARE NEEDED IN THE MEDICAL CARE SECTOR

To show that physician and patient attitudes are shaped by the delivery mode is an important first step taken by Professor Mechanic. He could

86

have profitably gone a step further and explored the ethical implications of his findings and the implications of his findings for medical ethics. What he might discover in an inquiry of this sort would depend very much on his vantage point.

Here the perspective of the economics profession is employed. Medical care delivery is examined in its role as a productive process. In this context, there is a natural first question, "Why do we care so much about ethics and ethical behavior in relation to the production of health?" In most other industries, say wheat or shoes or nails, issues of ethics hardly arise. The logical inference is that the production process for health and/or the way we value health outputs must be of a nature that ethics can play a useful and important role. Two signal characteristics of the health production process support this inference.

1. Human intervention plays a relatively minor role in comparison with nature in affecting health levels. Further, an individual's health, broadly speaking the well-being and sanctity of his body, is not a commodity that can be reproduced through traditional productive processes. This pairing, nature's role and nonreproducibility, accords health special treatment when it is valued as a productive output. (Consideration of frequently expressed concerns in the ecology field provide a test of this hypothesized linkage. The opponents of actions that would irreversibly damage ecosystems produce arguments that have the ethical ring of pleas for more humane and considerate medical care.)

We find it perfectly acceptable for an individual to sell some possession or the product of his labor; but we do not feel it appropriate for him to sell himself (or his family members) into slavery, or to place his bodily organs up for barter. The more commonplace aspects of health, of course, are personal to individuals. Even if there were no moral or ethical objections, physical limitations would prevent their trade.

Here the subject is medical care, a commodity that can be readily transferred from one man to another. Medical care is an intermediate good that promotes the restoration (nondeterioration) of health. It is through this relationship that medical care achieves a form of sanctity through proximity.

2. Health care is produced under conditions of massive uncertainty. This implies that consumer decisions should perhaps be relied on less heavily, since they are unlikely to be fully informed. The outcome of each medical encounter is a single point, or event, from a distribution of potential health outcomes. Just by judging his personal health outcome, a consumer cannot make an informed evaluation of the quality of his physician. If a consumer could gather accurate data on a large number of

medical encounters, he could make a statistically informed evaluation. But his own experiences are likely to be quite limited, and his most systematic mechanisms for sharing information with other consumers are likely to involve little more than personal gossip.

Not only are the outputs of the medical care process uncertain in nature, but there is an asymmetry in the ability of the producer and consumer to understand the factors that influence the probabilities that different outputs are produced. Yet there is an abiding need for the consumer to provide accurate information to the physician if an informed diagnosis is to be established and to convey to him his values and preferences if an appropriate treatment is to be prescribed. The production relationship that is most effective, and one that emerges naturally from this situation, is an agency process. Within it, for the most part, the consumer delegates decision-making authority to his physician. The physician in turn is expected to act in his client's behalf. This structure is characteristic of many agency relationships, with the more informed and sophisticated agent undertaking more favorable actions than the client could undertake for himself. (It is evident that if a doctor–patient relationship is to be successful, the client must be willing to reveal the information required for the physician's decision.)

An inherent difficulty remains. The client cannot assess whether his agent has performed effectively. This problem arises whether the agency relationship be in law, accounting, medicine, or in more mundane areas such as landscaping. Its virulence in the medical sector, as was suggested earlier, is due to the characteristic uncertainty of outcomes, the limited number of observable trials, and the inability of consumers to comprehend fully what information is available to them.

Having described some special features of the production process for health that might allow ethical codes to play a productive role, it seems appropriate to examine how ethics can influence the welfare of physicians, their patients, and society at large.

WHY PHYSICIANS IMPOSE ETHICS ON THEMSELVES

The primary force behind the development of ethical codes for medical practitioners has always been the physicians themselves. A cynic might ask, "To the extent such codes limit physicians' behavior are they not detrimental to physicians' interests?" If he determines that codes may prove beneficial, not detrimental, he may proceed to a second question. "If physicians find that self-imposed ethical behavior is desirable, why is it necessary to have codes?"

Ethical codes, which both producers and consumers can expect to be followed, play two related roles: (1) They ensure a minimum quality level for care on the part of the physician; (2) they inform the consumer that a minimum quality level is being maintained. The roles of ethical codes in many ways parallel those of licensing and certification procedures. Where licensing is, in effect, the prohibition against substandard service quality is enforced by the government through its legal arm. Certification, in contrast to licensing, is a voluntary procedure. Individuals choose to demonstrate some assured quality of service.

Individuals in a variety of occupations choose to be certificated. In industries subject to licensing, those who receive licenses have little incentive to complain; those who don't receive them usually find it difficult to organize. The ability to demonstrate competence and assure quality is likely to be of significant value to producers, particularly to high-quality producers, in a market where information on quality is difficult to monitor. An ethical code that is known to be followed plays this quality assuring role, among others.

Ethical codes are not needed to provide physicians with the exclusionary benefits that return to licensing and sometimes to certification (although individuals in some professions, realtors for example, may have restriction of competition as a motivation when they certify their ethics). Since codes of medical ethics supposedly gain universal adherence, the strictly pecuniary gains such codes offer to physicians must be reflected in the gap between the aggregate demand curves for ethically constrained and unconstrained medical care services. To stretch the market analogy to the limit, if physicians were operating as a "profit"-maximizing cartel, they would impose an ethical code upon themselves if it boosted their producers' surplus. (The introduction of ethics to an industry shifts both its supply and demand curves upward; thus, producers' surplus can expand or shrink. The shrinkage possibility suggests that there may be industries where, although the requisite coordination is available, ethics have not been self-imposed.)

Medical ethics can yield financial benefits to physicians quite apart from improving the market for physicians' services. Given the substantial entry barriers to the medical profession, we might expect that social pressures would be generated to have the government treat it as a cartel in restraint of trade. It would be somewhat unrealistic to expect the government to apply pressure against such anticompetitive devices as licensing arrangements; but more mundane regulatory tools, such as price controls, could be brought into play. Then again, if the government, not the profession, were defining acceptable behavior, we might discover that advertising prices was regarded as a desirable rather than an unethical activity.

By imposing ethics upon itself, as Thomas Schelling suggested to me, the medical profession may be engaging in the type of cliquish or restrictive activity that would prove attractive for any guild or manufacturers' group. It is announcing its capability to monitor and regulate its own activities. It creates for itself a climate in which it is allowed to operate independent of the regulatory procedures traditionally imposed on restricted-entry industries. This does not imply that the public is injured. If the poor performance of regulation in many nonhealth areas is indicative, more active regulation in the health care industry might hurt more than it helps.

Ethics can yield subtle, nonpecuniary benefits to medical care producers. Substantial reassurance may be gained from the guidelines ethics provides when a practitioner is facing difficult and delicate decisions. When he encounters a significantly unfortunate outcome, as surely each practitioner must at times, the knowledge that he has acted in accordance with established ethical norms may make it far easier for him to accept the mischance. (He may also gain protection from a malpractice suit.)

A profession's ethical code may also serve its practitioners as an image-enhancing public good. The members gain outside recognition, as well as self-esteem and stature, by being participants in an industry that abides by a more rigid code of ethical behavior than the one observed by society at large. It should perhaps be noted that the medical profession's actual image may differ significantly from the way it believes it is seen. Since it is the physicians who compose the "public" for this public good, it is the perceived rather than the actual image that is important.

This discussion provides an answer to a question raised earlier: "If self-imposed ethical behavior is desirable, why is it necessary to have codes?" First, if the code were adopted on a physician-by-physician basis, it would be difficult to inform consumers exactly who was and who wasn't subscribing to which standards of ethics. Enforcement would be more difficult. And the economies of scale reaped in present indoctrination procedures would vanish. Second, in a quite different vein, self-selected ethics would hardly provide the guidance, reassurance or self-perceived image enhancement that physicians now reap from codes that are universally or near-universally accepted.

ETHICS AND CONSUMER SATISFACTION

Patients benefit from adherence to medical ethics in two ways. First, it provides them some assurance of quality control, via mechanisms that have already been cited. In some circumstances the benefits to the consumer, though real, are not obvious. For example, in many instances the knowledge that medical ministrations are in accord with the ethics of traditional practice may lead physicians to accept errors of commission rather than risk errors of omission that would prove more costly on an expected-value basis. (Unfortunately, the support physicians garner by following the dictates of "quality medical practice" is a two-edged sword that can cut as well to the disadvantage of consumers. Surgeons have generated an atmosphere in which it is considered appropriate to perform what is sometimes alleged to be an excessive number of operations.)

Second, code adherence can promote aspects of medical practice that make patients feel better about the care they receive. Even if it would offer no improvement in medically measured outcomes, we would expect that consumers would find it desirable to know that ethical norms are guiding their physician's behavior. (This might suggest that the perceived ethics of the physician might count more than his actual beliefs or practices.) Ethics should hardly be thought of as prescribing decisions or decision procedures in each set of circumstances. But they do mold behavior patterns.

They can influence physicians' attitudes toward their patients, a most important observation implied by the Mechanic analysis. Though he does not make the proposal directly, Professor Mechanic would seem to be most receptive to reforms in ethics that would promote more empathetic attitudes in doctors toward their patients. His findings suggest, however, that such reforms will be limited by, and must be custom-tailored to, the delivery mode in which they are expected to operate.

Why are physicians' attitudes, about which Professor Mechanic informs us so effectively, so important? No one much cares, after all, what needle-workers think about the ultimate wearers of their clothes; neither do we worry about farmers' attitudes toward eaters. Once again the difficulty of monitoring information explains a phenomenon distinctive to the health care sector. Producer attitudes and manner are important to consumers, because other variables that consumers might prefer to monitor simply cannot be observed.

The physician's behavior and manner then become part of the treatment in many medical encounters. In some, they are the entire treatment. This observation suggests why we should be concerned about Professor Mechanic's finding that capitation-payment physicians frequently view many of their patients' complaints as trivial. If physicians communicate such an attitude to their patients, whether directly or indirectly, the patients will record an unsatisfactory rating on what by default must be one of their primary indicators of quality.

MEDICAL ETHICS AND THE WELFARE OF SOCIETY

It is not only the doctor and his patient who may be concerned with the ethics that guide his practice. It is quite possible, for example, that the personal welfare of the patient is in conflict with the common good—a possibility that arises most dramatically in considerations of medical experimentation. For example, the administration of a little-known and expectedly inferior treatment to one individual provides the benefit of increased knowledge to all future sufferers from this ailment. We are accustomed to compensating individuals for providing externalities to society. But most of us would feel quite uncomfortable merely providing monetary payment to individuals who undergo treatments of this sort. The offer of medical care superior to what otherwise would be received seems more acceptable, probably because health gained is the medium for health sacrificed. But, as the recently publicized experience of the Public Health Service's long-term syphilis-monitoring project makes clear, even payment in the health medium may not be adequate if there are substantial uncertainties in the outcomes. For then, the probability that a subject will be worse off for his participation is not inconsequential. (The current RAND health insurance experiment gives each participant lump-sum payments that assure that in any circumstance he will be better off for having joined the study.)

Ethical concerns for the individual may thus have generated restrictions on modes of experimentation that on an expected-value basis lead to an inferior medical outcome for society at large. Should this sacrifice be accepted? To answer this question we must look further into our personal preferences. If the externality that returns from injuries to individuals in the name of experimentation is sufficiently negative, we may find it beneficial to adopt and adhere to these (or some of these, or more of these) restrictions. This would suggest that where delivery of medical care is involved, welfare may be a function of process as well as outcome.

Perhaps the major externality associated with health care delivery is the substantial value we attach to the levels of health and health services received by other individuals. This is not the familiar contagion argument. It is simply that most of us feel better when our fellow citizens receive what is deemed adequate health care. We do not derive similar feelings of betterment when they receive more TVs, clothes, or beer. Much of the explanation for the unusual externality status of health care relates to the sanctity issues discussed earlier. Some ramifications of the agency nature of the production process may also play a role. In the vast majority of circumstances, middle-class citizens purchase health services when their physician/agent suggests that they need them. These citizens need conduct no delicate trade-offs between health services and other consumptive items. If health services are accorded this special status for middle class consumers, it becomes difficult for the middle-class to see why they should be viewed as other than necessitites, hence not subject to traditional consumer maximization operations, for less fortunate citizens as well. The slogan that has evolved from this pattern of thought is, simply, "Health care is a right."

It is interesting to speculate whether the special status of health would not be significantly diminished if we lived in a society with a relatively egalitarian income distribution. All citizens would then be in a financial position to purchase what by average standards would seem to be an adequate amount of health care or insurance coverage to provide such.

Health care in itself may not be so special as is its symbolic role in an unequal society. Providing equal access to medical services, like conscripting all classes of men into a draft army, may be a relatively inexpensive way to alter our perceptions of the distribution of welfare. Given their close relationship to many delicate issues, medical services, like army duty, stand out when we focus on distributional equity.

ETHICS AND MEDICAL DELIVERY SETTINGS

Upon reading Professor Mechanic's paper, one concerned with ethics would be led to at least hypothesize that different medical delivery settings will produce different ethical norms. This should suggest to us that there may be no unequivocal way to demonstrate that one delivery system and its accompanying values and norms is superior to another. If our experience with fee-for-service practice makes us attach great weight to producer–consumer relationships, we may end up choosing present methods even though we would have chosen prepaid capitation had we started with such. Similarly, changes in other areas of society may impinge on medical values and practices and vice versa.

This would suggest that to evaluate a medical care mode operating in a sphere where another is predominant may be a procedure fraught with difficulties. Thus, for example, the attitudes of United States physicians who are practicing in health maintenance organizations have been shaped by the fee-for-service world that surrounds them. Moreover, these physicians are a lot that has self-selected itself for its comparatively rare mode of practice.

Cross-system evaluations of complete medical care delivery modes suffer the additional peril of parochialism. Whenever attempting such a comparison, we should be particularly careful to assess the ethical norms and behavior patterns that will emerge along with any delivery mode. In his exploration of these issues, Professor Mechanic has been a pioneer. We are in his debt for providing us with so many helpful, policy-relevant examples.

If formulation for policy is our goal, warned as we have been, we must still be prepared to engage in the treacherous business of cross-system evaluation. Perhaps the best we can hope for is to arrive at a system that by its own standards is the most preferred. It would seem likely that some mixed system could best perform this job. In a democratic society, where we accept the persistence of individual differences, we might wish to allow each individual, whether physician or patient, to select the medical care delivery mode that is most responsive to his personal values and needs.

ACKNOWLEDGMENTS

The author gratefully acknowledges the helpful comments of Richard Light, Pamela Memishian, Frederick Mosteller, Milton Weinstein, and other Public Policy Program colleagues.

PETER H. SCHUCK*

Director, Washington Office, Consumers Union

A Consumer's View of the Health Care System

It has been certified on the highest authority that America is in the throes of a "health care crisis." Several years ago, President Nixon made it official. And if Watergate has rendered even such noncontroversial presidential pronouncements suspect, the blue-blood, blue-ribbon Committee for Economic Development has recently produced the ultimate incontrovertible evidence that the "crisis" does indeed exist—it has issued one of its reports.[1]

ONE, TWO, MANY HEALTH CARE CRISES

The precise nature of this crisis, of course, depends upon who is performing the analysis. From the perspective of the nonrural, private physician, the "crisis" consists of the rapid transformation of health care delivery from a decentralized, face-to-face, personalized, and independent economic function—in which the physician possessed all of the perquisites of a seller of a scarce but essential good—into an increasingly bureaucratic, impersonal, "rationalized," and extensively regulated function—in which the individual practitioner is sustaining a

* The views expressed in this paper are those of the author and do not necessarily represent the views of Consumers Union.

95

diminution in status, power, and autonomy. Like the free-wheeling small businessman gobbled up by the large conglomerate, the traditional physician finds himself an anachronism. The health care universe is increasingly dominated by what has been called the "medical empires"[2] — the large medical schools and other biomedical research centers; hospitals; large insurance companies; public health planning bodies; federal and state regulatory agencies; and corporate giants supplying drugs, equipment, and managerial expertise. Each of these entities is committed to the modern dogma of organizational "rationality"—systems analysis, bureaucratic structure and controls, coordination, and intimate interdependencies. The sole practitioner understandably regards the rapid expansion of these constellations as constituting a "crisis," in both the personal and professional sense.

To the institutional providers—hospitals, nursing homes, outpatient facilities, clinics—the "crisis" is one of swiftly rising costs and the resulting organizational, public, and governmental pressures. In recent years, the price of health care has been increasing at more than twice the rate of other consumer expenditures. This escalation corresponds closely with the beginning of Medicare and Medicaid in 1966. Between 1961 and 1966 physicians' fees increased at an average annual rate of only 3.2 percent, while between 1967 and 1969 the rate was almost 7 percent. Similarly, daily hospital charges during the 1961–1966 period averaged an annual increase of 6.4 percent; from 1967–1969, the increase averaged well over 15 percent.[3] This increase is particularly significant since hospital costs now constitute 39 percent of total consumer health expenditures, the largest single element.

Newhouse and Taylor[4] attribute these increases primarily to increased demand that derives from the extension of medical insurance to the poor and the elderly (there is, of course, a great deal of overlap) for the first time through Medicaid and Medicare and to the resulting stimulation of demand. Other contributing causes of spiraling health care costs include increased salaries of professional and nonprofessional employees, the colossal cost of many new medical technologies, increased building costs, and the strong incentives for inefficiency and overcharge built into Medicare and Medicaid reimbursement practices. To the institutional providers, these growing costs constitute a crushing burden, unless they can be passed on to the consumer.

But consumers are also taxpayers and voters. And so governments at all levels are experiencing their own health care crises of two distinct kinds. First, all levels of government are themselves direct providers. A municipality operating a hospital or clinic, a state operating a mental institution, and the federal government operating veterans hospitals are all public agencies caught in their own cost squeezes. Second, consumers confronting high and ever higher health care costs increasingly demand protection from government, particularly at the federal level. The various proposals for national health insurance, continuing price controls on certain health care services, the Medicare reforms embodied in the Social Security Amendments of 1972, and the efforts to emasculate Medicaid reflect the anxiety of governments as providers and funders of health care.

To consumers, the health care crisis has at least five dimensions. First, as the Nixon Administration recognized,[5] many consumers, particularly the inner-city poor and those in rural areas, lack access to primary health care services and particularly to services that could *prevent* illness.

The variation in physician/patient ratio between different regions of the U.S. is far more dramatic than that between the U.S. and, say, Pakistan. In the United States as a whole, there are 165 physicians per 100,000 people, but as Harry Schwartz points out in *The Case for American Medicine*, in Washington, D.C., there are 371 doctors per 100,000, while in Mississippi and Alaska the figure is 78. At latest report some 130 counties have no doctors at all practicing within their borders.[6,7]

Nathan Glazer[8] has noted the striking absence of doctors in many inner-city and smaller communities:

In Watts before the start of the OEO-funded community health center, there were eight physicians for 35,000 people. . . . In New York State, with the best doctor-patient ratio in the country, 56 municipalities with populations of more than 2,000 have no doctor.

Glazer also points out that nurses are in even shorter supply: In 1967, three quarters of the positions for professional nurses in New York City's municipal hospitals were vacant. Those who require hospitalization, on the other hand, normally can get it. But municipal and county hospitals, which primarily serve the poor, are notoriously inadequate, overcrowded, and tend to be staffed by physicians with inferior medical training. Indeed, foreign-trained doctors provide the slim margin preventing collapse of the entire public hospital system.

Second, consumers increasingly perceive a crisis in the *quality* of health care. To the extent that the quality performance of the system has been evaluated in the past, it has almost always been in terms of "input" or "process" criteria, rather than "outcome" criteria. The difficulties in employing "outcome" measures appear to be very formidable, indeed, and may yet prove insuperable as a practical matter.[9] What evidence there is on outcomes, however, suggests considerable quality variation and substantial inadequacy. The National Halothane Study, for

example, found threefold variations in postoperative mortality among
34 distinguished teaching hospitals, after all significant variables were controlled. Lembcke found enormous variations in the proportion of objectively justified hysterectomies among hospitals. Many other examples of
extraordinary variations have been documented.[10] Data developed by
the President's Commission on Medical Malpractice suggest that certain
physicians and hospitals may offer disproportionately low quality care.
Thus, 15 percent of the hospitals accounted for more than half of the
claims against hospitals, while 68 percent of the hospitals had no claims
asserted against them during the survey year. A limited study conducted
for the Commission concluded that some "medical injury" was sustained
by as many as 7.5 percent of the patients in the two (supposedly representative) hospitals studied.[11]

Third, consumers perceive a crisis in health care costs. Expenditures
for health care now exceed $83 billion annually and account for approxi-
mately 8 percent of our gross national product. Health insurance premiums are constantly rising. While between 84 and 93 percent of Americans
under 65 enjoy some health insurance coverage,[12] existing insurance
coverage is typically "shallow." Feldstein notes a 1963 study showing
that, of insured families with medical expenses of over $500, only one
third received benefits exceeding half of their expenditures, while another
third received benefits of less than one fifth of their expenditures.[13] And
as recently as 1968, some 36 million Americans under the age of 65 possessed no health insurance at all.[14] Similarly Medicare and Medicaid patients are not immune to the escalation in health care costs. Medicare
beneficiaries are required to "co-insure" themselves for certain health expenditures, and the Nixon Administration proposed that these fees be
increased. In the case of Medicaid, increased costs have caused many
states to expel many poor families from the program, thus leaving them
with no protection other than the already overcrowded public or charity
hospitals. Moreover, many jurisdictions have imposed clinic and other
fees on Medicaid patients, fees that have been steadily increased. These
fees have apparently reduced clinic utilization by the price-sensitive
poor, with uncertain consequences for their health.[15]

For a number of reasons, some of which are discussed below, consumers
face ever-increasing prices for health care whether or not we manage to
increase the supply of services available to them:

Utilization and prices for health care typically have risen with additions to resources.
When extra personnel or equipment are added, whether they are needed or not,
utilization adjusts to the increase in resources, and the fees and charges rise accordingly; insurance and government payments follow suit. An excess of surgeons, for
example, does not bring down the fees for surgery. On the contrary, in the four years

through 1971, the prices charged increased by about 25 per cent for the two surgical procedures—a herniorrhaphy and a tonsillectomy and adenoidectomy—that are monitored by the consumer price index. When ordinary housing is overbuilt there may be vacancies and cost concessions, but when hospitals are overbuilt the cost of hospitalization has not gone down.[16]

Hospital beds are indeed in oversupply except in some ghetto areas (the national surplus is roughly 300,000 beds on an average day). And, as often has been noted, if the beds are empty, doctors will tend to fill them.

A fourth "crisis" from the consumer's point of view flows from the emerging configuration of health care services in America, principally the drastic decline in primary physicians (particularly general practitioners) and the corresponding growth in the specialties and subspecialties. Consumers clearly desire the accessibility and familiarity of a personal physician, even at the expense of some technical expertise. Yet the last decade has witnessed a decline in primary physicians from 59 to 41.5 per 100,000 population.[17] The unfortunate effects of this continuing decline on the practice of low-cost, preventive medicine are likely to be very great indeed. Only 2 percent of medical school graduates in 1970 became general practitioners.[18] At the same time, surgeons are in great surplus, so much so that a past president of the AMA, Dr. Walter Bornemeier, has urged reducing the number of surgical residencies by half.[19]

Finally, a health care "crisis" exists for consumers in the sense that the health level of the American public is quite low relative to that of other industrialized nations. Life expectancy among men and women is lower, and infant mortality and, indeed, virtually all age-specific mortality are far higher in the United States than in many other developed countries; yet Americans spend far more per capita for health care. Indeed, Odin Anderson has found that "the Swedish mortality rates are lower than in any state of the United States"—even hale and hearty Utah.[20, 21]

ILLUSION OF CONSUMER SOVEREIGNTY

One might argue that if consumers are dissatisfied with the availability, quality, cost, and configuration of existing health care services, their remedy is simple and direct. As purchasers in an undeniably decentralized health services market, consumers may allocate their health dollars in such a way as to maximize their utility, thus reforming the health care system through their purchasing decisions. If enough consumers want general practitioners, this demand will elicit an enlarged supply of GPs. If consumers receive incompetent service, they may take their business elsewhere, rewarding the able and penalizing the incompetent. Consumers of health care, like consumers of shoes, may call the tune. Or so the argument runs.

This argument, however, assumes the existence of the elements of a competitive market mechanism for the expression of consumer preferences and values. Yet it is a fundamental premise of this paper that the basic prerequisites for such a mechanism do not exist in the health care subeconomy as it is now organized. In this section, I shall examine those conditions peculiar to the health care industry that have disabled "consumer sovereignty" from performing either its allocative efficiency or its equitable functions. In the following section, I shall consider some alternative reforms to increase the expression and satisfaction of consumer values with respect to health care.

Consumer Ignorance

Some 20 years ago, economist Tibor Scitovsky[22] analyzed the effects of consumer ignorance on the structure of a market, showing that such ignorance erodes price competition and the consumers' ability to make meaningful value comparisons. Consumer ignorance, he concluded, is a rich source of monopoly power, even where an industry is, like the health care industry, ostensibly decentralized and competitive.

In few consumer purchasing decisions does ignorance play so large a factor as in the purchase of health care. Consider a common example. A woman is advised by her gynecologist that a hysterectomy is "needed." She may or may not go to other gynecologists in order to test this advice. Her gynecologist may have indicated that the operation should be performed as soon as possible. Locating and visiting other specialists will take precious time and will be costly. And even if she consults a second gynecologist who advises her against the operation, she may well prefer to err on the side of conservatism and proceed with the operation. Whether she does or does not submit to the operation, she will almost certainly never know which advice was correct. If she submits to the operation and a malignancy fails to materialize, she knows little more than she knew before about the necessity or value of the operation; that is, she may not have needed it in the first place. Similarly, if she rejects the operation and ultimately contracts cancer, she remains equally ignorant of the wisdom of her choice; an operation might not have made any difference.

In the area of medical care, the concept of "need" to a considerable extent replaces the core concept of consumer sovereignty, "want." "Need," however, is a professional concept defined by professional standards. As Stevens[23] puts it:

The medical profession defines a certain "ideal" state of his [sic] client as a state of "health" which he has a professional interest in maintaining. The client is then said to "need" whatever medical services professional judgment deems efficacious for maintenance of this state.

Our patient, then, must decide not whether she *wants* this type or level of service, but how badly she *needs* it. Her doctor's credibility has become the issue; her preference as a consumer is little more than the outcome of this question of credibility. Yet in determining this question, she finds that not only is information difficult to obtain but sometimes is systematically withheld from her.

Her gynecologist may have a reputation in the medical community as one who operates precipitously, or even as a "butcher," but she is unlikely to learn of this. Canons of medical ethics discourage doctors from disparaging each other, either truly or falsely. Similarly, her gynecologist may be overpriced relative to others; yet she may learn of this only with difficulty. Medical ethics do not permit doctors to advertise price or anything else about their service, and few doctors will quote a charge over the telephone. The competency of her doctor will be certified, to be sure, but that certificate may be 35 years old, and she will have no way of knowing what the doctor has learned or forgotten since then. If the doctor should operate negligently and if this fact should somehow come to her attention, it will be little comfort for her to know that a very small number of persons have occasionally collected large judgments in malpractice suits. The cost of a lawyer and the difficulty in proving professional negligence will probably dissuade her from seeking judicial relief.

Nonpurchasing Consumer/Nonconsuming Purchaser

Even if the patient were well informed, some of the most important and costly purchasing decisions would be entirely out of her hands. Instead, these decisions are normally made by one who usually has some personal interest—often financial—in them. To continue with our example, if our thoroughly confused friend opts for the operation, she will be hospitalized, probably incurring costs of well over $100 per day (insurance aside). Yet while she will *consume* these costly hospital services, including routine laboratory tests, pathology services, x rays, anesthesiological services, food, nursing care, etc., she will not *purchase* a single one of them. Her consumer sovereignty, her "dollar votes," will consist of tendering her proxy to her doctor, carrying with it full control over her pocketbook. The doctor may be as saintly as Kildare; nevertheless, he is unlikely to be a careful shopper. He probably enjoys admitting privileges at only one hospital and is anxious to maintain good relations there. The hospital laboratory to which our friend's tissue samples and urinalyses will be sent is probably the well-guarded preserve of a pathologist whose compensation (sometimes well over a quarter of a million dollars annually) is based upon a percentage of gross revenues and whose contract with the hospital assures him a monopoly over laboratory work for its patients.[24] Similar arrangements probably exist between the hospital and its radiology and anesthesiology departments. The hospital's administrator is probably struggling heroically not so much to run an economically efficient facility as to maintain the goodwill of the fiercely independent, entrepreneurial department heads without whom the hospital cannot function. The trustees of the hospital, often answerable to no one but themselves, may well have personal or institutional interests in certain inefficient, costly, and occasionally improper hospital practices reflected in patient costs.[25] Our friend's doctor may not only maintain close ties with this hospital; if it is proprietary, he may also own stock in it.

There is nothing sinister about most of this; it is simply the way in which middle-class health care is predominantly organized in America. Consumers are encouraged to remain ignorant, entrusting critical purchasing decisions to their doctors, who frequently have personal stakes in these decisions, who have no particular stake in economy or efficiency and whose professional ethical norms mask the existence of potential conflicts of interest. It is in the nature of such a perverse system, of course, that the conscientious provider may suffer for his adherence to ethical canons, while his less scrupulous colleagues prosper.

Third Party Payers: Hiding the Waste

As we have seen, consumer ignorance makes quality and value comparisons (i.e., "economizing" behavior) by consumers in the health care field nearly impossible. And the anomaly that consumers of the most expensive health care services often do not purchase them, while the purchasers of these services do not consume them renders the notion of consumer sovereignty a cruel and costly hoax with respect to these services. But it is the combination of these factors with the pervasiveness of third party payment that makes this perverse "system" truly irrational, resistant to reform and largely indifferent to consumer pressures.

In fiscal 1972, almost $47 billion, or two thirds of the approximately $72 billion in personal health care expenditures, were made not by consumers, but third parties acting "on their behalf."[26,27] Insurers paid approximately 40 percent of this $47 billion, the federal government paid about 38 percent, state and local governments paid about 19 percent, and charities and industry paid about 3 percent.[28]

In theory, at least, a system of third party payment is neither beneficial nor harmful to consumers in and of itself. In theory, the third
party (usually an insurance company) could force the consumer to
"economize" by adjusting the consumer's insurance premium to reflect
the consumer's propensity to use health care resources; the consumer
would have an economic incentive (i.e., reduced premiums) to seek preventive care, avoid unnecessary doctor visits, use nurses rather than doctors where possible, use ambulatory rather than hospital facilities where
possible, shorten hospital stays, etc. In fact, however, this model is
wholly unrelated to the reality of the existing health care system. First,
as noted above, the most expensive health care facilities and services
are in fact purchased not by consumers but by providers, often having a
personal stake in high prices, overutilization, and inefficiency and rarely,
if ever, having a personal stake in their opposites. Indeed, since the patient will not usually be paying the bill, the most conscientious doctor
will be encouraged to spare no expense in selecting the form and provider of service for the patient. Thus, even a consumer anxious to reduce
his premium would find it difficult to do so; such expenditures are
simply out of his control. Second, also as noted above, consumers have
little evidence, other than anecdotal, upon which to make price and
value comparisons. They are, to this extent, unable to respond to the
economic incentives. Third, consumers often do not pay the insurance
premiums directly and so are insulated from a sense of what the system
is costing them. For example, many insurance plans are negotiated by
labor unions as a small part of a large package of benefits. The worker
will probably never see the money that is being utilized to pay his premium. Similarly, Medicare patients do not pay for their basic coverage
directly; it is paid for out of social security trust funds.

A fourth reason why third party payment entrenches perverse economic incentives is that the insurance companies, recognizing that the
consumer cannot, under the present circumstances, be counted upon to
"economize" and monitor quality, nevertheless rarely impose discipline
upon the only people and institutions that can—the providers. To begin
with, the insurers' economic incentives to do so have been systematically
weakened. Perhaps the clearest example of this is the fact that Blue
Cross has traditionally reimbursed hospitals on a "cost-plus" basis; that
is, it compensates the provider for all "reasonable" costs.* Under this
standard, it routinely reimburses the costs of grossly inefficient manage-

---

* The Social Security Amendments of 1972 introduced the concept of costs "found to be unnecessary in the efficient delivery of needed health services" as a restriction on reimbursable
costs under Medicare. PL 92-603, Sec. 223(a). How this standard will be applied in practice
remains to be seen.

ment practices, extravagant and underutilized equipment, unnecessary surgical operations, and overutilization of hospitals and passes the costs on to the consumer. Its sensitivity to the interests of the hospitals is not surprising. Blue Cross plans originated as the creatures of voluntary hospitals seeking to ensure financial stability through a guaranteed source of payment. Indeed, Blue Cross took its name from the American Hospital Association's trademark, a dramatic symbol of its traditional provider trademark. Until recently, the composition and selection of Blue Cross governing boards have assured provider control of the plans. Subscribers were not permitted to vote for the trustees, and the boards were composed wholly or predominantly of providers. In the last few years, adverse publicity and consumer pressures have goaded Blue Cross into the beginnings of change. Yet, according to recent data, only 6 out of some 74 Blue Cross plans permit subscribers to vote for the "public" members of the board. And of the board members designated as "public" representatives, the great majority were business executives, physicians, and bankers. Only 7 percent were labor leaders.* Fears of boycotts by providers have also kept insurers from asking too many embarrassing questions about costs.[29]

Efforts by consumers–subscribers to introduce competition and arm's length relationships into this cozy interlock have been notably unsuccessful. Because Blue Cross plans are regulated by state insurance departments, they have been held to be immune to liability under the federal antitrust laws. Consumers Union discovered when it sought without success to examine the reimbursement contract between the Washington, D.C., Blue Cross plan (in which it was a subscriber) and the local private hospitals, subscribers possess no rights apart from those in the insurance contract itself. And Blue Cross rate increases tend to be approved with little or no consumer participation in the process.

If the insurers have shown no inclination to discipline the providers (self-discipline is always most difficult), government has answered the eternal question quis custodiet ipsos custodes? with resounding silence. The regulatory inadequacies of insurance departments in all but the largest states are well known and continuing.[30] Small budgets, limited auditing or investigatory capacity, personnel interchange with industry, and powerful insurance company and insurance agent lobbies ensure that these departments cannot effectively represent consumer interests.†
At the federal level, the Social Security Administration has turned over the administration of reimbursement and other regulatory responsibili-

---

* From forthcoming book on Blue Cross by Sylvia Law, New York University School of Law.
† Only 4.2 percent of the $1.2 billion collected in state insurance premium taxes nationwide in 1972 were expended in regulation of the industry (Dean Sharp, Counsel to Senate Antitrust and Monopoly Subcommittee, personal communication).

ties under Medicare to Blue Cross, Blue Shield, and other insurers. The law contains few substantive standards to limit the discretion of the insurers and, apart from an occasional General Accounting Office audit, these standards are rarely enforced. It is an astonishing fact that Congress has never investigated the "Blues" on a comprehensive basis;[31] yet it has permitted them to expend $8.34 billion dollars a year in federal funds* in an essentially uncontrolled manner.

The incentive effects upon consumers of the coverage limitations built into third party payment programs greatly compound the indifference to cost exhibited by the insurers and providers. Feldstein[32] has noted:

A substantial body of research has shown that, because of the structure of insurance coverage, patients obtain expensive (but covered) in-hospital care when much less expensive (but uncovered) ambulatory care would have been effective. Insurance has also accelerated the rising cost of in-hospital care. Ironically, although the hospital patient with a large bill often finds his insurance grossly inadequate, the *average* patient stays a relatively short time (the 1968 mean stay in community hospitals was 8.4 days) and has almost his entire hospital bill paid for by insurance. . . . Because hospitals are able to pass almost all cost increases on to insurance companies and the government, there is neither internal incentive nor external pressure from patients to moderate cost increases.

In short, to the extent that the health care system responds to economic incentives, the incentives are socially perverse. Public and private health insurance, far from encouraging economizing behavior by consumers and providers, simply subsidizes extravagance, overutilization of expensive services, and underutilization of inexpensive services.

Provider Control of Licensure, Accreditation, and Professional Discipline

If consumer sovereignty is illusory with respect to the price of health care, it is equally so with respect to quality. Providers control the licensure, accreditation, and disciplinary mechanisms that purport to obviate the necessity for consumer sovereignty. Hospitals, for example, are accredited to assure quality of care, but the accreditation is conferred by an organization [the Joint Commission on the Accreditation of Hospitals (JCAH)], which is financed and controlled by providers.†

* Informal communication from Social Security Administration.

† JCAH's insistence that it does not assess quality of care seems somewhat disingenuous, in view of the fact that JCAH accreditation is a prerequisite for institutional eligibility under many Blue Cross plans, for an institution's acceptability for the training of residents and interns, and for qualification for reimbursement under Medicare and Medicaid.

Of the 20 seats on the JCAH governing board, 7 are occupied by representatives of the American Medical Association, 7 by representatives of the American Hospital Association, and the other 6 are split between the American College of Surgeons and the American College of Physicians. JCAH standards tend to be exceedingly vague, which is hardly surprising since the identical standard is intended to apply to the small rural facility and the large urban hospital. When consumer groups challenged the legality of HEW's reliance upon compliance with JCAH standards as a criterion for reimbursement under Medicare,[33] Congress amended the statute to abandon this minimal criterion.

To test the rigor of JCAH accreditation standards, consider the case of D.C. General Hospital, a notorious dumping ground for patients on welfare and Medicaid whom private hospitals do not want to treat. In 1970 numerous deplorable conditions prevailed at D.C. General, some of which are the subject of a pending lawsuit by a consumer group.[34] For example, it was often true that no licensed physician would be on duty in the emergency room at night; a patient was known to have died there after waiting 7 hours to be seen by a physician. The number of nurses was egregiously inadequate; on many nights, there would be one registered nurse for 70 patients. Record-keeping was a shambles; doctors failed to receive 25 percent of the charts they requested. Laboratory tests were notoriously inadequate. Yet the JCAH renewed D.C. General's accreditation both in 1970 and in 1972, when little had changed other than the staffing of the emergency room. Other city hospitals with comparable or worse conditions are also routinely accredited by the JCAH. Within the last year, the JCAH routinely accredited Bethesda Naval Hospital, notwithstanding the existence of a major fire hazard.[35]

The medical specialties are also accredited entirely by their own, and their ability to include and exclude practitioners for reasons of their own constitutes a paradigm of irresponsible and unaccountable power. For example, the Department of Justice charged the College of American Pathologists with conspiring with its members to, among other things, commercially boycott all doctors of all medical laboratories not owned and operated solely for the profit of pathologists; to refuse to accept positions with any medical laboratory not owned by or operated solely for the profit of pathologists; to refuse to accept salaried positions with any hospital or clinic unless the entire profit from the medical laboratory went solely to a pathologist; and to fix prices for laboratory services. All are in violation of the antitrust laws.*

---

* The College of American Pathologists entered into a consent decree in 1969, agreeing not to engage in these practices in the future.[36]

When viewed in light of this experience, the vigorous and increasingly successful efforts of numerous subprofessional groups in the health care and related fields to wrest licensing and certification authority from the state legislatures assume an ominous aspect. Unless this trend is reversed, we can expect these groups to use such authority just as their professional predecessors have always done in the past—i.e., to create entry barriers by new competitors and "paraprofessionals"; to raise prices; to control and restrict the terms of service to consumers; to prescribe quality standards of a minimal sort, which will tend to be maximal as well; and to use those standards to insulate the group from consumer pressures, malpractice suits, public controls, and advances in technology.[37]

There is nothing in the least bit unusual about all this. Adam Smith warned us 200 years ago that competitors rarely engage in cooperative ventures except as a means to conspire against the public interest. Yet countless occupational groups, led by my own, have persuaded legislators of the contrary. The medical profession has simply been the most successful of all the occupational monopolists. It is only recently, however, that consumers and taxpayers have begun to recognize some of the staggering costs imposed by that monopoly: the tragic shortage of primary care practitioners, a direct result of unnecessarily rigorous, AMA-imposed medical school admissions criteria; the painfully slow growth of innovations in the delivery of health care, due to the bitter hostility of the AMA*; the overbuilding of expensive inpatient facilities, subsidized by federal taxpayers and consumers; gross inefficiencies and featherbedding in the delivery of health care, jealously guarded by the providers who profit†; the retarded development of paraprofessional use and ambulatory care facilities, at the behest of their competitors; and

---

* So bitter was this hostility that the AMA was prosecuted and convicted of a criminal conspiracy to destroy the Group Health Association of Washington, D.C., one of the earliest HMOs in the nation.[38]

† An interesting example has recently come to light in the District of Columbia, where a suit has been filed charging that the Blue Cross health plan for federal employees violates the antitrust laws by refusing reimbursement for therapy by a psychologist unless the patient is sent to the psychologist by a physician who "consults" with the therapist at least every 90 days and sees the patient again at least once a year. Several characteristic features of this restriction should be noted. First, it is justified by Blue Cross on the ground that it will assure "quality" care; yet there is no requirement that the "consulting" physician be a psychiatrist. Second, the restriction is imposed by Blue Cross, which theoretically should be opposing just such restrictions but is disabled from doing so because of its provider orientation. Finally, chief plaintiff in the suit is the Council for the Advancement of the Psychological Professions and Sciences, seeking redress principally for professional disparagement. One wonders what restrictions *this* group will be able to impose in the interests of "quality" care once *its* professional status is vindicated against Blue Cross.

the continuing delay in the creation of some form of national health insurance, for decades the *bête noire* of the AMA.

By relinquishing to the organized medical profession and cognate institutions the power to define the "wants" and "needs" of consumers for health care, the appropriate "quality" of such care, and the nature of the system for organizing, delivering, and compensating for such care, the American public has managed to obliterate consumer sovereignty in health care markets and create instead a market utterly controlled by and for producers. Indeed, consumer sovereignty in the health care field has so atrophied and provider dominance has so securely entrenched itself, that few reforms are likely to be equal to the task of regeneration.

PUTTING THE CONSUMER BACK IN CONSUMER SOVEREIGNTY

If the remedy for this costly, wasteful, unresponsive, and self-serving system is difficult, the fundamental cause is rather simple and universal. Producer groups, as Milton Friedman[39] has observed, tend to be more concentrated politically than consumers. Nowhere is this principle more evident than in the health care industry. Provider groups, with relatively well-defined economic and professional interests, are well organized, well respected, and very well financed. They are positioned to extract from government the perquisites of the medieval guilds, to shape governmental programs to serve their interests, and to plunder the public fisc. Indeed, America's hospitals, nursing homes, medical equipment suppliers, biomedical researchers, pharmaceutical manufacturers, health care consultants, and the like have been able to transform the federal health care programs of the last decade into a bonanza of unprecedented proportions.

Consumers, on the other hand, are poorly organized. Their interest in health care policy is diffuse, occasional, and unpredictable. Because of this and because they are so numerous, consumers are organizationally debilitated. Economist Mancur Olson[40] has explained the apparent paradox between numerical strength and organization weakness:

... there are now three separate but cumulative factors that keep larger groups from furthering their own interests. First, the larger the group, the smaller the fraction of the total group benefit any person acting in the group interest receives, and the less adequate the reward for any group-oriented action, and the farther the group falls short of getting an optimal supply of the collective good, even if it should get some. Second, since the larger the group, the smaller the share of the total benefit going to any individual . . . the less the likelihood that . . . any single individual will gain enough from getting the collective good to bear the burden of providing even a small amount of it. . . . Third, the larger the number of members in the group, the greater the organization costs, and thus the higher the hurdle that must be jumped before any of the collective good at all can be obtained. For these reasons, the larger the group the farther it will fall short of providing an optimal supply of a collective good, and very large groups normally will not, in the absence of coercion or separate outside incentives, provide themselves with even minimal amounts of a collective good.

Olson's analysis, which is confirmed by the paucity of effective voluntary consumer organizations in the health care field, suggests several significant implications. If consumer interests in an efficient, varied, innovative, competitive, responsive, and accountable health care delivery system are to be represented, there are only two ways in which these might be advanced: (1) breaking provider sovereignty over the delivery of health care services through the strengthening of competitive market forces; (2) confronting the monopoly power exercised by providers with countervailing consumer power, through collective, organizational pressures on provider groups or on the macrocosmic policymaking process. Each of these two mechanisms for dealing with monopoly power is defective at present. Indeed, the burden of this paper has been to demonstrate why consumer sovereignty in the health care market is virtually nonexistent and why consumer organizations are impotent. Yet no one has ever devised an alternative to market power and organizational powers as means to promote consumer interests. Ultimately, even the visionaries who hope to create "a wholly new American health care system"[41] will find that they cannot possibly do so without first strengthening these mechanisms. What, then, can be done?

Revivifying the Health Care Marketplace

Several major structural defects of health care markets—consumer ignorance, the disjunction between consumption and purchasing, the third party payment system, and provider control over licensure, accreditation, and professional discipline—have been discussed. To these must be added lack of purchasing power for the poor. Any meaningful reforms must address these defects. I shall briefly list some possibilities.

Health Maintenance Organizations There no longer can be much doubt that various forms of prepaid group medical practice described under the general rubric of health maintenance organizations (HMOs) are singularly efficient and responsive delivery systems. While HMOs have been severely hobbled in the past by AMA attacks and legislative restrictions, they have clearly demonstrated in the only arena that ultimately matters—the marketplace—that they constitute a viable alternative to fee-for-service care.[42] The AMA attacks have not ended,[43] and many of the legal restrictions remain,[44] but the effectiveness of both obstacles in preventing HMO growth has abated considerably in recent years.

I shall not undertake a detailed review of the growing body of data concerning HMO performance relative to conventional delivery systems. Suffice it to say that HMOs have achieved remarkable success in dramatically reducing patient out-of-pocket costs, particularly for hospitalization. Thus, the most celebrated comparative study concluded that while Blue Cross–Blue Shield, commercial insurance, and individual practice plans resulted in 924, 987, and 471 hospital days per 1,000 persons covered, respectively, during 1968, related group practice plans (essentially HMOs) averaged 422 hospital days. Some of the largest HMOs were considerably lower. Group Health Cooperative of Puget Sound averaged 364 days and Kaiser Foundation Health Plan of Oregon averaged 254.[45] Low utilization rates in HMOs were experienced even by the elderly, a high-risk group.[46] In 1966, federal employees in HMO-type plans had half as many appendectomies, one fourth as many tonsillectomies and adenoidectomies, and half as many female surgeries, as those in the fee-for-service system.[47]

In stark contrast to the traditional fee-for-service–*cum*-insurance systems, HMOs, by contracting with a particular enrolled population of consumers to provide them with broad-scale (often comprehensive) care at a fixed prepaid fee, employ economic incentives to operate in an efficient and relatively inexpensive manner. Preventive care is stressed, paraprofessionals are used more readily, unnecessary operations are reduced, services that can be performed on an ambulatory basis are not performed in the hospital, and economies of scale are sought. The cost savings to HMO subscribers are apparently considerable. One study,[48] using national data, concluded that "a typical HMO saves a family of two adults and three children $115 a year in out-of-pocket costs"; the HMO in Columbia, Maryland, saves the average family of 2 adults and 1.9 children $170 per year, or 32 percent of the cost of comparable care under typical health insurance plans.

Some have feared that these economic incentives will induce HMOs to overeconomize at the expense of the patient's health and to confine enrollment to low-risk populations. There is little affirmative evidence for this, however, and a survey of recent studies suggests that precisely the opposite may be true. Patient dissatisfaction with HMOs was found to be considerably lower than with commercial or "Blues"-type plans, and this was true not only with respect to financial aspects but with respect to "medical care received" as well (although some studies have found some dissatisfaction with doctor–patient relationships in HMO settings).[49] Two older studies comparing HMO and non-HMO care in New York City found that "the quality of care was higher in the [HMO] group as assessed by outcome measures."[50]

Needless to say, many questions remain to be answered about HMOs, including whether they do in fact *prevent* illness and to what extent. Moreover, the data concerning the performance of for-profit HMOs is not yet extensive. Nor are the questions of inequitable risk selection and overeconomizing, if any, yet fully laid to rest. What is clear, however, is that HMOs present an attractive alternative to fee-for-service care, tend to be particularly responsive to market incentives, and minimize the problem of consumer ignorance. O'Donoghue and Carlson[51] suggest why this last attribute is peculiar to HMOs:

First, consumers make their choice of providers when they are well rather than when they are sick, as is often the case at present. Second, consumers must choose one provider whom they will almost certainly use rather than eight to twelve providers whose services they may or may not require in the near future. Third, consumers may join together in groups (e.g., employee groups, neighborhood groups, etc.) and bargain collectively with HMOs and other organizational providers over at least benefits, fees and amenities, thus increasing the leverage of consumers in the marketplace. Fourth, it should be easier to provide consumers with pertinent information about large organizational providers than about individual providers. Concomitantly and related to reason two above, it should be less difficult for consumers to grasp information about a small number of organizational providers than about a large number of individual providers.

Consumers have a strong stake in ensuring that HMOs are given a chance to compete for their health care dollars on equal terms. While long-term public subsidization of HMOs cannot be justified, all state laws inhibiting their growth should quickly be overridden by federal law. The new provision in the 1972 Social Security Amendments permitting reimbursement under Medicare to HMOs[52] should be implemented in order to prevent any competitive advantage to fee-for-service providers or to existing HMOs over new HMOs. By the same token, neither comprehensive health planning nor peer review should be used as a pretext for thwarting HMO development in the interests of existing fee-for-service providers.[53]

Competition by HMOs can provide the incentive for efficiency in the fee-for-service sector, which has been so notably lacking. Indeed, the recent growth of foundations for medical care attests to the vitality of the threat of HMO competition.[54] In the end, the effect of HMOs on the cost and quality of fee-for-service care may be even more far-reaching than the effect of HMOs on their own subscribers.

Professional Licensure   There is a strong case to be made that the system of professional and subprofessional licensure and accreditation, controlled by providers for providers, may have ill-served consumers, depriving them of the fruits of technology and organizational innovation, dramatically reducing the supply of health care professionals, and inflating prices, while producing few, if any, offsetting benefits that could not be achieved by a less restrictive system. Serious consideration should be given to repealing all licensure requirements for nonphysicians, replacing them with a system of organizational licensure. Under such a system, licensed physicians and licensed health care organizations (HMOs, hospitals, group fee-for-service practices, etc.) would be free to deploy health care personnel as they saw fit, subject to the requirement of quality assurance reflected in the malpractice sanction (and/or the no-fault liability sanction discussed briefly below) and to public disclosure requirements concerning the professional training and certifications of such personnel.[55] Supplanting licensure of nonphysicians with such a system of organizational licensure would almost certainly increase the health care options of consumers, lower the costs of service, increase the supply of subphysician personnel, enhance routine preventive services, and reduce provider control over entry into the health professions.

No-Fault Insurance   As noted above, the quality of health care in America apparently varies widely and is often substandard. If providers are to have an economic incentive to provide competent, quality care, liability for actual negligence must be swift and certain. Given the spectacular increase in the cost of malpractice insurance—700 and 1000 percent for general practitioners and general surgeons, respectively, between 1960 and 1970, most or all of which is passed on to the patients— and given the magnitude of the resources wasted on the process of litigating "fault," the long delays in payment, and the uncertainties of malpractice litigation as a means of monitoring quality of care, experimentation with a system of no-fault medical practice insurance, recently the subject of academic attention, should be considered.[56]

Health Care for the Poor   Medicaid as a means for providing health care for the poor has been almost universally reviled. It has been hopelessly bureaucratic, has continued a two-class system of care, has not reached many of those in dire need, has been unusually vulnerable to political manipulation, and, like third party payment systems generally, has swelled the incentives in favor of inefficiency and waste. Most of these defects could be cured by the simple, but politically unpopular, expedient of putting dollars available for health care directly into the hands of the poor on a graduated basis, permitting them to make their own choices in the market. If only "in kind" redistribution is feasible, an experiment with a system of health care vouchers,* similar to a current experiment with education vouchers, should be launched, including requirements that all providers receiving federal funds accept a certain proportion of "voucher patients."

Consumer Information Insofar as possible, the federal and state governments should gradually get out of the business of legitimizing provider self-regulation and should get into the business of vastly increasing the amount of information available to consumers concerning health care alternatives, while redistributing health care dollars to those who most need them. Restrictions on truthful advertising should be repealed, and the government should require providers to disclose to consumers various categories of information, including service benefits, prices, financial data, personnel data, hospital utilization rates, facilities data, etc. Government regulation of providers should strengthen, rather than supplant, the play of competitive forces in the health care market.

Strengthening Consumer Representation in Decision Making

Clearly, revivifying the operation of the health care market will not suffice as a consumer remedy, if only because much of the delivery system will continue to function under a regime of governmental regulation, professional self-regulation, and third party payment. Thus, consumers will have to be organized to exert countervailing power upon the relevant public, professional, and commercial decision-making groups. While the difficulties inherent in consumer organization have been mentioned, several reforms are nevertheless possible.

Peer Review While peer review, primarily through the foundations for medical care, has had some major successes in imposing cost controls on fee-for-service providers[57] (thus filling the vacuum left by insurer indifference to cost), the utilization review activities mandated under Medicare have been ineffective:

. . . utilization review activities have, generally speaking, been of a token nature and ineffective as a curb to unnecessary use of institutional care and services. Utilization review in Medicare can be characterized as more form than substance.[58]

* Even a voucher system would not obviate the necessity for some sort of protection for the poor against extraordinary medical expenses.

Tissue review committees in hospitals have also had little impact on quality or cost, as one might expect from self-selected groups of colleagues immune from outside scrutiny.

The Professional Standards Review Organizations (PSROs) mandated by the 1972 Social Security Amendments have not yet been established. There is some reason, however, to be skeptical about their future efficacy. First, they are efforts to institutionalize self-regulation and are thus, for the reasons discussed above, to be embraced only with great caution. They are likely to be dominated by the conventional providers, wedded to fee-for-service care. Indeed, widespread professional support for PSROs, although not universal, suggests that this expectation is not unrealistic. If this is the case, PSROs may well use their authority to harass HMOs who need no additional incentives to institute utilization reviews. As Havighurst[59] has pointed out, this would produce "either regulation of HMOs in the interest of fee-for-service providers or an accommodation between HMOs and the fee-for-service sector" inimical to vigorous competition. Just as compliance with JCAH standards, for all of their inadequacies, have come to be a defense for hospitals under attack, so may PSRO standards, however minimal and unenforced, also have the practical effect of immunizing physicians who follow their recommendations from civil liability.[60] This possibility is particularly disquieting given the complete absence of consumer representation on PSROs. Finally, PSROs may be quite costly to implement.

Implicit in these speculations, then, is the need to ensure that PSROs are in fact representative of HMOs as well as fee-for-service providers,* that their standards are not simply the minimal ones that can command universal agreement among providers, that their records be subject to public scrutiny (with appropriate safeguards for patient confidentiality), and that consumer interests be represented in PSROs. Finally, since PSROs will affect only services rendered under Medicare and Medicaid, and even then will not concern themselves directly with questions of *cost,* they must not be relied upon as a substitute for other reforms designed to avoid the perverse incentives that characterize the existing and far wider system.

Blue Cross The broad functions performed by Blue Cross, which may well be expanded even farther with the advent of national health insurance, are simply too important to be left to control by interlocking provider and cognate groups. Serious consideration should be given to

---

* Better yet, the statute should be amended to exclude HMOs from the PSRO system, thereby ensuring that the HMO and fee-for-service sectors cannot exploit the PSRO mechanism to effect a cartel arrangement at the expense of consumers.

federal chartering of Blue Cross plans above a certain size participating in federal programs and/or to conversion of Blue Cross plans into subscriber-controlled entities. The objectives of such reforms would be to require Blue Cross to aggressively promote consumer interests in cost controls and quality care. All such plans should finance an independent "subscriber advocate" to challenge rate increase requests and other significant decisions before appropriate regulatory bodies.

Consumer Representation   The phrase "consumer representation" can be a meaningless slogan, having no effect on the way in which decisions are made, or it can be a fundamental reallocation of power over centralized decision-making processes. Even if implemented, of course, consumer representation provides no assurance that "correct" decisions will be made. Nevertheless, in the absence of certain knowledge of what constitutes "correct" social decisions, in the presence of much data that the existing decision process is controlled by providers in the interests of providers and in the knowledge that social decisions are "improved" when the interests of affected groups are taken into account, there is a strong presumption that consumer participation in the decisions of health planning agencies, insurers, institutional providers, health bureaucracies, PSROs, foundations for medical care, professional disciplinary bodies, and the like would make the system more efficient, responsive, and just. In view of the inherent organizational difficulties of consumers discussed above, it is essential that such participation be subsidized and have access to professional assistance.

In addition to consumer representation *on* decision-making bodies, consumer advocacy *before* such bodies must be institutionalized. A compelling model for this may be found in the proposed Consumer Protection Agency now pending before Congress. It would have no regulatory power, but would present arguments, facts, data, and testimony to regulatory agencies on behalf of consumers and invoke judicial review to redress errors of law.[61] Another such model is the consumer counsel established in certain jurisdictions to challenge utility rate and service requests before the public utility commission. All state and federal agencies with regulatory responsibilities in the health care field, such as the Social Security Administration and state insurance commissions, should have the benefit of such advocacy before making decisions of enormous significance to consumers.

CONCLUSION

No system of national health insurance, peer review, comprehensive health care planning, or any other sweeping change is likely to produce a more efficient, competent, innovative, or just health care delivery system unless the definition and control of consumer demand and the terms of supply, the pace of technological and organizational change in the delivery system, and quality standards of care are taken from providers and returned to an informed consumerate. This can only be accomplished by renovating the moribund health care market mechanism so that it may generate socially desirable incentives for efficient and quality care and by ensuring that centralized decision-making processes affecting the nature and terms of health care delivery be made fully responsive to consumer views and interests.

REFERENCES AND NOTES

1. Committee for Economic Development: Building a National Health Care System. Washington, D.C., Government Printing Office, 1973.
2. Health Policy Advisory Center: The American Health Empire: Power, Profits and Politics. New York, Random House, 1970.
3. Newhouse J P, Taylor V: How shall we pay for hospital care? Public Interest spring 1971, p. 79.
4. *Ibid.*, p 81.
5. Testimony of Frank Carlucci, Undersecretary of Department of Health, Education, and Welfare, before Subcommittee on Public Health and Environment, Committee on Interstate and Foreign Commerce, House of Representatives, 93d Congr, March 6, 1973.
6. Blumenthal D, Fallows J: The care we need and want. Wash Mon, Oct 1973, p 10.
7. To the extent that these regional disparities are particularly great in the United States, they may partially explain why Sweden and England, with lower overall doctor–population ratios, nevertheless apparently enjoy better health. See, Glazer N: Perspectives on health care. Public Interest, spring 1973, p 112.
8. Glazer N: Paradoxes of health care. Public Interest, winter 1971, pp 63–64.
9. For a more optimistic view, see Assuring the Quality of Health Care. Minneapolis Interstudy, 1973, pp 35 et seq.
10. See, e.g., collection of studies, *ibid.*, pp 33–34.
11. Markus RM: We report: President's Commission on Medical Malpractice. Trial, Mar/Apr 1973, p 32.
12. Committee for Economic Development: *op. cit.*, p 63.
13. Feldstein MS: A new approach to national health insurance. Public Interest, spring 1971, pp 94–95.
14. Committee for Economic Development: *op. cit.*, p 63.
15. Health Policy Advisory Center: *op. cit.*, p 172.
16. Committee for Economic Development: *op. cit.*, p 42.
17. Blumenthal D, Fallows J: *op. cit.*, pp 13–14.
18. Alford RR: The political economy of health care: dynamics without change. Polit Soc, winter 1972, p 137.
19. Bornemeier W: What makes Americans so operation happy? Med Econ, Jan 8, 1973, pp 67–75.

20. Anderson O: Health Care: Can There Be Equity? The United States, Sweden and England. New York, John Wiley, 1972, p 158.

21. I am not suggesting that the causes of America's relative ill health are obvious or are entirely related to the health care delivery system; they are not. There is some evidence that spending more on health care will not necessarily improve matters. First, as just noted, a number of countries, including Sweden and England, spend considerably less per capita for health care, yet achieve a far lower age-specific mortality. Environmental, genetic, and cultural factors undoubtedly play a significant but poorly understood role. For example, Glazer (*supra* note 8, pp 74–75) has pointed to the "remarkable differences between different ethnic and racial groups in health, even when we hold constant the amount of health care available to these groups." And finally, the incidence of so-called iatrogenic (i.e., physician-induced) ailments and unnecessary operations suggests that some segments of the American population are overdoctored to their great detriment.

22. Scitorsky T: Ignorance as a source of oligopoly power. Am Econ Rev 40: 49–53, 1950.

23. Stevens R: On "consumer participation" in medical-care markets. Health Care Policy Discuss Paper No 5, Apr 1973, pp 4–5.

24. See, e.g., Kessler R: The hospital business. Wash Post, Nov 1, 1972.

25. It is not uncommon, for example, for private hospitals to maintain their case balances, often quite sizable, in interest-free accounts at banks of which the hospital's trustees are officers and/or stockholders. See, e.g., Kessler R: Trustees' banks use hospital money. Wash Post, Feb 4, 1973.

26. Committee for Economic Development: *op. cit.*, p 40.

27. This is not to suggest that insurance coverage is comprehensive or uniformly distributed among the population. As noted above, typical coverage is "shallow." Moreover, the deprived segments of our population—the nonwhite, poor, disabled, unemployed, and service and farm workers—enjoy only very limited coverage. (*Ibid.*, pp 63–64.)

28. *Ibid.*, pp 28–29.

29. See United States *v.* Oregon State Medical Society, 343 U.S. 326 (1952).

30. See The Insurance Industry, Hearings before Subcommittee on Antitrust and Monopoly, Committee on the Judiciary, United States Senate, 91st Congr, Part 15.

31. Wilbur Cohen on health care. Wash Post, Feb 5, 1973, p C1.

32. Feldstein MS: *op. cit.*, p 95.

33. Self-Help for the Elderly *v.* Richardson, Civil Action No. 2016–71 (DDC).

34. Greater Washington Council of Senior Citizens *v.* Washington, Civil Action No. 275–71 (DDC).

35. See Congressional Record, Oct 18, 1973, pp H9286–90.

36. United States *v.* College of American Pathologists, Civil Action No. 66C1253 (ND Ill.).

37. See Friedman M: Capitalism and Freedom. Chicago, University of Chicago Press, 1962, Ch 9.

38. American Medical Association *v.* United States, 317 U.S. 519 (1943).

39. *Ibid.*, p 143.

40. Olson M: The Logic of Collective Action: Public Goods and the Theory of Groups. New York, Schocken Books, 1968, p 48.

41. Health Policy Advisory Center: *op. cit.*, p 28.
42. See, e.g., Roemer MI, Shonick W: HMO performance: the recent evidence. Milbank Mem Fund Q/Health Soc 51(3):271 (1973); The role of prepaid group practice in relieving the medical care crisis. Harvard Law Rev 84(4):921–933 (1971).
43. See, e.g., Kernodle JR: HMO's: can they maintain health? Wall St J, Aug 8, 1973.
44. See Harvard Law Rev, *supra* note 42, pp 960 et seq.; see generally, Lawyers Committee for Civil Rights under Law: Health Maintenance Organizations, Oct 1972, pp 82–89.
45. U.S. Health Services and Mental Health Administration: The Federal Employees Health Benefits Program. Washington, D.C., Government Printing Office, 1971, p 11.
46. Harvard Law Rev, *supra* note 42, p 923.
47. *Ibid.*
48. Rothfeld M B: Sensible surgery for swelling medical costs. Fortune, Apr 1973, pp 114–116.
49. Roemer MI, Shonick W: *op. cit.*, pp 48–55.
50. Interstudy: *op. cit.*, p 22.
51. O'Donoghue P, Carlson RJ: Actual and possible interrelationships between HMOs and CHP agencies. June 1972, p 16.
52. PL 92–603, Sec 226.
53. See *supra* note 56; see also, Havighurst CC: Government's increasing involvement in the health care sector: the hazards of regulation and less hazardous alternatives. Address to 1973 National Health Forum, March 20, 1973, pp 15–16.
54. Havighurst CC: Speculations on the market's future in health care. Paper for Conference on Health Planning, Certificates of Need, and Market Entry, American Enterprise Institute, June 1972, p 17.
55. Carlson RJ: Health manpower licensing and emerging institutional responsibility for the quality of care. Law Contemp Prob, 35: 849–878, 1970.
56. O'Connell J: Expanding no-fault beyond auto insurance: some proposals. Va Law Rev, 59, No. 5, 1973; Havighurst CC, Tancredi LR: Medical adversity insurance—a no fault approach to medical malpractice and quality assurance. Milbank Mem Fund Q/Health Soc, 51:125, 1973.
57. See, e.g., Hicks N: Nation's doctors move to police medical care. NY Times, Oct 28, 1973, p 52.
58. U.S. Department of Health, Education, and Welfare: Legislative History of Professional Standards Review Organization Provisions of the Social Security Act Amendments. Washington, D.C., Government Printing Office, 1972, p 2.
59. Havighurst CC: Foundations for medical care: an antitrust lawyer's perspective. pp 20–21.
60. *Supra* note 58, p 14.
61. See, e.g., testimony of author on the proposed Consumer Protection Agency before the Senate Subcommittee on Reorganization, Research, and Internal Organizations of the Senate Government Operations Committee and the Consumer Subcommittee of the Senate Commerce Committee, March 28, 1973, and before the Subcommittee on Legislation of the House Government Operations Committee, September 18, 1973.

PHILIP R. LEE, M.D.
Professor of Social Medicine, University of California, School of Medicine, San Francisco

Commentary

America's health care system is viewed with a discerning but highly critical eye by Mr. Schuck. His criticisms stem from his belief that consumer
sovereignty in the health care market is virtually nonexistent. He decries
what he calls the physician-provider sovereignty in the United States and
he emphasizes the need for consumer information, consumer participation, and consumer control.

Mr. Schuck's paper might more appropriately be called "One Consumer's View of the Health Care System" in that he appears to believe
that there is little or nothing good about health care in the United States.
Many statements he makes about providers are true. Others, however,
appear to be straw men. He fails to acknowledge that many physicians
can be trusted to put their patients' welfare ahead of their own or that
many are working hard to bring about constructive reforms to benefit
patients. It is easier to diagnose the defects in the health care system
than it is to prescribe solutions that will work and that are acceptable
to patients and providers. It is to Mr. Schuck's credit that he does not
shy away from this difficult task.

It has not been adequately recognized until recently that recipients
of services should be involved in decisions regarding their own health
care and in decisions about the organization, financing, and provision
of health care generally. The United States has an increasingly bureau-

119

cratic health care system. Direct patient influence has decreased markedly, while professional, third party and other bureaucratic influences have
increased. The reasons for this are numerous and include growth of
specialization, private health insurance, and government involvement in
the provision and financing of health care. Research advances, medical
technology, and the recognition of health care as a fourth necessity,
along with the other recognized necessities of life—food, shelter, and
clothing—have resulted in a variety of large and complex systems for
financing and providing health services. Large medical centers have replaced the doctor's office and the community hospital. Private health
insurance and government financing have joined the consumer's pocket-
book to meet the rising costs of care. The growing demand and increasing
complexity in health care happened in the absence of a national program
or policy on how to provide or pay for health care for the nation's
people.

Growth in numbers and complexity produces layers of organization
that are sometimes far removed from patients or doctors, private offices
or hospitals. The result has been a decline in consumer influence in decisions about care or about the system. The opposite of this is needed to
counter the powerful forces at work influencing priorities, programs, and
the provision of services.

One of the problems in discussing "consumer participation" is implied
in the term itself. Webster defines "consumer" as "one that consumes,
specifically one that utilizes economic goods." Patients, however, require
services—professional expertise and judgment—not economic goods. The
delivery of this service is built on trust, and the product is often intangi-
ble. The transaction is not carried out in a usual economic market, and
the needs of the patient can seldom be met by using boycotts or similar
actions that have traditionally been effective in bringing about desired
change in other areas of society.

A factor in this, as Mr. Schuck points out, is the difference between
want and need. Health services are needed, and they are supplied by
those who possess a knowledge the user does not have. This makes the
consumer an unequal partner in the transaction.

Because of this inequality, it is paramount that each patient have a
physician he or she can trust. Here it is interesting to note that, in the
last half century, the relationship of the professions to the public has
been changing from one of *caveat emptor* (let the buyer beware) to one
of *credat emptor* (let the buyer have trust). This has been brought about
by a number of factors, including the growing realization that members
of the health professions could be trusted to put the welfare of their
patients ahead of their own.

Trust has been an implied value of our health care system. Mr. Schuck and I agree that it is essential for a health care system to have defined and stated values and we would also agree that this has not been accomplished. He makes certain basic value assumptions about a desirable health care system when he states:

> If consumer interests in an efficient, varied, innovative, competitive, responsive, and accountable health care delivery system are to be represented, there are only two ways in which these might be advanced: (1) breaking provider sovereignty over the delivery of health care services through strengthening competitive market forces; (2) confronting the monopoly power exercised by providers with countervailing consumer power, through collective, organizational pressures on provider groups or on the macrocosmic policymaking process.

Are there not values for the consumer other than "efficient, varied, innovative, competitive, responsive, and accountable?" Are these values widely shared? Certainly, accountability is vital. But is cost control implicit in this? Is "competitive" a desired value? Responsiveness may encompass other values such as ease of access. Competence, compassion, availability, and appropriateness could certainly be added to the list. Although perceived differently by providers and consumers, quality is a value desired by both. Freedom of choice may also be valued by physician and patient. The list could go on, and it is possible that some of the values may be in conflict. What priority should be accorded these values by the physician, the patient, groups of patients, or the community at large, and how do we evaluate them? What and how can consumer participation and/or consumer control contribute to the development of a health care system that includes these values? How can we reach agreement in what the values should be?

In his analysis of the health care system, Mr. Schuck focuses primarily on the clients of the system, but he does describe some of the needs for the other groups, including individual patients. He analyzes the system in relation to his stated values and describes five major problems that are sufficiently severe to justify the term "health care crisis":

1. The lack of access to primary health care services, and particularly to services that could prevent illness;

2. The uneven quality of care and the difficulty of assessing quality, particularly as it relates to outcomes of care;

3. The high cost of medical care;

4. The emerging configuration of health care services, particularly the sharp decline in primary physicians in relation to specialty physicians; and

5. The relatively low health level of the American people as compared with other industrially developed nations.

In describing these five problems, he stresses what he considers to be the deficiencies of the health care system, including the self-serving role played by physicians individually and collectively as the principal culprits. He is also critical of the hospitals and the health insurance industry. He does not consider that separate but interrelated health care systems serve the American people, nor does he adequately relate the effects of the life styles of different groups to their health status.

In examining the problems and deficiencies of the health care system in the United States, it must be recognized that there are actually four subsystems serving different, but overlapping groups. The first subsystem serves the inner-city poor. It is based largely on public hospitals or publicly subsidized voluntary hospitals. Services are often provided by physicians in training. In many hospitals these physicians are foreign medical school graduates with vastly different cultural backgrounds than the people served. There are disproportionate numbers of aged, poor, and minority groups served by this system.

The second subsystem serves the urban and suburban middle and upper classes. Services are provided largely by specialists. Voluntary, nonprofit community hospitals are the base for inpatient care and most of the people served have health insurance. This subsystem has often been referred to as mainstream medical care.

The third subsystem serves the people living in rural areas. The general practitioner and the small, often modestly equipped, rural hospital form the basis for this subsystem. Many of the residents know their doctor. Many people have health insurance. Many do not, or they have inadequate coverage.

The fourth subsystem serves all federal beneficiaries—members of the armed forces and their dependents—veterans, merchant seamen, native Americans and Alaska natives. This subsystem includes separate organized services operated by the army, navy, air force, Veterans Administration, and Public Health Service. Inpatient and outpatient care are often separated. Specialty services, not primary care, are often emphasized. Hospital stays tend to be longer than in civilian institutions.

The consumers in these settings may have varying degrees of influence. Veterans organizations, for example, have been influential on behalf of both individual patients and clients of the Veterans Administration system. It is clear, however, that consumer participation would have to take different forms within these four subsystems. No one has determined what the approaches should be given the fact that there are four separate systems.

The wide-ranging criticisms Mr. Schuck makes of the health care system are shared in varying degrees by many who have analyzed the health care system. They are not, however, completely shared by either the general public or the medical profession.

The perception of the health care crisis, or lack of it, in this country and the priority accorded its solution is very much in the eye of the beholder. The patient may want easy access and a competent, concerned physician. The physician may accord a higher priority to the quality of care and freedom of choice, while the taxpayer, the legislator, and the employer who pay the insurance premium may choose cost control as their first priority.

In a recent survey analyzed by Dr. Stephen Strickland, a political scientist associated with the Health Policy Program, University of California, San Francisco, it was found that 84 percent of the American public had either a great deal or a fair amount of confidence in their ability to obtain good medical care. Although this figure revealed a strong vote of confidence in the medical profession and our medical services, it also revealed that 29 million Americans, mostly the poor and the aged, had little confidence in their ability to obtain the health care they needed.

Physicians were also surveyed and they had an even more critical view of health care than did the public. While 89 percent of the physicians had a great deal or fair amount of confidence in the health care system's ability to deal with medical emergencies or acute illness, only 66 percent felt that long-term illnesses were dealt with adequately.

The public and professional perceptions revealed in this survey are in accord with many other views that the poor, the aged, and the chronically ill do not receive the same quality of care as the great majority of the middle-aged and middle class whose needs can be more easily met.

The problems were thought to be of sufficient importance so that both the public and the physicians surveyed agreed on the need for change in the health care system. They did not agree on the nature of the changes needed or the priority that should be assigned to particular actions. The public ranked the physician shortage as the most urgent and important problem; cost of medical care ranked seventh. Physicians, on the other hand, ranked cost as the number one problem, followed by the physician shortage and the growing problem of malpractice.

The patients and physicians surveyed were both concerned, not only about the physician shortage but about the kind of physician or physicians needed to provide medical services.

After a careful review of the survey data, Strickland[1] observed:

Most Americans agree that a good general practitioner who will use specialists when necessary is the kind of doctor they want. But, beyond basic competence, people feel that a highly important consideration in choosing a doctor is whether he will be available to attend their needs whenever they arise. They want assurance that their doctor can be reached on short notice, and if necessary, that he will take care of them regardless of their ability to pay.

Physicians, in contrast, felt that the most important quality was the physician's willingness to treat the whole patient and his understanding of the personal and family circumstances of his patients. Next in order were knowing how to use specialists, affiliation with a good hospital, a high quality medical education and training, and the physician's ability to treat most illnesses. This last criterion had been ranked first by patients.

The results of this survey could be considered further evidence of the broad basis of support for change in the organization, financing, and provision of health care. Hopefully these changes will provide for all Americans comprehensive health care that is accessible and available when and where they need it, that is appropriate and responsive to their needs, that is within the financial means of individuals and society, and that is accountable to the public.

There is no question that we do not have an equitable health care system in the United States. Many do not have adequate access to care. The burden of cost, disease, and disability fall unequally. Many receive benefits who do not share equally in the costs. Equity is certainly one of the basic values we need to achieve in our health care system. What can consumer participation and/or consumer control contribute to the achievement of equitable care? What would be the best forms for consumer participation to take?

The answer depends on the problem. Mr. Schuck describes five structural defects blocking the consumer sovereignty he considers essential for the creation of a responsive, accountable, health care system:

1. Consumer ignorance;
2. The limited role of consumers in decision making;
3. The perverse economic incentives of the third party payment system;
4. Provider control of licensure, accreditation, and professional discipline; and
5. A lack of purchasing power for the poor.

A key to dealing with all of these barriers is participation. Like equality, this is a basic value in our society and one that is receiving increasing attention and recognition. Participation in our society has been limited in many areas. Women, minorities, the aged, the physically and mentally

handicapped, and many other groups have either been totally excluded
or offered little opportunity to participate in decisions that affect them
directly.

Participation in the health care system on the personal level includes
the right to be told about the cause, diagnosis, and prognosis for the
state of one's health. It also includes informed consent or the right to
be involved in decisions about one's care. There is participation at three
other levels as well: the national level where broad social policy decisions
are made on such matters as social security and national health insurance;
the national and state levels where decisions are made on allocations
within the health sector; and the local or institutional level where decisions may be made on what services are to be provided, where, how,
and under whose auspices.

In his paper, Mr. Schuck suggests the need for a somewhat different
approach to increase consumer power. His prescription calls for a series
of actions to deal with the five basic problems he identified. His proposals include:

1. The development of health maintenance organizations (HMOs);
2. Consumer control of licensing through institutional licensure and
accountability rather than professional licensing;
3. The providing of no-fault medical practice insurance;
4. Health care vouchers for the poor;
5. Improved consumer information about the health care system;
and
6. Stronger consumer representation in peer review, third party
payers, and perhaps in the creation of a new federal consumer protection
agency.

He cites the usual arguments in favor of HMOs and also points out
the often overlooked fact that:

In the end, the effect of HMOs on the cost and quality of fee-for-service care may
be even more far-reaching than the effects of HMOs on their own subscribers.

He does not describe possible adverse effects of the development of
HMOs, especially those that operate for a profit. Research is needed on
these questions, and they should be examined as HMOs begin to develop
in a variety of settings.

His arguments in favor of institutional licensing do not consider the
problems institutions would have in establishing and evaluating criteria
for competency, nor do they consider the predictable lack of mobility,
or the possible results of institutions using unqualified personnel. His

arguments for no-fault medical practice insurance are more persuasive. I believe that neither of these, however, is as important as some of the other proposals he makes.

The implications of a voucher system for the poor are not discussed at all. The major question of equity remains: Who decides? How do they decide? What kind of voucher is necessary for a chronic diabetic, compared with a patient with catastrophic illness? Even if such problems of equity were solved, it is not reasonable to assume that providing purchasing power will guarantee access, or affect the possibilities for provider–consumer interaction. In addition, he does not deal with the trade-offs that may be necessary or the possible losses that may occur with the changes he proposes.

As Mr. Schuck points out, "the phrase 'consumer representation' can be a meaningless slogan, having no effect on the way in which decisions are made, or it can be a fundamental reallocation of power over centralized decision-making processes." If one of the issues to be addressed is participation versus alienation, the effect of implementing a "meaningless slogan" demands attention. It is not difficult to conceive of increased alienation of representatives and consumers if consumer advisory councils or consumer boards are not representative or do not function according to expectations. Meaningless slogans are not new in any area of our society, but to add this to the burdens of illness is a cruel hoax indeed.

The growth of third parties, the increasing complexity of providing and financing needed services, the growth of a host of programs to meet the needs of different groups have led to the growth of bureaucratic and professional influences. To counter these trends and to provide the consumer the opportunity for greater influence in the system, Mr. Schuck stresses the need to strengthen the consumer's interest at the professional and the administrative levels. This same point was made earlier by Professor Eliot Freidson[2] in his book *Professional Dominance*:

But since administration has its own needs independent and sometimes conflicting with those of the client and the professional, it too requires tempering. While the strengthening of administrative influence over the way a professional's work is performed is important, the strengthening of the influence of the client on both groups is more important.

In recent years, there has been a great deal of discussion in favor of consumer participation or consumer control of health care, but there has been little documentation of the benefits in terms of cost, quality of service, or other outcomes.

In spite of the lack of evidence, I agree with Schuck, Freidson, and others who support greater consumer participation in the planning and management of health care delivery systems. Recognizing the lack of evidence relating to health outcomes, Dr. Alberta Parker[3] has stated the case for consumer participation this way:

Encouragement and basic support of consumer participation need not wait, however, upon a detailed assessment of benefits and their costs. Citizen participation in activities and institutions is worthy of support because of a very basic American value, namely, the belief that individuals should participate in the determination of their own destiny.

Part of the evaluation problem, I believe, relates to the criteria necessary to demonstrate the value of consumer participation. Health outcomes are often too remote to relate in a cause and effect manner. Dr. Parker has listed acceptability and utilization of services, ease of access, scope of available services, types of services used, professional satisfaction, costs and efficiencies in operations, consumer communications mechanisms, legal problems, and community support among possible criteria.

Mr. Schuck's proposed solutions do not suggest a method for evaluating their impact on the problems described. Putting the consumer or a new organization into control may not change the motivations or methods of providers. This might, in fact, simply transfer them to a different setting with additional pressures. The point is that agreed-upon criteria can be established and studies of health care systems carried out. It would be possible, for example, to compare physician-controlled prepayment plans with those governed by consumers; it should be possible to evaluate the strengths and weaknesses of group practice versus solo practice, particularly from the standpoint of an agreed-upon set of attributes felt desirable by consumers.

If health care services are to improve health status through better utilization, health information, or action programs, they need the support and participation of individuals, groups of clients, and in some cases the community. This is particularly true in poverty areas where the people bear the greatest burden of disease and disability.

Consumer information is a key element in making the health care system more responsive and accountable. Informed consent is being broadened by the courts, and patients' rights are gradually being recognized in this area. Providers should take the initiative and not wait for others to tell them what to do in providing facts about diagnosis and treatment and about the health care system.

Although I agree with Mr. Schuck that there should be a consumers health care organization, I would broaden its proposed role to include education of consumers, providers, and policymakers, as well as the advocacy function. The health care constituency has had no effective organization because the issues have been too complex and too far-ranging. An additional problem is that health care is so fragmented; therefore, the solutions are fragmented. The problem is how do we make the structure more cohesive and care more accessible and responsive? How do we assure every citizen a personal physician?

A consumers health care organization could, as its first task, begin to define the areas where direct consumer participation is needed and suggest ways to get consumers into the process. The second task could be to suggest ways that the results of consumer participation can be evaluated in terms of better health. Yet a third, and extremely important task, could be researching areas that require consumer information or education and suggesting the most effective way to get the needed information to the public.

It is possible that an added benefit of such studies would be to provide consumer education not just on "how to beat the system" but on how to use health professionals and health services wisely. Other examples of issues that a consumer organization might address include:

1. Expanded duties of other professionals, such as nurse practioners or physician assistants;
2. The form of national health insurance;
3. Geographic restrictions on health professionals educated in state schools (in terms of manpower distribution);
4. Developing more community clinics;
5. What kinds of training programs most deserve funding.

The list could go on. The point is that members of the Congress as well as state and local legislators attempt to make reasoned judgments and a consumer group could assist in their decisions.

Finally, I share Mr. Schuck's view—without being able to provide the needed evidence to support my position—that for at least two of the values that should characterize health care, equity and participation, far more must be accomplished. It will not be accomplished easily, but the benefits should justify the effort.

REFERENCES

1. Strickland SP: U.S. Health Care—What's Wrong and What's Right. New York, Universe Books, 1972.

2. Freidson E: Professional Dominance: The Social Structure of Medical Care. New York, Atherton Press, 1970, p 211.
3. Parker AW: Consumer participation in health programs, Young Doctors, Health Care and the American Future. Proceedings of the Second National House Staff Conference, Institute for the Study of Health and Society, Atlanta, Georgia, March 3–5, 1972.

NATHAN MACCOBY, Ph.D.
Professor of Communication, Stanford University

The Effects of Mass Communication on Shaping Consumer and Provider Values in Health

We live in a society in which the mass media of communication play an increasingly important role. The broadcast media of television and radio, the print media of newspapers, magazines, books, leaflets, and billboards, and the movies provide us with a continually fuller stream of communication. The total number of hours per week spent by persons in this country attending to all media is growing and formidable. Wilbur Schramm[1] points out that on any weekday evening some 75 million Americans are likely to be watching television, and over 90 million people read newspapers. Radio listening has been on the rise in the last decade after being badly cut into by the development of television. In other words, as new media of communication develop—and let us not forget that still further new media are coming along—they tend replace old media initially. Over time, however, there is an increase in the total amount of exposure to mass media. Television sets are turned on an average of about six hours a day, but radio listening and newspaper, book, and magazine reading are also up. Only movie attendance is going down, but movie watching is increasing because movies constitute the largest single fare offered on TV.

It is clear enough that of all these media, TV is the most prevalent. Furthermore, on TV, approximately 15 percent of all broadcast time is devoted to advertising. In addition, of course, the contents of a great

130

many telecast hours may really constitute indirect influence on the consumer. For example, what physicians are like and how they interact with patients is even more likely to be communicated by "Marcus Welby, M.D." than by ads for pharmaceuticals.

How potent is all this material in influencing people? To what extent are people learning how to protect themselves from illness and disease via the mass media? To what extent are they being induced to engage in activities and pursuits that are harmful or damaging? How about children? Are they peculiarly defenseless in the face of the onslaught of purchasing and other behavioral instructions?

These are very difficult questions to answer with scientific validity. The ideal method for ascertaining the effects of a communication is like the ideal way of measuring the effects of anything; namely, the controlled experiment in which the independent variable(s) is (are) manipulated under controlled conditions, and changes in the dependent variable(s) is (are) measured against those, if any, in the control(s). Experiments of such classic design can be and are done to measure communication effects. However, when carried out under laboratory-type conditions, they leave something to be desired in terms of understanding what happens under ordinary conditions of exposure. When the effectiveness of a film in influencing information and/or attitudes—say about smoking cigarettes—is measured by a controlled evaluation experiment, the audience is necessarily a "captive" one. Audience members did not select themselves to be viewers as is the case in "real life." If they did, the condition of random assignment to cells would not be met. This problem of self-selection of exposure is in itself a complicated problem, and a good deal of work has been done in this area.[2] Hypotheses on who elects to expose himself to a given type of communication can also be tested experimentally. Random subpopulations can be subjected to such treatment as sensitizing with particular kinds of information prior to being given the opportunity to elect exposure to a given communication.

One group can be sensitized to a given problem or issue, with a comparable group held as a control. The effects of such sensitization can be assayed by giving both groups an opportunity to elect exposure. For example, in a major study designed to discover effective ways of getting people to change their behavior in particular ways so as to reduce risk of heart disease, we have intensively interviewed and medically examined samples of people in three communities. We are concerned with attempting to change habits via differing communication patterns in the several communities. We strongly suspect that people interviewed and examined in this way are likely to elect to pay more attention to our mass media material than comparable others not so treated. The extent to which such is the case is being assessed (at least in part) by selecting a comparable sample not interviewed until after the communication intervention is over. This is dubbed an "after only" control group.

In measuring television effects on general populations who view TV in their own homes under ordinary everyday circumstances, such elegant designs are generally not feasible. In recent years, considerable improvement in designs aimed at teasing out causal connections in the absence of controlled experimentation in the laboratory have been developed. McGuire[3] points out in a recent paper that there is a definite need for field experiments and sophisticated correlational analysis in naturalistic settings. Campbell[4] has pioneered in the development of such methods. Parker[5] some years ago used cross-lagged correlations to test the effects of television on library usage.

Eventually, the logic of these methods is to rule out potential falsifiers, i.e., possible alternative explanations, one by one. In any case, there is an increasing amount of research on communication that is aimed at assessing effects with some precision in field or naturalistic settings. Some of the relevant recent research on communication effects, as it pertains to health-related matters, will be discussed below.

CONSUMER SOURCES OF INFORMATION, ATTITUDES, AND BEHAVIOR

In a certain sense, it is an incredible state of affairs that by far the overwhelming amount of information about health matters is communicated via advertising by profit-making producers and purveyors of drugs and goods. The marketers of products sell these to more or less unsuspecting consumers. They push vitamins, laxatives, pain relievers, cures for hemorrhoids, arthritis, hypertension, and a host of other cure-alls for what does and does not ail one.

While the evidence on the extent of harm to individuals who follow the health instructions of product advertisers has not been fully reviewed, it is clear that little if any good can come from such prescriptions. Evidently, the need for supplementary vitamins for most Americans is absent, and laxatives have been shown to be generally harmful. (Bowel movements do not need to occur at least once a day with everyone, and artificial stimulation, at least, interferes with normal habit formation and maintenance and, at worst, can contribute to cancer of the colon.) Hemorrhoids, arthritis, and hypertension are not generally cured by advertised drugs, suppositories, and pills; and so it goes.

In a recent survey by National Analysts of Philadelphia for the Food and Drug Administration many public misconceptions were uncovered.

Almost three quarters of the population, for instance, believe that by taking extra vitamins a person can gain extra pep and vitality. Even before Linus Pauling's advocacy of vitamin C hit the national press, 58 percent of the survey respondents expressed the belief that the vitamin can prevent colds. Two thirds of those interviewed felt that a daily bowel movement is essential to good health. Americans revealed an enormous faith in the power of drugs in curing their ills. One third of the subjects interviewed by National Analysts said that, as long as they themselves were benefiting, they would continue to use a medicine even if their doctor told them it was worthless. This willingness to try anything, coupled with the placebo effect and the notion of uniqueness (It will work for *me*!), has led a huge number of Americans to put their trust in useless drugs and sometimes to avoid the less zealously promoted advice of their doctors.

The mass media, especially in advertising, have fostered the belief that there is a medicine for every ailment. The survey reported above also found that a great many people believe that advertisers are so well regulated that they dare not make false claims. Yet a recent analysis of advertising content in television conducted by Wayne State researchers and reported in the *New England Journal of Medicine* shows that, of the 7 percent of the ads that were health related, 70 percent were unsatisfactory or misleading. It is not too surprising, then, that the attitudes and opinions of most Americans tend to be similar to the distorted and inadequate information provided by their mass media. Before examining the information available to the health-seeking consumer, let us review the dynamics of advertising's contribution to consumer knowledge.

During fiscal year 1969–1970 drug companies invested almost 10 percent of their sales dollars in advertising. Manufacturers of tobacco products used a little over 5 percent and food packagers and processors around 3 percent of their total sales revenue in the same manner. For the purveyors of these products the money was well spent. National advertising, especially in health-related products, is an enormous boost to the legitimacy of any ordinary product. Bayer aspirin provides a good example. There are numerous other brands that are equally effective and cost much less. Why will most Americans spend more than necessary for the privilege of buying Bayer aspirin? One answer is that they trust it more. Having seen its quality attested to on an almost nightly basis, usually in the context of network news reports, consumers come to believe that Bayer is more dependable than other less well-known brands might be. Thus to gain a reasonable share in a competitive market, many firms selling health-related products are forced to advertise.

Often, however, simply having a product legitimized by the media is not enough. There may be other, equivalent products that were there earlier and have thus previously accrued considerable legitimacy. To sell the product in a competitive market, the advertiser must present the consumer with some reason why his product is newer and better and should be chosen over its competitors. This leads to a clamorous cacophony of claims and counterclaims, added and extra-added ingredients.

Such frenzied economic competition has unfortunate effects on the values of both consumers and providers. Consumers are led to develop unrealistic notions of the power of pills. They come to believe that there is a "miracle" or "wonder" drug for every problem. Providers in this competitive situation are led to value expensive and marginally excusable additives for which they can make exaggerated claims. It is more profitable for them to present the public with the puffed-up rhetoric of advertising, a modern version of the old medicine shows, than with the reliable information needed for intelligent decisions.

Advertising in the mass media has the effect of legitimizing the product advertised. For example, if a product is regularly advertised on TV, people tend to think that the advertising must be reasonably truthful or it would not be permitted.

Apparently, advertising medicines goes back at least to Roman days. Brown[6] in his book *Techniques of Persuasion* refers to the small stone printing stamps used by quacks to impress messages on their salves and ointments. Some of these printing stamp stones are in the British Museum. (The relationship between what is claimed in the ads for remedies for disease and what they actually accomplish doesn't seem to have changed much over the centuries.)

Brown refers to a green salve named "Chloron" (even the names sound familiar) advertised by the Roman merchandisers in Britain as an unbeatable ointment. With the advent of the mass medium of communications made possible by the invention of the printing press, medical advertising really got going. Daniel Defoe in his *Journal of the Plague Year* describes posters inviting people to come to doctors for remedies during the 1665 plague.

However, the real bonanza in the drug business came with the discovery of the wonder drugs and their marketing in the years since World War II. Penicillin, Aureomycin, the sulfas, and the steroids have produced fortunes for a number of pharmaceutical manufacturers and distributors. It should be pointed out that the marketing of so-called ethical drugs is not done so much via mass media advertising as via practicing physicians who are called upon by detail men and in more recent times are simply flooded directly by mail with samples and literature. An excellent set of studies mainly by Katz and Lazarsfeld[7] and Coleman and coworkers[8] have documented the manner by which drug prescriptions by physicians are adopted. Style setters among physicians play a critical role in which drugs become fashionable for particular ailments at particular times in particular locales.

It is a curious phenomenon that when attempts are made to market helpful health practices on a wide scale, little is currently known about how to do it successfully. It has been almost 20 years since the Surgeon General officially pronounced that smoking cigarettes is likely to be injurious to health, that it might well be a major source of alarming rises in lung cancer and a significant cause of heart disease, a really big killer.

While there have been variations from time to time in the rate of cigarette smoking in this country, certainly cigarette marketing and cigarette smoking have not been materially reduced. The most that can be said of all the efforts to reduce or eliminate cigarette smoking is that they have succeeded dramatically in convincing people that cigarette smoking may be indeed bad for their health. However, such beliefs do not mean people quit smoking. For example, in a recent study we are conducting in three central California small towns referred to above, over 85 percent of all smokers report believing that smoking is bad for their health, but over a third have continued to smoke nonetheless. National sample data are consistent with this finding. The statement on the back of a package of cigarettes that the Surgeon General has found that "smoking may be hazardous to your health" has been fully accepted but has done very little, if anything, either to deter new smokers from beginning or veteran smokers to stop, except for selected groups, notably physicians.

The drug market is not the only public health area that has been damaged by the competitive fervor of advertising. The *Journal of Nutrition Education* recently published a report that indicated that the "dietary habits of the American public have become worse, especially since 1960." Their study also found that children in higher income families—targets of most advertisers—were often less well nourished than those in lower income families. Action for Children's Television (ACT) spokesmen have reported, as an example of the total situation in food advertising, that a child watching Channel 7 in Boston from 7 am to 2 pm on Saturday, October 4, 1972, would have seen 67 attractive messages urging him to eat or drink sweetly flavored products. Robert Choate, Chairman of the Council on Children, Media and Merchandising, has been a most vocal critic of children's food advertising. In an article in *Nation* he[9] states that, "With no accompanying warnings, a child is invited ten times per hour to establish food habits which his dentist or doctor will later deplore. . . . Nutrition is human ecology and television is a master polluter."

All the broadcaster and advertiser can say is, "Nutrition just doesn't sell." This trend shows signs of reversing, at least in cereal advertising. Note the recent upsurge of ads for "health" cereals such as Quaker's "Granola." In competing for the food dollar, manufacturers find it most profitable to offer people what they want, not what they need. But for young children the gap between wants and needs in food products is, as any mother will attest, considerable. The willingness of food providers to cater to immature tastes has grave consequences for the values of young consumers and for those who provide them with sustenance. Children are reinforced in their desire for sweets and their mothers led to believe that flavored synthetics (with vitamins added) are sufficient for their children's nutritional needs. Providers emphasize only the most superficial notions of what a good diet really is both in the products they sell and the sketchy information they provide.

A solution that is often offered to the advertising problem in public diet and drug consumption is the same one that was recently used in attempting to eradicate the public health menace of tobacco advertising. The Fairness Doctrine is a Federal Communication Commission requirement that broadcasters provide rebuttal time for their editorial opinions. John Banzhaf[10] was able to convince the courts to extend that doctrine to require public service announcements warning of the health danger of cigarette smoking as a rebuttal to the many ads promoting smoking that appeared on television every day. Though the courts originally held that the situation was unique and that the doctrine would not be extended in the case of other types of advertising, more recent court decisions have held that it may be applied in a wide variety of circumstances. Consumer advocates concerned with the advertising problems discussed on the previous pages have thus proposed that such counteradvertising be used as an antidote to misleading food and drug information promulgated by commercial messages.

If such a system were adopted, consumers might learn that pills are not the final solution to their ills and that cereals and candy pseudo-meals do not provide the nutritional benefits they seem to promise. Public awareness on these issues might then lead the providers of food and drugs to value true dietary usefulness and sensible views of drug effectiveness, but some voices argue that counteradvertising will destroy the economic foundation of broadcasting and leave consumers worse off than they were to begin with. It remains to be seen if a policy of counteradvertising can be applied judiciously enough to accomplish appropriate results.

Cartwright[11] some 25 years ago found that, in order to alter behavior, people must not only be prepared cognitively and emotionally to change but also willing to learn new behavior. This acquisition of new knowledge (in our present example that smoking is hazardous to health) and the desire to quit sets the stage for change (to stop smoking), but is not sufficient to actually effect the change. The behavior indicated must be initiated in some way. People need to learn new habits that are often incompatible with the old ones (in our example, doing something else when smoking a cigarette is the indicated act). There are a variety of ways of instigating this new behavior. B. F. Skinner[12] has developed the concept of behavior shaping, a form of training in which the learner is rewarded as he gets closer and closer to performing the desired response. C. B. Ferster, a former protégé and collaborator of Skinner, and many others, including my colleague Dr. A. J. Stunkard, have applied Skinnerian ideas on schedules of reinforcement and Bandura's on modeling to the health field. Rewards are administered for behavior of the desired sort. In the process of getting people to perform the correct or desired responses, responses close to the desired ones are initially rewarded and then only responses even more similar to the desired ones are rewarded in subsequent instances. One of the most interesting aspects of this kind of training is the means used to maintain the change. Mark Twain once cogently observed that quitting smoking was easy; he had done it hundreds of times. This is precisely the problem with getting people to quit smoking. Leventhal* has pointed out that there are several techniques that have been attempted to get people to stop smoking and that all seem to be about equally effective; namely, they all seem to result in getting about 25 percent of smokers to quit. Few, if any, however, seem to be very effective in keeping people from resuming the habit.

Reward during training, instead of being administered on the occasion of every successful response, could be administered only some of the time. For example, every nth successful response could be rewarded, with the number of successful trials between rewards randomly varied around n to control for "expectancy." This procedure has the interesting effect of producing a response that is more resistant to extinction; that is, it will continue to be elicited long after all reinforcement is stopped in contrast to the response learned via 100 percent reinforcement. Thus, in training people to quit smoking, one could apply these so-called operant conditioning techniques involving random ratio reinforcement and hope thereby to reduce the frequency of backsliding. If, in training people to stop smoking cigarettes, one reinforced "not smoking" with decreasing frequency, one could expect "not smoking" to last longer.

---

* Personal communication with the author.

There are other approaches to learning to change undesirable health habits that have been used. Research on persuasion seriously began during World War II, which was continued at Yale by the late C. I. Hovland and his associates. Since then, it has become a major area of investigation by experimental social psychologists and other communication researchers. While it would be inappropriate here to attempt an exhaustive summary of this area of research, a brief description of some of the most relevant approaches may be indicated. Most work in this field is done via controlled experimentation, although some has been based on correlational field studies. The methodological problems are of the sort discussed earlier. If the hypotheses about attitude change are tested under controlled conditions with captive audiences, the communications responsible for the changes might or might not be attended to by the relevant people in real-life settings. Thus, if a particular kind of communication is effective in getting smokers to stop when applied to captive audiences, will it be effective when presented over television or some other mass medium? Will heavy smokers expose themselves to the communication and really attend to it, or will they avoid it?

Another even more serious problem is the measure of verbal statements as dependent variables in most studies on attitude change. These measures may or may not involve changes in actual behavior. We have already seen that campaigns on smoking have had much more effect on people's attitudes toward the hazards of smoking than on smoking itself.

In spite of problems of this sort, I feel confident that there is a great deal to be learned from the research literature on persuasion. There have been a great many experiments testing a variety of hypotheses about persuasion. While there are many ways of grouping these studies, a simple way is to employ a neo-Lasswellian model of "Who says what via what channel to whom?" Thus some experiments deal with characteristics of the *source* of the persuasive message; some with the *content* of the message; some with the nature of the *media* or *channels* through which the message is sent; and finally some are concerned with the role of the characteristics of the *receiver*. To illustrate, Hovland and Weiss[13] did a study in which exactly the same message was attributed to different sources. Four different messages were used as replications, but the one of most interest to us here was one dealing with the issue of whether or not antihistamines should continue to be sold without the prescription of a physician. In one condition, the *New England Journal of Medicine* was stated as the locus of the article; in the low credibility condition a mass circulation monthly pictorial magazine was the attributed source. As might be expected, the high credibility source worked better than the low one. However, two other interesting findings occurred. First, even the low credibility source was influential; second, and more important was the finding about how enduring the effects were. After four weeks subjects were retested in order to assess the duration of the change. The differences between the effects of the communications attributed to the high and low credibility sources disappeared completely. Subsequent experimentation demonstrated that this finding was due to the dissociation of the source from the message. Clearly, as the authors conclude, to the extent that such dissociation occurs, the acceptance of the message will be independent of the source. In other words, people will tend to accept a message even if the source providing the content of the message and who said it get separated.

Of course, advertising is not the only content of the mass media that affects consumers and providers in health-related areas. Entertainment, journalism, and news, as well as formal health education are all part of the media content, and each has its own way of affecting health care in America. Though its contribution to public attitudes concerning health matters is often overlooked, the entertainment content in the mass media can exert a profound influence. People tend to be easily persuaded by information that has no obvious or overt persuasive intent. It has been demonstrated that more attitude change results when a message is prefaced by a statement disclaiming persuasive intent than when the same message is presented without a disclaimer. Similarly, overheard communications are often more persuasive than are those obviously intended to persuade.[14] Dramatic television programs, especially those taking a serious approach and attempting to create an air of verisimilitude in dealing with health care matters, can color the viewers' perceptions and future evaluations of health care in real life.

A whole series of experiments deal with questions pertaining to the nature of arguments included or omitted from the message. The first study was done by Sheffield of the Hovland group in World War II. He used the issue of how long the war with Japan would last, given that the war in Europe was about to end. In one experimental condition, he cited arguments advocating that the war would end soon (opposing arguments) prior to stating his intended message as though it were refuting the opposition. In other conditions, no opposing arguments were mentioned. Interestingly enough, both treatments proved equally effective, but there were important differences depending on the receiver. Of greater interest to us is that subsequent experiments first by Lumsdaine and Janis[15] and then a long and highly systematic series by McGuire[16] demonstrated that while the *initial* impact might not vary by whether or not opposition arguments were included, backsliding did. Those trained

by the positive arguments only were easy victims of subsequent communications advocating the opposing point of view. However, those
originally exposed to a communication containing opposition arguments
(or even references to the fact that opposition arguments existed) re-
sisted to varying extents the blandishments of the opposing communication. It was as if mentioning the opposition position in some way had
an innoculating effect on the receiver of the communication that the
one-sided presentation lacked.

Another and perhaps equally relevant problem area in this rubric is a
series of experiments begun by Janis and Feshbach[17] on the effects of
fear arousal in achieving persuasion. Is strong fear more effective than
moderate or mild fear in producing attitude change? While common
sense would seem to argue that strong fear arousal would be superior,
some consideration of the possible interference effect caused by strong
fear, such as avoiding paying attention, might lead to a different prediction. In any case, the researchers found that strong fear-arousing communications were less effective in getting people to brush their teeth in
prescribed ways than were milder fear-arousing messages. Subsequent
research has, I am afraid, clouded the picture considerably. Sometimes
results replicated the above ones, and on occasion they have been contradictory. Leventhal[18] has presented a systematic account of the state
of theory in fear-arousal communications. Chu[19] has posited a model
that takes account not only of the intensity of the fear aroused by the
communication but also of the direness of the threat, how soon the
blow would strike, and how effective was the proposed remedy. Taking
these variables into account, Chu has helped make sense out of what
appeared to be conflicting research results. One of the important findings that emerges is that strong fear arousal is most effective when the
threat of bad consequences appears to be imminent and when the proposed remedy is likely to be highly effective in dealing with the threat.
Clearly these findings do not give much aid and comfort to those concerned with getting people to change their ways in order to reduce the
likelihood of their getting heart disease or cancer.

The channel or *medium* through which the communication is sent
has been the least systematically studied. H. M. McLuhan, a humanist
who writes a great deal about communication theory, has made the
channel or medium through which the communication is transmitted
the central point of his analysis. McLuhan argues that technological
change in the media of communication—such as the development of the
printing press, movies, radio, and television—are critical to the processes
of human communication and tend to shape the way people perceive
and react to their environment. Very little theory-based empirical re-

search has as yet, however, employed the medium of communication as its main focus. Salomon has done some research involving varying simultaneity versus successive observation, but it does not involve attitude change. The many experiments comparing mediated versus live instruction have generally shown no differences. However, these studies for the most part lack any conceptual base. If exactly the same information is transmitted via a sound television receiver as in the live, and there is an equivalent captive audience in both instances, there is no reason to expect a difference in learning and, of course, none occurs.

Finally, the area of characteristics of the *receiver* of the communication is proving to be a productive one for attitude change research. The self-esteem of the person to whom a communication is directed is, for example, a very important factor in whether or not the communication will be persuasive. The extent to which an individual is initially committed to his position affects his resistance to persuasive communication. There is evidence to suggest, however, that—once such a committed person is changed—he is more likely to stay changed than is a more easily influenceable noncommitted receiver of a persuasive message. One could characterize the latter person as "easy come; easy go"; the former, although hard to change, once changed stays changed.

In the last decade or so, attempts have been made to systematize theory in the scientific study of persuasion. Early attempts at formulating hypotheses for testing and at explaining experimental results usually grew out of applications of learning theory derived primarily from studies of animal behavior to this more complex area of human social behavior. We have seen the application of Skinner's operant conditioning. Many students of persuasion continue to employ this approach. Other varieties of learning theory have also been applied. Hovland himself was a student of Hull, and Hull had developed perhaps the most sophisticated approach to reinforcement theory. Learning for Hull, as for Skinner, was conditioning via reinforcement. However, unlike Skinner, for Hull the stimulus had to be specifiable, and he was willing to infer a set of intervening stimulus–response units that are not directly observable. This author was a student of Guthrie's and has attempted to develop theoretical principles and hypotheses about persuasion growing out of Guthrie's contiguity theory of learning. Guthrie posited a model based on the simultaneous occurrence of conditioning or substitution of a new stimulus for an old one when that new stimulus happened to accompany a response. Roberts–Maccoby[20] report theory and experiment on the nature of the persuasive process along these lines.

Another widely used approach to persuasion has been a theory developed by Festinger[21] to apply to a wide range of social behavior known as cognitive dissonance. Festinger points out that, when two cognitions are held simultaneously and if one is the obverse of the other, motivation to reduce this dissonance occurs. If one designs an experiment such that changing one's attitude is the most feasible way of reducing such dissonance, one can achieve persuasion. Researchers in attitude change have been attracted to this approach, among other reasons, because it frequently leads to nonobvious predictions.

Particularly, it may lead to predictions that are contrary to what simple reinforcement theory would lead one to expect. For example, Festinger and his student Carlsmith, in one of the earliest studies stemming from this approach, predicted and found that smaller rewards could lead to more persuasion than larger ones. They had subjects who had performed a boring task tell their successors that the task was highly interesting. If they were not paid much, people would tend to believe that the boring task actually was interesting; if they were paid a great deal, however, they knew they were lying.

There are a number of other additional theoretical approaches to attitude change that may have some relevance to the persuasion process as it applies in "real life" settings. One more approach is perhaps important enough to mention here. It is called social judgment theory, which grew out of the work of Sherif and Hovland, and has been continued by the former, his wife Carolyn, and their students. It is a perception-based formulation that posits there are anchors in making judgments. Positions being advocated that are in part not too different from the one the receiver of the communication already holds tend to be perceived as being more or less synonymous with that attitude. As Sherif and his colleagues put it, such positions in communications tend to be assimilated by the recipient. On the other hand, when the communication advocates a point of view that differs considerably from the receiver's initial position, the latter tends to perceive that point of view as being even more different than it really is; it is said to be contrasted. This type of reasoning and research has led to a number of interesting predictions about persuasive communications.

For example, Hovland, Harvey, and Sherif[22] used this approach to account for the fact that in many persuasive communications—even those that are effective with many receivers of the message—there is often a boomerang effect. Thus while many people may be persuaded to adopt the position being advocated in the message, some will actually move in the opposite direction and be even more against the point of view of the communication than they were prior to being exposed to it. They found that this is particularly the case when the message receiver holds his initial position very strongly. In such cases the assimilable distance between the initial position held and the one being advocated shrinks and the zone of contrast expands to cover points of view not so very different from one's own.

The application of such kinds of research to public education on preventive health practices is clear. People who strongly hold erroneous views on such matters as diet, drugs, exercise, and smoking are more likely to be influenced by communications advocating positions not too far from their own. Communications urging extremely different points of view could well boomerang. There is one more important lesson here. People may differ considerably from one another not only in the initial points of view on an issue, but they may also differ greatly from one another on how strongly they hold that point of view. Addressing the same communication to everyone, which is what the use of the mass media usually involves, may have its drawbacks.

I have only been able to touch briefly here on the state of theory and research in the area of persuasive communication. I do want to mention one other experiment because it may help to focus a serious ethical problem posed by this type of research. Almost a decade ago, Festinger and Maccoby[23] reported an experiment whose published report we entitled *On Resistance to Persuasive Communications.* Actually we were concerned with ways of overcoming resistance. We reasoned that when people are exposed to a communication that strongly advocates a point of view that is anathema to them, they would tend to resist. We predicted further that this resistance would, among other means, take the form of engaging in debate or counterarguing against the advocated position. In a mass media setting in which there was a large live audience, this counterarguing would have to take place by thought rather than by overt word. We therefore designed an experiment in which two visual versions of a film carrying a persuasive message were made, both with the same sound track.

One visual version was straightforward, showing the speaker in front of a red velvet backdrop after some campus scenes used as establishment shots. The alternative version consisted of an edited version of a diverting film about a hippy painter. The message advocated the abolition of college fraternities. Fraternity members—assumed to be strongly opposed to the message—who were shown the "distracting" version of the film were more likely to be convinced by its message than were comparable undergraduates shown the "normal" version. Furthermore, this did not happen with nonfraternity members. Evidently, the "painter" film was not diverting enough to keep people from receiving the message; indeed, it was engineered to have precisely enough redundancy in the message to make sure the arguments were clearly received by audiences. The film evidently did serve to distract people from engaging in covert counter-arguing and thus penetrated their defenses. Subsequent research by Roberts and Maccoby[24] substantiated that, when people have counter-arguments available and are involved or committed to their initial point of view and are given the opportunity to counterargue, they will do so as a way of defending themselves against persuasion.

My colleague, social psychologist Darryl Bem, and his associates have formulated a somewhat different approach to persuasion. If a person can be induced to change his behavior, the perception of this changed behavior as originating with that individual can result in a change of his attitude. Instead of the paradigm information–attitude–behavior, the order goes information–behavior–attitude. Particularly in the area of prejudice, it has often been noted that it is sometimes easier to get people to engage in nonprejudiced behavior than it is to get them to change their verbal statements or attitudes.

Clearly, some very serious ethical problems arise. Persuasion is usually done without the permission of the person being changed. While presumably the changed behavior may be more beneficial to that person being changed than his old habit—say cigarette smoking or diet or exercise changes—does anyone have the right to impose his will in this way on another? Certainly, our Stanford Chicano students raised serious questions with us in the Stanford Heart Disease Prevention Program about this issue. They were concerned about several implications of our research on behavior change. Suppose, they said, people whose motives were not as noble as ours learned from our work how to change people. Suppose advertisers interested solely in selling their products without regard to the welfare of the purchasers studied our research and applied our findings to their activities. Certainly, the advertisers whose activities we discussed above would not be above using such applications.

Another question these students raised was, "What were we doing to the life styles characteristic of the culture, particularly in the area of diet?" After all, when researchers from one culture study another, and this was particularly relevant to this study, diet is especially likely to be different, and its values are difficult for an outsider to understand. I should point out that we had taken considerable pains to consult with and obtain the cooperation of Chicano leaders in the communities we were studying. With their cooperation, we had developed a comprehensive media campaign in Spanish and had pretested all materials carefully prior to their use. In fact, as one highly vocal and powerful Chicano labor leader put it to us when we told him of the student objections—since this research was supported by the federal government and since Chicanos' taxes were being used to finance it, they insisted on being included in the research.

How might current medical drama programs affect the consumer's image of health care? What millions of people see every week on "Marcus Welby, M.D.," "Young Dr. Kildare," "Medical Center," "The Bold Ones, and others is an idealized version of the medical world. When they see doctors who take very close, often intensely personal interest in their fictional patients, viewers may be frustrated when they do not receive such personal interest from their own doctors. From programs like "Emergency!" they learn methods of dealing with traumatic situations that they may attempt to apply in emergencies in their own lives. Viewers with real-life concerns with various diseases see these diseases dramatically handled in television dramas and get ideas as to how they should approach their own real problems.

These considerations make it apparent that great caution must be taken in dealing with medical affairs in dramatic television programming. Toward that goal the Physician's Advisory Committee on Television, Radio, and Motion Pictures recruits members to review medical dramas for "medical accuracy, medical plausibility and upholding of professional ethics." But such a negative, censoring approach is not the only one available. While taking care that nothing dangerous appears in these programs, an effort should be made to see that every possible positive educational opportunity is taken. Harold Mendelsohn[25] has suggested that in the context of dramatic entertainment it may be possible to present health-related information for the public benefit that has much greater impact than information presented in the traditional channels. Not only will people be happy to devote time to information packaged as entertainment, but they may also be more willing to accept that information if it is not in the traditional context of a persuasive appeal. Perhaps a viewer may even be more likely to overtly model a dramatic heroine's example.

Such a communication system could be easily developed. A set of public health experts could be drafted to recommend information to be disseminated. Each coherent bit could be given to the scriptwriter of the dramatic series for which it is best suited and incorporated in an upcoming program.

News reports also have strong effects on the health-related values of consumers and providers. Information presented in news presentations is probably the single greatest media determinant of consumption behavior. News scares concerning contaminated canned goods, for instance, have succeeded in nearly wiping out entire industries despite vigorous advertising campaigns to counteract them. When they are poorly or inaccurately handled, news reports in the health sphere may have grave results. An example occurred in 1972 when irresponsible reporters puffed up a routine cancer research news item from the National Cancer Insti-

tute and led people to believe that BCG, an organism previously used as
an antituberculosis vaccination, was 100 percent effective with animals
in eradicating cancers and that experimentation and therapy with hu-
mans was just around the corner. Hundreds of people began to call, and
some poor cancer victims went all the way to the Tennessee research
center asking to be treated. With thousands of people desperately wanting to believe that a cure for cancer was imminent, it was very difficult
for researchers to clear the air and get out the truth.

Such poor handling of health-related news is starkly contrasted by
the American Cancer Society's style of dealing with the news media.
Each year the Cancer Society holds a seminar for science writers at
which the latest factual information about cancer research is presented
by experts. Though the Society has been accused of managing the news
in its favor at these seminars, the information presented is accurate, and
the reporters are schooled in preventing fiascoes of ignorance like the
cure panic described above. The American Heart Association holds similar meetings. Such formal, systematic handling of news in health care
should be encouraged by the establishment of clearinghouses and autho-
rization or review boards that would make health news available and ensure its accuracy.

Closely related to health journalism are the numerous magazines and
paperback books that are available with health information. Such material has very high readership, especially among women. Many magazines take care to include only sensitive and accurate treatment of health
topics and should be congratulated for the informational service they
provide. Some sources are very expert. Other information sources, especially some in the paperback book market, are somewhat less credible
sources of medical information. In the diet fad area a few books offer
health information of questionable or negative value. While flagrant examples are generally repudiated in the press, consumers might be well
serviced by some kind of professional review service that grants or with-
holds approval according to the merits of the information provided.

Another mass media source of consumer information in health-related
matters is the formal educational system that operates through government or private public interest funding. This source of information has
been responsible for most of the increases in general health knowledge
in recent years. In 1940 only 38 percent of the population knew a symptom of cancer. By 1955 nearly 70 percent of the nation had that knowledge, largely as a result of national information campaigns in magazines
and newspapers, on radio, and even on billboards. But such programs are
not always successful in attaining their goals. Many of the recent drug
education campaigns have included film materials that may actually

incite rather than discourage drug abuse. Great care should always be taken to see that such unwanted, dysfunctional effects are avoided.

A more general problem with health education programs in the mass media is the tendency not to reach those individuals who need them most. Media exposure and comprehension are nearly always greatest among the social groups with the greatest income and education. Thus a middle-class youngster may be exposed to many different messages about venereal disease while his lower class counterpart, much more likely to come into contact with syphilis or gonorrhea, may have only sporadic contact with a single source of venereal disease information. There is no simple solution to this paradox in information dissemination. One would hope that media planners in information campaigns will take careful stock of the channeling options that are available to them in order to reach the audience for which their facts will be the most useful. Commercial advertisers are very conscious of the need to reach such target audiences. Perhaps public health agencies can learn from them.

Yet, in and of itself, the presentation of information is often not enough to accomplish the goals of a public health campaign in the mass media. Simply providing target individuals with information in a health-related area may not have any real effect on their behavior in the segments of their life to which it pertains. An example previously noted is the recent antismoking campaign. While nearly everyone is willing to agree smoking is bad for one's health (opinions were not nearly so unanimous a decade ago), many individuals continue to smoke in spite of that information. In other words, while the media campaign has been highly successful in changing attitudes, it has done little to alter actual behavior. An example of this lack of effect on behavior is reported by Auger *et al.*[26] The amount of cigarette smoking was surreptitiously measured in an office complex before and after gruesome antismoking posters were placed on the office walls. The introduction of the posters had no effect on the number of cigarette butts that were found in ashtrays at the end of a day.

The problem here is that it is often not enough merely to educate individuals about health hazards. They must also be persuaded to take action on the basis of that education. Current research employing behavior modification is having some success. However, it is difficult to apply behavior modification techniques on a wide-scale basis. We hope to discover ways to train people to modify their risk-increasing habits via mass media in the present Stanford Heart Disease Prevention Program.

We have discussed some of the problems arising from various kinds of efforts to get individuals to change their health-related behavior. We have seen the emergence of serious ethical problems arising even when the efforts that are being made are made with the best of intentions and with the aim of scientific discovery whose target is learning how to help prevent disease. Tentative efforts at the solution of these problems have been discussed.

Far more serious ethical problems arise from the attempts to market products when the marketer's aim is primarily profit making. While federal law and regulations of the Federal Trade Commission (FTC) and the Federal Communications Commission (FCC) can make some contribution toward alleviating the problem, the very nature of the system of advertising militates against simple truth telling. Theory and research on persuasion suggest that in the long run the only real defense against illegitimate attempts at persuasion lies in knowledge on the part of the receiver of the communication. I trust that few if any physicians are taking daily laxatives or are succumbing to other wiles of the other drug advertisers. A well-informed population is the best defense. Meanwhile, perhaps strengthening the hands of the FTC and FCC and other regulatory efforts to contain false claims in advertising can be of help.

Finally, I think we can learn a great deal from studying how other countries deal with these problems. In such a study we should examine not only societies that are organized politically and economically in a similar fashion to ours but also, and perhaps even more importantly, what differently organized societies are doing. We might well learn a great deal in this way if we can successfully avoid ideological stereotypes and study empirically how various so-called communist countries deal with advertising and consumer education in health matters.

ACKNOWLEDGMENTS

The assistance of Alfred McAllister, Institute for Communication Research, Stanford University, is gratefully acknowledged.

REFERENCES

1. Schramm W: Men, Messages and Media: A Look at Human Communication. New York, Harper & Row, 1973.
2. Freedman J, Sears D: Selective exposure. Adv Exp Soc Psychol 2: 57–97, 1965.
3. McGuire WJ: The yin and yang of progress in social psychology: seven koan. J Pers Soc Psychol 26: 446–456, 1973.
4. Campbell DT, Stanley J: Experimental and quasi-experimental designs for research and teaching. Handbook of Research on Teaching. Revised edition. Edited by NL Gage. Chicago, Rand McNally, 1972.
5. Parker EB: The effect of television on public library circulation. Public Opin Q, 27:578–589, 1963.

6. Brown JAC: Techniques of Persuasion. Baltimore, Penguin Books, 1963.

7. Katz E, Lazarsfeld PB: Personal Influence. Glencoe, Ill., Free Press, 1955.

8. Coleman S,Katz E, Menzel H: Indianapolis Medical Innovation: A Diffusion Study. Indianapolis, Bobbs Merrill, 1966.

9. Choate RB, Chairman, Council on Children, Media and Merchandising: Statement before the Federal Communications Commission, January 9, 1973.

10. Banzhaf J: Pages 188-191 in How To Talk back to Your TV Set. Edited by F Johnson. Boston, Little Brown, 1967.

11. Cartwright D: Some principles of mass persuasion. Human Relat, 2:253-267, 1949.

12. Ferster CB, Skinner BF: Schedules of Reinforcement. New York, Appleton-Century-Crofts, 1957.

13. Hovland CI, Weiss W: The influence of source credibility on communication effectiveness. Public Opin Q, 15:635-650, 1951.

14. Allyn J, Festinger L: The effectiveness of unanticipated persuasive communications. J Abnorm Soc Psychol 62:35-40, 1961.

15. Lumsdaine AA, Janis IL: Resistance to "counterpropaganda" produced by one-sided and two-sided propaganda presentations. Public Opin Q 17:311-318, 1953.

16. McGuire WJ: Inducing resistance to persuasion. Adv Exp Soc Psychol 5:191-229, 1964.

17. Janis I, Feshback S: Effects of fear-arousing communications. J Abnorm Soc Psychol 48:78-92, 1953.

18. Leventhal H: Findings and theory in the study of fear communication. Adv Exp Soc Psychol 5:120-186, 1970.

19. Chu, G. Fear arousal, efficacy and imminency. J Pers Soc Psychol 4:517-524, 1966.

20. Roberts DF, Maccoby N: Information processing and persuasion: counterarguing behavior. Sage Communication Research Annuals. Vol. II. Edited by F Kline, P Clarke. New York, Sage Publications, 1973.

21. Festinger L: A Theory of Cognitive Dissonance. Evanston, Ill., Row Peterson, 1957.

22. Hovland CI, Harvey OJ, Sherif M: Assimilation and contrast effects in attitude change. J Abnorm Soc Psychol, 55:242-252, 1957.

23. Festinger L, Maccoby N: On resistance to persuasive communications. J Abnorm Soc Psychol 68:359-366, 1964.

24. Roberts DF, Maccoby N: *op. cit.*

25. Mendelsohn H: Which shall it be: mass education or mass persuasion for health. Am J Public Health 58:131-137, 1968.

26. Auger TJ, Wright E, Simpson RH: Posters as smoking deterrents. J Appl Psychol 56:169-171, 1972.

BIBLIOGRAPHY

Bem D: Attitudes as self-descriptions: another look at the attitude-behavior link, Psychological Foundations of Attitudes. Edited by AG Greenwald, JC Brock, TM Ostrom. New York, Academic Press, 1968, pp 197-215.

The boy who cried cancer cure: raising false hopes in the news media. Sci News Sept 30: 102-214, 1972.

Brecher R, Brecher E, et al.: The Consumer's Union Report on Smoking and the
    Public Interest. Mount Vernon, N Y, Consumer's Union, 1963.
Brennan RE, Anderson L, Joslyn MA, Briggs GM: A book-shelf on foods and
    nutrition. Am J Public Health 58:621–637, 1968.
Butler, BB, Erskine EAG: Public health retailing: selling ideas to the private practi-
    tioner in his office. Am J Public Health 60:1996–2002, 1970.
Cannell CF, MacDonald JC: The impact of health news on attitudes and behavior.
    J Q 33:315–323, 1956.
Cassidy JE, Barnes FP: Organization and operation of a military preventive denistry
    program. Am J Public Health 62: 1072–1076, 1972.
Choate RB: Sugarcoated children's hour: advertising of inferior foods by television
    commercials. Nation 1972:146–148.
Cone FM: With All Its Faults. Boston, Little Brown, 1969.
Culliton BJ: Cancer news: cancer society makes it with style. Science 1973: 722–224.
Dennison D: Social class variables related to health instructions. Am J Public
    Health 62:814–820, 1972.
DiCicco L, Apple D: Health needs and opinions of older adults, Sociological Studies
    of Health and Sickness. Edited by D Apple. New York, McGraw-Hill, 1960.
Feldman J: The Dissemination of Health Information. Chicago, Aldine, 1966.
Festinger L: A Theory of Cognitive Dissonance. Evanston, Ill., Row Peterson, 1957.
Festinger L, Carlsmith JM: Cognitive consequences of forced compliance. J Abnorm
    Soc Psychol 58:203–210, 1959.
Griffiths W, Knutson AL: The role of the mass media in public health. Am J Public
    Health 50:515–523, 1960.
Hovland CI, Lumsdaine A, Sheffield F: Experiments on Mass Communications.
    Princeton, Princeton University Press, 1949.
Howard JA, Rulbert J: Advertising and the Public Interest. Chicago, Crain Com-
    munications, Inc., in press.
Hunter BT: Consumer Beware. New York, Simon and Schuster, 1971.
Jeffers JR, Boganno MF, Bartlett JC: On the demand versus need for medical ser-
    vices and the concept of "shortage." Am J Public Health 61:46–59, 1971.
Leventhal H: Fear appeals and persuasion: the differentiation of a motivation con-
    struct. Am J Public Health 61:1208–1224, 1971.
Maccoby N: Communication and learning. Handbook of Communication. Edited by
    W Schramm, et al. Chicago, Rand McNally, 1973.
Maccoby N, Roberts DF: Cognitive processes in persuasion. Proceedings of the
    Fourth Annual Attitude Research Conference of the American Marketing Associa-
    tion, 1971.
McLuhan HM: Understanding Media: The Extensions of Man. New York, McGraw-
    Hill, 1969.
Review of studies of vitamin and mineral nutrition in the U.S. 1950–1968. J Nutr
    Educ 1:39–57, 1969.
Salomon G, Suppes JS: Learning to generate subjective uncertainty: effects of
    training, verbal ability and stimulus structure. J Pers Soc Psychol 23:163–174,
    1972.
Schwartz JL, Dubitsky M: Maximizing success in smoking cessation methods. Am
    J Public Health 59:1392–1399, 1969.
Sherif M, Hovland CI: Social Judgment. New Haven, Yale Press, 1961.
Spencer FJ: A paperback bookshelf on public health. Am J Public Health 58:639–
    646, 1968.

Smith FA, Trivax G, Zuehlke DA, Lowinger MD, Nghiem LN: Health information during a week of television. N Engl J Med 286:516–520, 1972.

Stanton F: Counteradvertising. Vital Speeches 38:526–528, 1972.

Suchman EA: Sociology and the Field of Public Health. New York, Russell Sage Foundation, 1963.

Skornia H: TV and Society. New York, McGraw-Hill, 1965.

Swinehart JW: Voluntary exposure to health communications. Am J Public Health 58:1265–1275, 1968.

Toch HH, Allen TM, Lazer W: Effects of the cancer scares: the residue of the news impact. J Q 38:25–34, 1961.

Turner ES: Shocking History of Advertising. London, Michael Joseph, Ltd., 1952.

Udry KJR, Morris NM: A spoonful of sugar helps the medicine go down. Am J Public Health 61:776–785, 1971.

Wackman W: Family and media influences. Am Behav Sci 14(3):415–427, 1971.

Wade N: Health fad underworld surveyed. Science 1972:178–379.

ROBERT MICHELS, M.D.

Associate Professor, Department of Psychiatry,
College of Physicians & Surgeons, Columbia University

Commentary

The greatest impact of modern medicine on the health and life of our citizens has not resulted from the improved treatment of specific diseases. Rather it has followed advances in hygiene, sanitation, public health, and alterations in behavior and life style that have had a secondary impact on morbidity and mortality. Naïvely, one would think that the medical profession would direct its attention to those factors that are the primary determinants of health, but on the whole this has not been the case, and it is only in recent years that medicine has defined its subject matter as broadly as the public health data suggest is appropriate. Indeed, this very conference is indicative of the growing professional awareness of this issue. Every medical student today learns that, even for the most specific of physical illnesses, the critical determinants of the patient's prognosis often rest not on the availability of a suitable remedy, but rather on the likelihood that it will be employed and that the patient will seek it, find it, and use it. The epidemic proportions of venereal disease, the incidence of unwanted pregnancies, and the difficulty in bringing individuals with early symptoms of cancer or asymptomatic hypertension to treatment all attest to this problem.

This means that if we are to understand and influence the nation's health, we must look beyond our understanding of disease processes and their treatment to the social and cultural institutions that shape our

152

citizens' lives and mold their behavior. The mass media are one such institution, and television in particular is a major determinant of contemporary life styles. Everyone has a television set, and it is turned on an average of six hours a day!

Thus health is intimately related to patterns of behavior and the psychosocial factors that influence them, and television is an important determinant of these patterns. Further, the explicit content of television, reflecting the interests of advertisers, producers, and audience, has a high percentage of health-related material. Over 7 percent of all television time—25 minutes of those six hours—is related to health. This includes material designed to influence behavior (advertising and public service programming), to inform (news), and to keep the set turned on (entertainment). The time devoted to health in this last category is astounding. Ben Casey and Dr. Kildare are more well known than Sir William Osler and, while many physicians over their lifetimes have practiced medicine in several of the United States, Marcus Welby, M.D., practices in 60 different countries each week.

This emphasis on health in the media reflects the economic and psychologic importance of health-related activities in our society. In 1972 the nation's medical bill was $83.4 billion, 7.6 percent of the gross national product (almost exactly the same percentage as that of television time devoted to health subjects). The drug industry devotes 10 percent of its sales dollars to advertising. The emotional significance of health is even greater than the economic. Our awareness of our bodies and our own mortality is a central theme of our fantasy life, the mental background that filters and determines the impact of the various communications we receive from others and from the media. The popularity and success of mass advertising or entertainment is based on an understanding and exploitation of universal mental fantasies. Thus while the advertising of medical products is related to the economic interests of the drug industry, the ubiquity of doctors and medical themes in television entertainment is largely unrelated to the economic importance of the health industry complex; rather it reflects the prevalence of health themes in the psychologic preoccupations of the audience.

To summarize, we find that general attitudes and behavior patterns are important determinants of health, that the mass media play a major role in shaping these attitudes, and that the mass media and society, in general, devote a significant proportion of their resources and attention to health matters. Further, we find that there are two distinct motives behind the health-related material observed on television or other media. First is the desire to influence health-related behavior, usually for economic gain, whether in the narrow sense such as advertising to encourage the sales of pills or in a broader sense such as public service programs providing health education. The second motive is to hold the audience's attention, presumably so that it will stay tuned in and be kindly disposed to advertising messages that may be unrelated to health. Ben Casey and Marcus Welby are examples. Both types of television content may have a strong impact on the health of the audience, that is, of all of us. However, the nature of this impact is likely to be different.

Commercial advertising is linked to the consumption of things, usually medicines, and usually involves exaggerating the efficacy and range of indications of a drug while minimizing its side effects and at the same time suggesting that it is preferable to all available alternatives. This is in no way different from other commercial advertising, unless one wants to argue that drugs and health are different from soap and laundry, but that would take us beyond the realm of this discussion. A side effect of this type of advertising is to encourage a "drug orientation," an attitude that taking drugs is average expected behavior and that there is likely to be a desirable drug solution for one's problems, just as advertising cosmetics not only encourages the purchase of brand A over brand B but also the notion that women should use cosmetics.

In contrast, entertainment health programming is more likely to influence life styles related to health and expectations in the treatment situation and the attitudes about doctors and hospitals that the patient brings to his contact with the medical establishment. For example, on the great majority of the medical television programs that I have observed, the patient has a specific illness, the doctor makes a diagnosis, and treatment is instituted leading to a definitive result. In real life, of course, it is otherwise. Patients have problems that are not usually encompassed by the categories of illness taught in medical schools. Treatment programs often precede definitive diagnoses and may at times seem almost unrelated to them. The results are difficult to specify, and patients usually neither die nor recover but continue to have problems more or less related to the problems that brought them to the doctor in the first place. If he is a good doctor, they are somewhat better off as a result of the contact with him. Now this real story wouldn't make a very successful plot for a television drama because it doesn't correspond to the wishful fantasies we all have about doctors. However, the wishful fantasies are largely unrealistic, and television dramas, by supporting and gratifying them, may contribute to attitudes and expectations that interfere with the optimal utilization of the health care system. A typical undesirable result are patients who insist on specific treatments when none are available and shop until they find charlatans who, like television, play on the wishful fantasy of the audience.

Furthermore, the media influence doctors and doctors-to-be as well as patients. In teaching freshmen medical students, one repeatedly observes their disappointment and feeling of betrayal when they learn that the practice of medicine, as they see it in the hospitals and clinics of the medical school, is not what they had anticipated. The expectations they brought with them were largely shaped by personal experiences with physicians, most often pediatricians who treated and "cured" the acute diseases of childhood, and by the doctors they had observed on the media. However, the practice of medicine on television is different from that seen in the teaching hospital. Television patients tend to be young or middle aged, attractive, articulate, appealing, clean, and to have well-formulated problems. Television doctors have time, few interruptions, little sense of conflicting demands on their resources and, although usually in private practice, are unconcerned about fees. The medical students, dissatisfied by the reality when contrasted with this fantasy, select practice settings and specialties that allow them to recreate their fantasy. They avoid the old, inept, disabled, chronically ill, and "incurable." Television medicine shapes the attitudes and expectations of both providers and consumers, encouraging a model of medical practice that is suboptimal for society.

To further contrast the impact of intentional behavior shaping—that is, advertising—and unintended influence through entertainment, the deleterious effects of the former are largely purposeful, although their extent may be unintended, while the deleterious effects of the latter are largely unintended, although they may be integrally related to the basic strategy of holding the attention of the audience by giving it what will make it happy. However, I suspect that this differentiation is more important in discussing strategies of regulation and control than in understanding the psychologic basis of the effect.

As Professor Maccoby has pointed out in another context, people tend to overemphasize immediate and certain results when compared with deferred and problematic ones. An evening's security with a charismatic doctor on the screen is more potent than the slight probability of an uncomfortable change in behavior leading to a decreased morbidity many years hence. I have discussed this as the difference between subjective and objective probabilities. To an individual, one in a thousand and one in a million are almost synonymous; to someone making national policy decisions, they are not. To complicate the problem, the average patient may actually be better off, or at least not much worse, with a charlatan, although to a significant minority charlatans are a disaster. Similarly, television doctors may comfort and even help most; certainly, they may educate and encourage some to seek help, while seriously injuring only a few. The commercial interests paying the advertising and entertainment bills may find this acceptable. Whether there is a more basic question of conflicting rights involved is an issue for discussion.

The problem of the impact of the media on behavior may be seen as analogous to the recent concern with the ecology of our physical environment. We live not only in a physical world but also in a psychologic world of information and meaning. For years we considered the physical world to be virtually infinite and had little concern for the indirect impact of what we ejected into it. Today we recognize that this was short-sighted and that we quite literally live in our refuge, with the corollary that we acknowledge a right and responsibility to regulate, police, and tax the refuge production of our neighbors in order to safeguard our survival. If we consider the world of information to consist of all of those meaningful stimuli that impinge on us and determine our behavior, we must recognize that it is also finite. Furthermore, television, at six hours a day, occupies a rather large segment of it. The deleterious effects of casual ejections of information into this system are a kind of pollution of the mind, and the drug advertisers may be analogous to smokestacks blighting our horizon while the Marcus Welbys and Ben Caseys may be likened to those apparently innocuous or even praiseworthy substances that had unforseen and long unrecognized but dangerous effects, the DDTs and detergents of the environment.

The metaphor is admittedly flawed, but the problem is still immense. I am afraid that my diagnosis is too preliminary to suggest the definitive treatment; perhaps, however, like the real doctor I mentioned before, It might help us to progress somewhat more adaptively than we could have without it. Of the nation's $83.4 billion annual medical bill, 39 percent. is public tax dollars, a proportion that is likely to increase. Our nation has an urgent economic as well as ethical concern with its citizens' health. The mass media may be an important means of influencing the health of our citizens, as well as an important area to examine for negative influences that might be regulated or controlled. The Children's Television Workshop idea for a Sesame-Street-like health information series for adults is an example of the former; vigorous interpretation and application of truth-in-advertising laws to drugs and the development of anti-drug public service advertisements is an example of the latter. The most difficult problem, and to me the most interesting, is how a free society entertains itself without injuring its more vulnerable members. Again, I regret not having a remedy, but it is often helpful to track down the symptom of the more pervasive problem of which this is only a manifestation.

IV

Professional Values

The process of admission to medical colleges, as well as the training that students undergo, can influence the values of the provider of health care. Those partici-pating on admissions committees have their own no-tions of qualities that an applicant should possess to be successful in medical school and practice. The values of the entering student are either reinforced or modified through formal medical or dental training and specialty work. The papers presented on this topic examine the extent to which the values being intro-duced in the socialization process are compatible with those of the society at large with respect to the func-tioning of the health care system.

JOHN S. WELLINGTON, M.D.
Associate Dean, University of California Medical Center, San Francisco

Changing Values and the Selection Process for Medical School

The main purpose of this paper is to explore the values used in the selection of medical students. The data and the perceptions herein derive largely from the author's own experience with the admissions committee of one school. While it may be argued that this experience may be atypical, the fact remains that the students ranked highly by the committee to be described are with few exceptions ranked similarly highly by one or more other medical schools to which they have applied. Presumably, if the outcome in selection is similar, these other schools are looking for a similar set or subset of values upon which to base their selection.

IDENTIFICATION AND RANKING OF THE VALUES OF THE PROFESSION

Whatever definition of value is used, it still applies to a belief, standard, criteria, or preference that is held by an individual. Within the context of this paper the term refers to those beliefs[1] held by, perhaps shared by, members of medical school admissions committees that bear upon decision making in the selection process for medical students. The act of selection requires evaluation and decision making, processes that require judgment. Judgment in turn requires data, and these judgment

159

data include personal value commitments, educational and professional aims, goals, objectives, priorities, perceived norms, and standards.[2] These judgment data are applied in the selection process to two broad categories of characteristics of the individual applicant: academic ability and personality qualities.

It seems important to try to identify the values of admissions committee members. Since, for all practical purposes, admission to medical school is tantamount to entry into the profession of medicine, the selection process becomes a focal point for the application of the values of the profession. These values may relate to two classes of applicant characteristics. The first, academic ability, refers to a set of characteristics that can be expected to predict that the selectee can adequately master the technical and scientific aspects of the profession. The second includes those personal characteristics that indicate that the applicant holds a set of personal values consistent with those expected by the profession. It has been pointed out that the value systems of individual administrators provide the key to operational values of an institution.[3] In the case of a medical school admissions committee, interest should be focused not only on the values of the committee members themselves but on the values of the next layer of administrators who appoint them. This point is illustrated by observation of the result of one example of a change in committee membership in a medical school. In the course of substantially increasing the size of the admissions committee of the school, an effort was made to include as many women as possible in the expanded membership. In the first class admitted by this new committee, the number of women increased from about 16 percent, where it had been for three or four years, to nearly 25 percent, where it has remained since. Values of individual committee members certainly contributed to the selection decision as did values of the administrators who appointed the new members.

RELATIONSHIP OF SELECTION PROCESS TO HEALTH CARE SYSTEM

To examine professional values relating to the selection process for medical school, it is desirable to have a conceptual framework in which to view them. A health care system will include the profession of medicine as one of its component parts. If optimal health care is to be the major goal of the system, the values of the profession must be consistent with this goal and supportive of it. The subsystem that is the profession of medicine may be viewed in terms of its own input, throughput, and output. The first of these, input, or the selection process for the profession, is the subject of this presentation.

In a logically designed system the values governing input are dictated by the goals of the system and are subject to feedback control based on the extent to which the selection process promotes these goals. The selection process for medicine has always been shaped by value systems that have held optimal health as as a goal, but this does not necessarily mean that these value systems have remained unchanged or that the values and attitudes affecting selection decisions have not changed.

The hypothesis to be tested in this presentation is that there is a change taking place in how the multiple criteria used in the selection process are being applied and that this change has arisen from a re-evaluation of how these different criteria may be related more closely to the long-term goal of the system—i.e., provision of optimal health care. Admissions policymakers are being made more aware of the ways in which both cognitive and noncognitive factors may or may not play a part in determining the physician's future role in health care provision. Propensity for different geographic locations, interest in primary care, attitudes toward new definitions of roles for health care providers may all be important factors in constructing a new equation for selection criteria.

The insistence that these factors be heeded has come largely from outside the profession. To establish what these multiple criteria for selection are and how they have come into use, we need to know something of their background.

Development of Selection Procedure

Admissions committees are a relatively recent addition to American medical education. Prior to the twentieth century, there was no overt selection process. If a prospective student wished to pursue a course of medical study, he could do so, provided that he had sufficient money to pay tuition and (with few exceptions) was male and white. So in reality, from the beginning of U.S. medical education, there was only a kind of covert (or inadvert) selection system in operation that resulted, however, in medical student bodies similar in three important characteristics to every subsequent entering class since then in that they were predominantly male, white, and from the upper economic class. Did these characteristics reflect values held by medical school proprietors and teachers? Perhaps so, but from whatever its selection or nonselection process stemmed, nineteenth century American medical education turned out to be an academic disaster.

The extent of this disaster must have become apparent to U.S. medical educators largely by comparison with European medical schools, especially the German ones. How much of the motivation to improve American medical education in the early twentieth century may have

come, on the other hand, from consideration of the quality of health
care delivered by American physicians is a question that has received
very little attention.

Academic Ability

The reforms that American medicine was to make in the first two decades of this century are epitomized in Abraham Flexner's[4] report on
medical education. Flexner's contribution to the selection process was
to recommend that students of medicine be required to have an academic background sufficient for them to perform adequately in the
basic science courses offered in medical school. This background was
most frequently two or more years of college, including courses in physics, chemistry, biology, mathematics, and French or German.

In these recommendations of Flexner can be recognized the introduction of the notion of academic ability as a value that dominated the selection process for medical school for the next 60 years. It might be
noted that even what surely must have been one of the minor recommendations of the prophet—that no medical school enroll a student who
had failed in another medical school—has remained as one of the com-
mandments of admissions committees today. No points for persistent
motivation here!

But certainly Flexner's values did not remain unmodified and un-
challenged until now. First of all, what were Flexner's contemporaries
who were medical educators (which, of course, Flexner was not) saying?
Richard Pearce, then Professor of Research Medicine at the University
of Pennsylvania, said in an address at Harvard in 1911, that ". . .our
product, our graduate in medicine, has been found wanting by the German finishing school."[5] He made a strong argument for the scientific
rather than the practical physician. Much of what Pearce proposed,
Welch, Minot, Bowditch, and others were instituting at Harvard and
Hopkins. Proficiency in the sciences was stressed. Welch, in a convoca-
tion address at the University of Chicago in 1907, complained that the
development of American colleges made them almost unadjustable to
the needs of professional education and urged the requirement of college laboratory training in the natural sciences. At the same time he allowed that, "a liberal education and broad culture raise the influence
and standing of a physician in the community, enhance and widen the
intellectual pleasures of his life, instill an interest in the history of medicine and give him greater joy in the pursuit of a noble profession."[6] He
warned, though, to take care lest this liberal education for physicians-to-
be "blunt man's innate curiosity for the facts of nature."[7] Still during
this period of the beginning of academic reform in American medicine,

Charles Minot of Harvard, in a commencement address at Washington University in St. Louis, said that "Medicine is a profession which only men* of exceptional ability should enter. Men of moderate gifts should seek other occupations."[8] Schools should select students to the exclusion of not merely the bad ones, but also the mediocre. "Examinations should have their main use, not as a means of admission, but as a means of exclusion, and the more men of low and middle rank that are excluded the better."[9]

Minot in the same address spoke also of other essential qualities of a physician. These were a faculty of exact observation, combining intelligence with concentrated attention and judgment; intellectual endurance expressed as the habit of lifelong learning; and loyalty and devotion shown in faithfulness to occupation, purpose, and person.

During the next decade or two after the Flexnerian watershed of 1910, the selection process began to take shape. In 1926–1927, there had been only 8,500 applicants for 6,000 places in U.S. schools; by 1929–1930, the ratio of applicants to places was 2:1, and in 1973, 3:1. How was the selection being made? While in 1909 only 17 U.S. schools went so far as to require two years of college work for admission, among the matriculants of 1930, nearly half already held university degrees.[10] The growing preference for the bachelor's degree must have been a major factor in the process.

With the limiting of places in medical schools, academic qualifications began to be used in more systematic ways in the selection process. An aptitude test was developed and has undergone numerous refinements. (Another is currently in progress.) Success in selection procedures was measured by diminution of the dropout rate. Measures aimed at other than academic values were slower in coming.

The extent to which academic ability dominated the admissions process into the 1960s can be seen in the responses of more than 500 admissions committee members to a 1957 questionnaire asking the importance of intellectual characteristics of applicants to medical school.[11] Nearly 90 percent of the respondents assigned great importance to this aspect of the candidate's qualifications; all regarded it as of at least some importance.

Personal Qualities

A structured list of personal characteristics, together with scales by which they might be measured (such as Jackson's list of measures of impulse expression and control, orientation toward direction from other

---

* He, of course, did not mention women.

people, intellectual and aesthetic orientations, degree of ascendancy, and degree and quality of interpersonal orientation[12]), was not conceived of at the time when the selection process was first being developed. This is not to say that personal qualities were not valued by medical educators concerned with student selection. Minot's qualities of "loyalty and devotion shown in faithfulness to occupation, purpose, and person"[13] were a rather elegant expression in 1909 of what has now come to be called "high motivation toward medicine, and personal responsibility both for the integrity of the profession and for direct relations with patients."[14] Some insight into the values applied to the selection process in 1930 is expressed editorially in the *Final Report of the Commission on Medical Education*[15]:

> Studies of successful practitioners emphasize that there are factors other than training which are the essential elements in later success, chief among which are character, personality, industry, native ability, alertness, devotion, thoroughness, judgment, constant study, and good health. Greater weight is being placed upon these factors in the selection of medical students.
>
> Medical schools employ various means to assist in the selection of students from the large number of applicants and are giving more weight to considerations other than scholarship, although this is likely to remain the chief criterion. Among the methods used may be intelligence, reading vocabulary, essay, aptitude, and similar tests, interest analyses, personal interviews, recommendations (particularly from previously reliable science instructors), age of student, length of preparation, nature of extra-curricular activities in college, and information regarding character and personality. There is agreement that the most important requirements for admission to medicine are character, ability, personality, a mind prepared by a sound plan of general education, and a grasp of the sciences upon which medicine is dependent.

Concern with personality qualities of individuals continued to grow. In the *Report of the Fourth Teaching Institute of the AAMC*,[16] only 23 pages were devoted to the intellectual characteristics of applicants, while 81 dealt with nonintellectual characteristics. A more recent bibliography[17] lists 52 reports dealing with measurement of qualities of personality. These figures are indicative of the concern of medical teachers with personal qualities and suggest a growing conviction that they are important in the selection process; unfortunately, these figures tell us little about how these qualities may be identified in candidates or how they may be ranked by admissions committees.

Admissions Committees

Systems of selection began to develop as the numbers of applicants outstripped the available places. The dean, in the days when there was only

one per school, probably first exercised the function of selection. By
1956, when 20 percent of U.S. schools still had fewer than 250 applicants each, 93 percent had admissions committees with four or more
members, while only 38 percent had more than seven members. In two
thirds of the schools the committees were appointed by the dean; in one
tenth, they were elected by the faculty.[18] Presidents, deans, and department chairmen comprised 37 percent of the committee members in 1956,
while in 1972 the figure was 9 percent.[19] Admissions committees by
1972 included more women (8 percent), more students, and more minority members (10 percent).[20] More than half the schools in 1972 had
student members; and, in half of this subset, student bodies exerted some
formal influence in the selection of committee members.

Identification of Characteristics in Applicant Indicative of Values of Profession

What are the tools with which admissions committees work? Academic
ability is an important value to medical educators concerned with selection of students. In the immediate post-Flexnerian period it was measured in terms of college work completed, especially with regard to
attainment of (1) the bachelor's degree and (2) completion of courses,
preferably with laboratory, in chemistry, biology, and physics. Mathematics and French or German were often included. By 1930, when there
were two applicants for every place, the selection process included
grades, and a scholastic aptitude test for medical schools has been developed.[21] Overall college grades, as well as subsets of grades, such as those
in the sciences or those attained during the last year of college attendance, continue to be major data used in the selection process as has the
Medical College Admissions Test (MCAT). Personality qualities have been
sought with increasing vigor. The search for appropriate indicators of
these qualities has been hampered by two things: lack of a clear idea of
the relative or hierarchical value of the personality qualities; lack of a
way of measuring whether selection of candidates on the basis of some
or other personal characteristics had or had not resulted in selection of
a better group of doctors. A very wide range of existing psychological
devices and instruments have been administered to incoming students,
and their predictive value measured in terms of later performance. The
criterion value of later performance, however, has most often been class
standing on the basis of grades achieved in the basic science subjects of
the first year of medical school. There are probably three reasons for
this choice: First, it is the earliest criterion to become available after
the initial testing (and in any case correlates well with later grades); it

is capable of being measured precisely; and it is a good indicator of whether the individual will eventually enter the practice of medicine, since most academic failures occur in the first year.

The dropout rate between matriculation and graduation in U.S. medical schools has for a number of years been in the vicinity of 10 percent, of which perhaps half might be identified as academic failures. This attrition rate is exceedingly low in comparison with that for students in other professional and graduate programs. It is unlikely that further refinement of admissions criteria can significantly affect the dropout rate.

Still, the principal instrument for assessing personal qualities in the candidate remains the interview. The interview has long since been stripped of any status as a valid predictor of any behavior that can be measured subsequently; yet the relative weight given to it in the selection process has increased, rather than decreased, in the 30 or more years it has been in general use. Why is this so? The answer is probably that it represents the only way in which admissions committee members feel that they can test for and apply their own individual value system to selection. While it is rather doubtful that committee members think specifically in precise psychological terms, it is likely that they look toward the interview in their attempt to gather judgment data for decision making.

AN ADMISSIONS COMMITTEE

A medical school admissions committee was studied in an attempt to identify values of the committee members and to determine how these values affected the intake process of the school. The structure of the committee in question during the most recent year of operation comprised four subcommittees of 14 members each. Three members of each committee were students in their second, third, or fourth years, and the remainder were, with the exception of one subcommittee, all faculty members, in the ratio of about three full-time faculty to one volunteer. Each committee chose students to fill one fourth of the 146 places.

There were some differences in the subcommittees. One considered all applicants with advanced science degrees and/or those with an expressed interest in the "medical scientist pathway." Its makeup was heavily weighted with basic scientists and science-oriented clinicians and students. Another considered all minority applicants and was mainly made up of Black and Latin or Chicano members. Its membership included two community nonprofessionals. Two other subcommittees had no specialized function. In all subcommittees some care had been taken to achieve a mixture of ethnic backgrounds and of basic science/

clinical, full-time/volunteer, and male/female members. Women comprised 28 percent of the total membership.

Operation of the Committee

Approximately 3,500 applications were screened by a subset of committee members made up of three experienced members from each subcommittee. Screening was in multiple stages and was preceded by assignment of standard scores for various academic and nonacademic attributes of the applicant. Initial screening was based on academic attributes but permitted educationally or socioeconomically disadvantaged candidates to pass through to the next stages. Subsequent screening took into account a number of nonacademic attributes, scores for which were derived by the screeners by reading the application form, personal statement of the applicant, and letters of recommendation. This multistage screening procedure then led to the decision whether to invite the candidate for interview. About one fourth of the total applicants received such an invitation. None of the three quarters of the applicants whose applications did not survive this screening procedure were rejected, however, without a review of their entire file by an experienced committee member. A mechanism was provided whereby this final review could result in the decision to proceed to the interview stage and consideration by a subcommittee, and approximately 10 percent of those applicants initially screened out were retained in the selection procedure. The criterion for reinstatement was the individual judgment of the committee member reached after review of the whole application, including the written statement of the applicant.

Each admissions committee member shared in the interviewing and was asked to rate each individual who was interviewed in each of the first nine categories listed in Table 1, as well as to give an overall rating based on all of the nonacademic qualities observed during the interview.

After the candidate had been interviewed, his application was brought to the subcommittee to which the two interviewers belonged, and a "case presentation" was made by each interviewer. After discussion, each member then rated the acceptability of the applicant on a scale of 0 to 4. The arithmetic mean score given by the subcommittee then determined the rank order of that candidate among all others who were reviewed by that subcommittee during the year.

In this way, about one fourth of the candidates, or nearly 900 applicants, were judged to be not only acceptable but in one or more ways desirable by the school. Very few were judged unacceptable by the interviewers. Many more than this one fourth were acceptable on the basis of their record, but were screened out because there was no one particularly

TABLE 1   Committee's Rank Order of Importance in Selection Process of Selected
Personal Attributes of Applicant

---

1. Humanitarian beliefs and sincerity
2. Evidence of psychological maturity
3. Initiative, perseverance, enthusiasm
4. Ability to communicate effectively
5. Interest in and knowledge of medicine
6. General intellectual interest and cultural development
7. Imagination, creativity
8. Level of awareness of modern society
9. Interest in and knowledge of research
10. Professionally appropriate appearance and demeanor

---

strong characteristic or combination of characteristics that carried them
through the process to the interview stage.

After interview, selection among the approximately 900 applicants
left was by individual assessment of each candidate by each member of
the subcommittee. Each subcommittee selected one fourth of the class.

Historical Development

The structure and function of the 1972 committee were quite different
from what they had been in the past. In 1946, a seven-man committee
included the dean of the school of medicine, two deans from undergraduate colleges of the university, a zoology professor from the undergraduate campus, the university admissions officer, and two medical
school faculty members, one of whom served as premedical adviser on
the nearby undergraduate campus of the university. This committee
made policy regarding admissions, and a committee of 15 faculty members from clinical departments, including two women, interviewed and
made selections. Candidates were interviewed by two faculty members.

By the mid-1960s, the policy committee had disappeared, and the
same 15-person selection committee reported directly to the dean. With
increasing numbers of applicants, two 15-person subcommittees were
appointed in 1967, each to fill half the class. The reason for this was to
permit adding more members to interview and process the ever greater
number of applicants without losing the capability of small group discussion and evaluation of them.

Minority Admissions

In 1968, growing pressures for recognition of the needs and aspirations
of American minorities resulted locally in demands for greater minority

representation in the health professions schools. To meet these demands (one definition of demand is to ask for that which is due), a subcommittee of 15 members had been appointed with the goal of filling one fourth of the places in the incoming class with minority students. This subcommittee included faculty, students, and community professionals and nonprofessionals, nearly all of whom were themselves members of racial or ethnic minorities. At the same time, students were appointed to the other two subcommittees. Subsequently, to accommodate the still increasing number of applicants, a fourth subcommittee was appointed by the dean. As new appointments were made, increasingly large numbers of women became members of the committee. The result of increased numbers of minority persons and of women on the committee was an increase, by nearly the same percentage, of minority and women students in the entering class.

Each year the committee established its own guidelines and procedures for the screening of applications, building on its experience in previous years. The changes were consistently in the direction of placing greater emphasis on the nonacademic characteristics of applicants. Greater weight in screening formulas was placed on personal characteristics, and by the year in question the committee had formally assigned numerical scores to a variety of personal qualities. This sounds as if the committee were moving away from the previous heavy emphasis on academic achievement, and it was just this that the committee members verbalized in the annual discussions of change. But it happened that every year as the number of applicants increased, so did the number with outstandingly good academic records and test scores. The committee responded to this by raising the cutoff point for assigning a "superior" score for grades and MCAT scores. The result was that the committee continued to select from a limited pool of students with the highest academic records.

It was in an effort to apply criteria other than grades and MCAT scores that a mechanism for processing the applications of minority students was developed. In 1969, when strong concerns for minority opportunities developed, there was no large pool of minority applicants with high grades and MCAT scores. Had there been, there would in all likelihood already have been larger numbers of minority medical students. Therefore, for students from the small minority pool to compete, a wider range of characteristics had to be evaluated.

Minority Subcommittee

How was the selection made in this subcommittee? Did the committee have a widely different set of values that were employed in the decision process? Discussions within the committee centered again and again upon the desirability of selecting students with a strong sense of commitment to providing health care for their own ethnic group, as well as a strongly felt self-identification with their own ethnic group. External evidence of this strong identification, such as a past history of personal exposure to the injustices of a racist society, was often sought by interviewers. In the case of Latin or Chicano applicants, fluency in Spanish was often taken as *prima facie* evidence of an upbringing that included exposure to the culture of the barrios. The point was sometimes proposed, though not necessarily accepted, in these discussions that physical appearance—the presence or absence of physical traits characteristic of an ethnic minority—should be taken into consideration as judgment data in the selection process.

More generally, the difficulty that an individual had experienced in gaining a college education was given a positive weight. The further the individual had had to come to get where he was now, the more credit, it was felt, should be given him. Poverty, lack of parental education or lack of positive parental orientation to education, attendance at poor elementary schools, a history of receiving negatively oriented education and counseling, having had to support himself and sometimes his family as well tended to be accepted as evidence that an individual had experienced unusual difficulty in obtaining an education and that by achieving it against odds had demonstrated uncommonly strong motivation, determination, and ability.

This latter cluster of values was not limited to minority students, but spread to the other three committees as well and was weighed there in decision making, albeit to a lesser degree.

The question, "What kind of student are we trying to select?", of course, arose frequently in all four subcommittees. Bright, humane, concerned, strongly motivated—these and similar terms were often used to describe the ideal. In some of the subcommittees there was frequent discussion of the applicant's attitudes toward medical care, for example, regarding fee-for-service vis-à-vis prepaid health maintenance organizations, or regarding the applicant's interest in health care for underserved groups and areas. Since a wide range of views was represented in the membership of each subcommittee, the outcome of the application did not correlate with the applicant's perceived views in any discernible way. There were strong defenders on the committees of the most divergent points of view about medical care. In this final part of the selection process, then, the values of each individual committee member were expressed, but the outcome depended on the arithmetic mean of the score given by each member.

The interview, of course, played an enormously important role at this stage. The interviewers, depending on how strongly they supported a candidate, usually exerted great influence on the outcome of the ranking, especially if both were in agreement.

Questionnaire Study of the Committee

Since the system in its operation placed such weight in the final selection process on each committee member's evaluation of the individual, an attempt was made to determine how these committee members ranked the importance of those characteristics of the individual they were trying to evaluate. A questionnaire was distributed to committee members wherein they were requested to rank a number of items in a way that best reflected the relative importance of the criteria that they personally found themselves using when selecting applicants. Forty-seven questionnaires (82 percent) were returned.

Respondents ranked three general categories of attributes, personal characteristics, academic performance, and socioeconomic conditions, in order of their importance in the selection process. The results are shown below:

Characteristic	Mean Rank
Personal characteristics	1.4
Academic performance	1.8
Socioeconomic conditions	2.7

An applicant evaluation summary had been completed as part of the routine processing of each applicant whose application came before the committee for final ranking. Twenty specific attributes listed in Table 2, half of them academic, were listed on this summary, and each applicant had been assigned scores. For the purposes of this study, committee members were asked to rank these 20 factors on a 5-point scale according to the importance they attached to each item when selecting applicants. The percent of respondents indicating each value is shown in Table 2; Table 3 rearranges these results to show relative ranking.

Respondents in this study were also asked to rank the relative importance in decision making for selection of 10 clusters of characteristics. All of these characteristics, except "professionally appropriate appearance and demeanor," had been given scores earlier by interviewers as part of the regular application procedure. The results are shown in Table 1.

If the ranking of the three broad classes of applicant characteristics in order of their importance in the selection process is examined in each of the four subcommittees studied, some differences appear. The uniquely identifying features of these four subcommittees may be summarized as follows:

I	no special makeup or characteristics
II	Chairperson female
III	90 percent of respondents Black or Chicano
IV	Medical scientist oriented

	Subcommittee			
	I	II	III	IV
Respondents				
Student	3	2	3	1
Full-time faculty				
Basic science	1	2	0	4
Clinical Dep.	3	4	3	3
Volunteer faculty	4	3	2	2
Community representative	0	0	2	0
Male:female	7:4	6:5	8:2	7:3
Ranking				
Personal characteristics	1.5	1.2	1.5	1.5
Academic performance	1.5	2.0	2.1	1.6
Socioeconomic conditions	2.9	2.8	2.3	2.9

Subcommittees I and IV ranked personal characteristics and academic performance equally, or nearly so; subcommittees II and III clearly ranked personal characteristics higher (especially subcommittee II).

Subcommittee III ranked socioeconomic conditions higher than the other three committees; it was still third, but not far behind academic performance. Since subcommittee III, the minority subcommittee, had been given the explicit charge of considering a wider range of criteria, including those that could be included under the rubric socioeconomic, it is not surprising that their ranking of this factor was higher.

In the assignment of relative weights to 20 items considered in the selection process shown in Table 2, there are again some differences among the subcommittees. Subcommittees I and IV again appear to share certain values, while subcommittees II and III share others. I and IV give greater weight to MCAT scores, both science and overall, to science GPA, to recommendations by faculty and legislators, and to the applicant's written statement. Subcommittees II and III place slightly more weight on the interview, although all committees give it a high rating.

The individual subcommittee rankings of the 10 personal attributes

TABLE 2 Relative Importance Given by Committee to Types of Information Used When Selecting Applicants

		Percent of Respondents Indicating Each Value[a]				
	1	2	3	4	5	Mean Score
1. Overall GPA	0	5	42	44	9	3.6
2. Last year GPA	0	7	10	62	21	4.0
3. Science GPA	0	5	32	44	20	3.8
4. MCAT	5	35	40	21	0	2.8
5. Science MCAT	7	21	31	36	5	3.1
6. School	7	33	42	19	0	2.7
7. Course work	12	9	44	35	0	3.0
8. State of residency	72	14	9	0	5	1.5
9. Major	30	40	23	7	0	2.0
10. Advanced degree	33	28	37	0	5	2.1
11. Socioeconomically disadvantaged	12	19	42	14	14	3.0
12. Extracurricular activities: work	2	5	36	36	21	3.7
13. Extracurricular activities: research	0	17	38	36	10	3.4
14. Special interest in student by dean	69	21	7	0	2	1.2
15. Special interest in student by faculty, legislators	33	19	19	19	10	2.5
16. Applicant statement	2	14	35	40	9	3.4
17. Letters of recommendation	0	0	28	40	33	4.0
18. Interviews	0	0	9	33	58	4.5
19. Interviewers	0	2	10	46	41	4.3
20. Personality attributes	0	4	12	50	35	4.2

[a]Scale: 1, of little or no importance; 2, of rather limited importance; 3, important; 4, quite important; 5, extremely important.

listed in Table 1 showed no such pattern. If on the basis of their make-ups we regard subcommittee III as the most likely to have different values and subcommittee I as the most like a traditional committee, comparison between I and IV shows them to be very similar in their ranking of six of the attributes, differing in only four. Subcommittee III gives somewhat higher ranking to ability to communicate effectively and level of awareness of modern society and a lower one to initiative, perseverance, and enthusiasm and to interest in and knowledge of medicine.

If there is a pattern in this, it reflects a tendency of the new and different committee to weigh society-oriented or other-oriented values more highly.

The comparison of the four subcommittees, insofar as it reflects differences between older and newer sets of values, indicates that while there are some differences, there are more similarities than might be expected.

TABLE 3 Committee Member's Ranking of the Importance They Attach to Different Types of Information in the Selection of Applicants[a]

4.5 – –|	Interviews
–	
–	Interviewers
–	Personality attributes
–	
4.0 – –	Strength of letters of recommendation; GPA in preceding college year
–	
–	Science GPA
–	Extracurricular activities: work
–	Cumulative GPA
3.5 – –	
–	Written statement of applicant; extracurricular activities: research
–	
–	
–	Science MCAT score
3.0 – –	Quality of courses completed
–	Socioeconomically disadvantaged
–	Overall MCAT score
–	Academic rating of school attended
2.5 – –	Special interest in student by faculty members or legislators
–	
–	
–	
–	Possession of advanced degree
2.0 – –	College major
–	
–	
1.5 – –	State of residency
–	
–	Special interest in student by dean

[a]See Table 2 for scale values.

Application of Values in Selection

It may be helpful to consider different ways in which values held by several different groups might be applied to the selection process.

There is application at the formal, institutional level. Legislative or administrative policies—for example, relating to state residence, basic levels of academic performance governing admissibility, prerequisite courses, hours, degrees—may provide a framework of values within which selection must operate. Such institutional constraints or lack of them may also bear on the selection of the admissions committee itself, in that its composition may be firmly fixed by institutional rules, or left more open for discretion in choice of committee membership.

Values may be applied at a personal level. Few would argue against the notion that a committee chooses in its own image; as such committee members are selected because they hold given sets of values, these values will very likely be reflected in the choice of candidates.

A third level at which values may operate to influence decisions is in the process of group interaction within the committee. To the extent that group interchange of ideas occurs, there exists the likelihood that individual sets of values will compete for sharing by the committee. For example, if students sitting as a small minority on a committee have different sets of values, these will, if they are to become operative, do so by persuasion of other nonstudent members to share them.

The purpose in stating the above is to provide the background for saying that each of the specific subcommittees described above has, in its ground rules and in its makeup, already set the stage for application of certain sets of values. Subcommittee III, the minority selection committee, is a case in point. An institutional mandate was given to the committee to select individuals from among groups who because of socio-economic conditions had experienced undue difficulty in achieving their education. Committee members were nominated and selected with consideration of their commitment to this idea of equal educational opportunity being a factor in their appointment. Before this subcommittee even considered an applicant, a screening process had already occurred that limited the applicants to be considered to those who were considered socioeconomically disadvantaged. A major set of values had already been applied.

In interpreting the committee answers, it is important to keep in mind that the individuals are responding in terms of the values they apply in a specific situation—that of selecting students out of an already highly selected group. Prior screening, based to a large extent on academic scores, had resulted in deletion from the pool of many applicants with lower grades and MCAT scores. At the level of the final selection process, the committee was considering a group of students with scores for intellectual characteristics restricted to the higher ranges. Even so, while the committee, as shown in Table 3, rated interview assessments, personality attributes, and letters of recommendation most highly, grades were still not far behind in importance.

Committee Responses to Questionnaire

The committee members tended to look at the cognitive characteristics of the applicant in a rather selective way. They ranked science grade point average higher than cumulative GPA, and GPA during the college year just preceding application still higher. The latter recognized the positive aspects of an upswing in performance. Similarly, science M C A T scores were considered more important than overall M C A T performance, but any aspect of the M C A T was held far less important than grades or personal characteristics. Again, the restricted range of M C A T scores of the population under consideration should be kept in mind. Most would agree with the committee that the M C A T was never designed to discriminate in its upper ranges.

The committee members responded that they did not attach much importance to the college major of the applicant, or whether he had earned an advanced degree. They attached the least importance of all to the state of residency of the applicant and to interest expressed in individual applicants by the dean. It is not hard to recognize a division of values here; that is, the latter characteristics reflect values held by administrators, not committee members.

The weight given to socioeconomic disadvantage fell in about the middle range of those characteristics being ranked. The weight given to disadvantage by the subcommittee selecting minority students was much higher than that assigned by any of the other three subcommittees. The minority subcommittee ranked interest and experience in research, the academic rating of the undergraduate school, and M C A T scores lower in importance than did the other committees and indicated that they placed greater importance on who had interviewed the candidate. They were in close agreement on grades and personal characteristics in all other categories.

The committee's ranking of the importance of the personal attributes of applicants listed in Table 2 showed relatively little difference in any of these characteristics except the two called "interest in and knowledge of research" and "professionally appropriate appearance and demeanor," both of which were ranked very low. The minority subcommittee's rankings were very similar to the others except with regard to "ability to communicate effectively," which was given a higher ranking by this subcommittee.

Study of Relationship of Criteria to Outcome

Another method of exploring the values of the committee, which might be termed policy capturing, consists of looking at the characteristics of those individual applicants given the highest overall rating by the committee. Which characteristics had the committee apparently prized the most when actually making its selection?

In an attempt to answer this question, two groups of applicants were compared. All 94 candidates who had received unanimous highest endorsement from their committee and had been given a maximum overall score by the committee were compared with a group of 40 candidates who had been given an overall score that placed them in a category called "middle priority," meaning that they were too good to reject but not ranked nearly high enough to stand any chance of receiving an acceptance; too many other candidates were ranked above them. The two groups, one high and the other low, were chosen to allow comparison of scored characteristics of candidates with the outcome of the selection process. The results are indicated in Table 4, where these groups are identified as "accepted" (A) and "rejected" (R), and the percentages of each rated in "highest category" are compared. Higher percentages of the unanimously accepted applicants were rated in the highest category, and higher percentages of rejected applicants in the lowest category of every cognitive and noncognitive characteristic measured with but one exception—state of residency. The greatest spreads between accepted and rejected groups were in the quality of course work completed, in the scores assigned by interview, in the strength of the letters of recom-

TABLE 4   Committee's Ranking of Importance of Selected Characteristics Compared with Their Importance as Indicated by Outcome of Selection Process

| Characteristic | Committee's Rank | Percent of Applicants Scoring in Highest Category | | Ratio A/R | Rank of A/R Ratio of Candidates in Highest Category |
		Accepted	Rejected		
Interview ratings	1	55	12.5	4.4	3
Personality attributes	2	76	30.0	2.5	5
Letters of recommen- dation	3	68	12.5	5.6	2
GPA in preceding college year	3	52	37.5	1.4	9
Science GPA	5	40	35.0	1.1	11
Extracurricular activities	6	66	37.5	1.8	6
Cumulative GPA	7	36	12.5	2.9	4
Written statement of applicant	8	56	40.0	1.4	9
Science MCAT score	9	69	37.5	1.6	7
Quality of courses completed	10	15	2.5	6.0	1
Academic rating of school attended	11	66	42.5	1.6	7
State of residency	12	67	87.5	0.7	12

mendation, in cumulative GPA, and in the assessment of the personal characteristics listed in Table 1.

The difference between accepted and rejected applicants was less pronounced in respect to the applicant's statement, various other aspects of GPA, and MCAT scores, but still favored the accepted applicants.

In summarizing the committee members' statements about themselves as well as the outcome of their actions, several points should be kept in mind. First, the model for admissions described above is a multistage procedure. At each stage a decision is made whether to reject the application or to proceed further with its consideration. The judgment data on which the decision is made was different at the differing decision-making points. Early, the data are derived from (1) academic performance and (2) socioeconomic status. Either category can provide data for a proceed decision.

Later, after the first screening stage in the admissions process has been passed, decisions are made on the basis of a wider range of judgment data that include measurements, or at least assessments, of personal characteristics such as those indicated in Table 2. It is in the ranking of the importance of these personal qualities that the values of individual decision makers are expressed.

It was with regard to these later stages of the selection process that the committee was asked to assess the importance of the criteria they employed in ranking. Students at this stage had already been screened on the basis of prior academic performance and were within a range that the committee regarded as fully acceptable.

Comparison of Outcome with Committee Ranking of Values

The outcome data with which the committee's estimate of its own weighting of applicant criteria may be compared are derived from the comparisons of the scores of two groups of candidates in this pre-screened group. It can be seen from Table 4 that the applicant's cumulative GPA and his scores for the quality of course work completed appeared to be a greater factor in the decision to reject or accept than the committee thought they were. Conversely, the committee in its responses assigned greater importance to applicant's grade point average in the year just preceding application and science GPA than seems warranted from the relatively small effect these factors seemed to have on the final outcome of the selection process.

A great deal had been said in committee meetings about the relatively greater significance of academic performance in the sciences and of how an applicant should not be penalized for a bad freshman or sophomore year, if his most recent performance had been very good. In spite of this, cumulative GPA outstripped any other measures of academic qualities in their correlation with the outcome of selection. Keep in mind that this was within a group already selected for high grades and high MCAT scores.

Similarly, the academic rating of the applicant's undergraduate college played a greater role than the committee seemed to think it did. Perhaps committee members were experiencing a conflict in their own values between academic excellence and unfashionable elitism.

All available data do confirm that, at this stage of decision making, personal attributes outweighed academic ability of candidates in influencing the decision or selection. Academic ability had exerted stronger input earlier in the screening process and was still not wholly without influence even in the later stages.

A Psychologic Test for Committee Members

In a further attempt to identify the values of the committee, the members were asked to indicate on a list of 300 adjectives[22] those that would describe a candidate to whom they personally would give the highest ranking. Forty-six members (81 percent of the committee) responded.

Individual adjectives endorsed by 75 percent or more of the whole committee were adaptable, alert, capable, clear-thinking, confident, conscientious, considerate, dependable, energetic, enthusiastic, friendly, honest, imaginative, intelligent, interests wide, mature, responsible, sensitive, sincere, stable, and warm.

Adjectives given unanimous endorsement by the four separate subcommittees described previously are as follows:

  I   alert, conscientious, enthusiastic, honest, responsible
 II   alert
III   conscientious, sincere
 IV   dependable, energetic, friendly, honest, intelligent, responsible

These descriptions were scored on the 23 scales described by Gough and Heilbrun, the authors of the test. The mean profiles bear a striking resemblance to the mean profiles Gough had obtained 8 to 10 years earlier when he administered the test to three entering classes in the same school.[23] The description Gough derived from the testing is of "a planful, conscientious, dependable individual, somewhat conservative and inhibited, resourceful and independent, and able to cope well with both physical and intellectual stress."

The committee's description of the ideal student differs only in that scores for the scales upon which this description was based deviate even further from the norm than did the older self-description.

SUMMARY

With the development of highly science-oriented medical education in the United States, increasing emphasis has been placed on academic capability in the selection process. Quite understandably, use of academic criteria as the only, or nearly the only, characteristic for selection of students resulted in constriction of the range of many other individual qualities in medical students—sex, race, urbanity, and economic status to name a few. Changing values in society in recent years have resulted in increasing demand for diversification of the human input of the medical profession, particularly with regard to increasing representation for ethnic minorities, women, and individuals with qualities that will ensure better geographic distribution of doctors.

Medical schools, through the action of admissions committees, have responded to these demands. Even so, traditional values held by the profession as they relate to scientific competence and responsibility may not have changed greatly. Study of one admissions committee suggests that academic capability and traditional personal qualities are the characteristics most heavily weighted in the selection process.

This ministudy of one committee in one year does point out that noncognitive as well as cognitive attributes are held to be of value in the selection process and that they were used by the committee as judgment data. The attributes conform rather closely to fairly traditional professional norms, even in the case of a subcommittee newly conceived and comprising mainly minority members, students, and community representatives. In view of a specific charge to broaden the criteria for selection, ways have not yet been found to relate these selection criteria to future performance as a provider of health care in specific social situations. The selection process continues to seek bright, humane individuals who seem likely to develop into rather traditional professionals.

Social change, including new health careers and new ways to deliver health care, are in the air, but, back home at the medical school, the admissions committee continues to do business as usual.

REFERENCES

1. Rokeach M: Beliefs, Attitudes and Values. San Francisco, Jossey-Bass, 1968, p 160.

2. Stake RE: Objectives, priorities, and other judgment data. Rev Educ Res 40: 181–211, 1970.
3. Parsons T: Suggestions for a sociological approach to the theory of organizations. Admin Sci Q 1:63–85, 1956.
4. Flexner A: Medical Education in the United States and Canada. Bull. No. 4. New York, Carnegie Foundation for the Advancement of Teaching, 1910.
5. Cattell JM (ed): Science and Education. Vol. II. Medical Research and Education. New York, Science Press, 1913, p 89.
6. *Ibid.*, p 165.
7. *Ibid.*
8. *Ibid.*
9. *Ibid.*
10. Rappleye W, Director of Study: Final Report of the Commission on Medical Education. New York, Office of the Director of Study, 1932, Appendix, Table 123.
11. Gee HH, Cowles JT (ed): Appraisal of Applicants to Medical Schools. Evanston, Ill., AAMC, 1957, p 32.
12. Jackson DN: Recent developments in structured personality assessment: implications for medical education, Conference on Personality Measurement in Medical Education. Edited by HB Haley, AG D'Costa, AM Schafer. Evanston, Ill., AAMC, 1971.
13. Cattell JM (ed): *op. cit.*, p 286.
14. Friedson E: Profession of Medicine. A Study of the Sociology of Applied Knowledge. New York, Dodd Mead, 1970, Ch 8.
15. Rappleye W: *op. cit.*, p 272.
16. Gee HH, Cowles JT (ed): *op. cit.*
17. Schofield W: Research Studies of Medical Students and Physicians Utilizing Standard Personality Instruments: An Annotated Bibliography. Evanston, Ill., AAMC, 1972.
18. Gee HH, Cowles JT (ed): *op. cit.*, p 200.
19. Oetgen WJ, Pepper MD: Medical school admissions committee members: a descriptive study. J Med Educ 47:966–968, 1972.
20. *Ibid.*
21. Moss FA: Report of the committee on aptitude tests for medical schools. J Assoc Am Med Coll 15:249–255, 1940.
22. Gough H: The recruitment and selection of medical students. Psychosocial Aspects of Medical Training. Springfield, Ill., Charles C Thomas, 1971, p 32.
23. *Ibid.*

ANNE KIBRICK, R.N., Ed.D.
Professor and Chairman, Department of Nursing, Boston College

Commentary

Dr. Wellington's paper effectively describes the current state of the art with regard to admission of medical students and draws attention to some of the problems confronting admissions committees. He demonstrates convincingly the need for further studies in the procedures for selection of students. His paper also raises many questions.

How often have we examined the admissions procedure in terms of substance rather than process? How often do we assess the implications of our decisions? Do we take the long look in terms of the professional product or the short look in terms of academic success in the program? Have we delineated those particular personal characteristics that we say make so much difference? How often do we deliberate together and explore our own value systems? Does the application of our own value system to the prospective candidate have any referent base or is it primarily a subjective matter? Academic achievement has always been easier to ascertain than values, attitudes, and desirable personal qualities; thus, academic accomplishment has become, and still remains, the primary tool for the evaluation of prospective candidates.

Education has been, and always will be, a moral endeavor. We, as educators, select those students whom we will admit to our schools, based on our own system of values, and therefore those who will become the future practitioners. We select those experiences to which the students will or will not be exposed, those criteria by which they will be passed or failed, and those actions and behaviors that will or will not be rewarded. In short, we have the opportunity to decide on and delimit the type of practitioner to be produced. This is an awesome responsibility that demands thoughtful deliberation.

As far back as 1930, character and personality were identified as highly important characteristics in the evaluation of applicants, and yet the criteria used have remained intelligence, vocabulary, writing, and similar measurable parameters. The importance of character and personality were again cited in the 1957 report of the American Association of Medical Colleges. The basic problems in the implementation of these beliefs were, "how to identify and measure desirable qualities, lack of a clear idea about which qualities are most desirable, and lack of measurement as to whether selection on the basis of character or personality attributes is successful." We have been identifying the same problems for many years but have been slow in taking definite steps to alter the situation.

Dr. Wellington points out that a variety of psychological instruments have been administered to incoming students and indicates that their predictive value is measured in terms of later performance. Unfortunately, the criterion value of later performance is most often the class standing on the basis of grades achieved in the basic sciences of the first year of medical school. This criterion, while it may predict one's ability to succeed in medical school, does little to describe or identify those factors that make up the desired or successful practitioner. We need to define what we mean by success, or what we would like our product to be, before we can identify significant personal characteristics for admitting students or for determining what experiences we should provide for them during the educational process. Furthermore, such a criterion value is a totally inadequate measure of later performance in medical practice. The characteristics of those who rate high in basic sciences in the first year may be quite different from the characteristics of the optimally endowed practitioner. The problem may be not so much with the types of tool being used to evaluate later performance but rather how and at what point in the educational process we apply the results of the psychological measurements.

Dr. Wellington states early in his paper that attention should be focused not only on the values of the admissions committee members but also on the values of the administrators who appoint them. However, later on he demonstrates that the dean's recommendation regarding the admission of candidates counts for very little in the decision of the committee and attributes this to a difference in values. I feel it is more important that the values of the committee reflect the philosophy and views of the faculty. In most instances admissions committee members are appointed by the dean and, therefore, do not necessarily reflect the values of the faculty to whom the students will be exposed for their professional education.

While it is recognized that the interview is not a valid predictor of behavior, its relative weight in the selection process has increased. The interview permits admissions committee members to apply their own individual value system to selection. If admissions committees are to reflect faculty values, it becomes increasingly important that faculty deliberate together on the values that they feel are important to success. If faculty are able to identify the values and characteristics they feel are essential, the committee members should overtly test for these rather than depend on their own intuitive reactions for making such judgments.

I should like to comment on the organization of the four subcommittees for the admission of candidates. Each subcommittee was responsible for admitting approximately 37 candidates. The subcommittee responsible for all applicants with advanced science degrees and applicants interested in the medical scientist pathway was made up primarily of basic scientists and science-oriented clinicians and students. The subcommittee to consider all minority applicants was comprised mainly of faculty members representing minority groups and included community nonprofessionals. The remaining two committees reviewed all other candidates. This practice results, in this case, in three types of selection committees, each with their own separate set of criteria. The criteria for admission obviously varied among these committees. The academic qualifications of those admitted, therefore, covered a rather wide range. It appears that the values of the faculty in relation to their expectations for the products of the program embraces the broad spectrum of medicine—from general practice to advanced scientific investigation. Should one school attempt to be all things to all students? Maybe the faculty should clarify and specify its purpose and select students accordingly. Within the state system of medical education, it might prove more practical for one school to admit those students who want to pursue the "medical scientist pathway" and develop a curriculum to maximize their potential.

Doctors do not need to be all things to all people and maybe they should not be. If medicine would delimit what it can best do and work with other professional groups in deliberating on complementarity of roles, it would not have to be in the position of making trade-offs.

The shortage of physicians is particularly acute in areas of chronic illness, rehabilitation, psychological support services, counseling, follow-

up, and health teaching. All of these areas are included in the goals of
nursing education as it stresses health maintenance and disease prevention as well as acute care nursing. Physicians should learn to use other
health workers in providing health care on a collegial type of basis where
each one does what he wants to do and what he can do best.

I do not agree with the practice of a separate committee, comprised
primarily of members of minority groups, to review the applications of
minority group members. The criteria for selecting members of minority
groups tend to be different from those applied to candidates reviewed
by the other committees. It was pointed out that each committee, as a
result of frequent and long meetings, developed a "flavor" of its own.
The interview process played an "enormously important" role in the admission of students. Although there was a "wide range of views" on
each subcommittee, the enthusiastic support of an interviewer exerted
great influence on the outcome of the decision.

It is difficult to rationalize the committee's consideration of the
presence of physical traits and characteristics of an ethnic minority as a
basis for selection. The criteria of difficulty experienced in college as
well as an educationally and financially poor family background are regarded for the minorities as evidence of strong motivation and determination. Fortunately, these values are spreading to the other three committees. Criteria applied to members of minority groups, if different
from those applied to the total group of candidates, will result in isolation of the minorities who realize and resent that they are judged by
different standards.

Admissions committees that represent faculty opinion and whose
criteria are developed within the framework of an acknowledged concept of needs in the health care system should have criteria that apply
equally to all candidates and are reflective of the value system of the
faculty. This should hopefully include concern for a segment of society
whose disadvantaged early education militated against their subsequent
admission to medical school.

Under the four-subcommittee system, one could hypothesize that the
probability of students entering via the advanced science degree committee or the minority committee would be considerably higher than
for students considered by the other committees. If personal attributes
of the candidates are to determine the decisions of the committee, then
it becomes critical that these be more objective and less subjective.

In the judgment of the admissions committee, the hypothetical ideal
candidate had few nurturant and intraceptive qualities but was strongly
directed toward independence, achievement, and control. His attempt
to understand behavior was primarily an intellectual exercise rather than

a means of giving help and love to others. It would be interesting to explore whether those qualities identified as least desirable tended to be de-emphasized in the curriculum and those identified as desirable were rewarded and stressed. If so, it would be fairly easy to describe the type of practitioner for that program.

Dr. Wellington states that the selection process for medicine has always been shaped by the value systems that hold optimal health care as a goal. The public is not aware of this value as they have been complaining about the health care system for many years. Dr. Wellington points out that the impetus for change in admission criteria has come largely from outside the profession and that it is not a single voice. These outside voices demanding change will continue unless medicine evaluates its admission criteria in terms of the product they want to graduate.

Gottheil and co-workers,[1] at Jefferson Medical College, studied the attitudes of medical students and how they are formed. He was concerned with the low nurturance and intraception leanings of today's medical students. He found that they learned values and attitudes chiefly through the role models of the physicians with whom they came in contact. The student basically was influenced by how the faculty related to him, to each other, and to their patients. He stated that, "if the student perceives his medical school primarily as a scientific laboratory, we might expect him to behave toward his patients differently from the way in which he behaves if he sees it to be mainly a place in which he learns to care for sick people." Gottheil goes on to say that,

> ... in the selection of medical students, admission committees are often faced with the task of trying to balance a liberal, sociohumanistic education against achievement in the sciences. A broad cultural background is desirable but good grades and courses in the sciences are better predictors of success in the typical medical school curriculum. [To what extent should we be willing] to modify the traditional curriculum and atmosphere of the medical college in order to have the student acquire the attitude that the patient is not merely an interesting disease but a total person? Modifications in the academic and social atmosphere of the medical school could be made without compromising good teaching or professional goals.

Medical schools seem to pride themselves on their low dropout rate. As long as students are evaluated primarily on their intellectual capacity and ability to diagnose and institute proper treatment and emphasis is placed on treating the disease rather than on concern for the total person, dropouts will remain low. If criteria were concerned more with humanistic values, the dropout rate might be higher. Dr. Wellington states that it is unlikely that further refinement of admission criteria can affect the dropout rate. This is true if criteria and expectations for students remain as they are. Admissions committees must look more closely at the qualities they desire in the products of their programs, with an awareness of the needs of society. According to Wellington's Table 3, of the 12 values judged by the admissions committee to range from important to extremely important, six were concerned with academic accomplishments and one with interest in research. His Table 4 shows that the cumulative GPA ranked higher than personality attributes in the selection process. At this stage in the final selection process the committee was dealing with candidates who had survived earlier screenings and who were academically capable.

My own research in this area[2] was premised on the belief that when one enters into an occupational or vocational choice, there is, during the stage of induction, opportunity for discovery of incompatibility between presumed and actual job images, and of incompatibility between self-image and the self-image as modified by experiences provided by the role. This research was focused on an investigation of the effect of role and self-perception on the withdrawal of students from selected schools of nursing. The role segments included responsibilities, relationships, behavior, and attributes. The results showed that the greater the extent of conformance to the expectations of the role definers (faculty and supervisors), the more likely the student was to remain in the program. The study also indicated that when one chooses an occupational role, one is in effect choosing a means of implementing a self-concept. Thus, staying with an occupational choice is a measure of whether the role the individual has to play is compatible with his self-concept. However, more significant than the implementation of one's self-concept for occupational perseverance was the relationship between the student's self-concept and the faculty's expectations for role attributes. The more the student conformed to the faculty's expectations, the more likely she was to remain in the program.

Contrary to Dr. Wellington's assumption for medical schools, that other schools are using similar sets or subsets of values as admission criteria, there was relatively little consensus among the seven nursing schools in my study on role expectations of students. It should be pointed out that my schools represented different organizational controls, namely, municipal, community, Roman Catholic, and Protestant. The variability in administrative control was not part of the initial design but rather an accident. However, it does point out that educational systems reflect the values of the institutions of which they are a part and, with the exception of academic achievement, not all schools may be looking for the same characteristics in their students.

Certain personality characteristics were found to distinguish nursing students who left the program from those that remained. Students who withdrew resented authority and were more aggressive and independent and less willing to submit to the routines and practices of the school. Remaining students were more nurturant, more submissive, and more intraceptive.

Personality characteristics vary according to the occupational field and according to different roles within the selected field. It is interesting that the hypothetical ideal medical school candidate has low nurturant and intraception values and high achievement and control values, while nursing students have demonstrated the reverse. Given the personality structure of students who enter nursing and those who enter medicine and the expectations that faculty have had for the products of each of these programs, it is easy to see why nursing has been subservient to medicine rather than defining its own role. Faculty must reassess their values and expectations for the products of the programs if medicine is to become more humanistic and nursing is to become more self-directive.

The values that faculty and admissions committees have established have permeated the public so that those who select these professions have already done some self-screening or have been screened out by counselors or others in terms of the expectations of the role.

Rhoda Epstein's[3] doctoral study, currently in progress at Boston College, is concerned with the attitudes and values of nursing students. This study was less concerned with the selection process than with the results of that process. One of the major objectives of her study is to identify the type of product or practitioner the faculty wishes to produce and to design the educational process to effect this result. She found that those qualities most desired by the faculty included nurturance and intraception. The nursing students demonstrated extremely high scores in nurturance, intraception, and abasement and fairly low scores in autonomy and achievement. The faculty then decided that values of autonomy and achievement were the qualities that should be encouraged and that feelings of abasement should be decreased. Strategies to accomplish the results were then identified.

The qualities one desires in the professional must be encouraged and expected in the learner. The student cannot incorporate behavioral traits on the day of graduation if these characteristics have been discouraged during the educational process. The student cannot view a patient as a member of a total family if he has not experienced that orientation during his education. Students need role models of desirable behavior if they are to acquire the desired behavior as a result of the educational program. What is most important in this process is the interaction between educator and student. Faculty cannot state one behavior as desirable and then reward the opposite. Unless there is consistency and follow-through with a shared value set in all experiences, the student either is confused by changing value orientations or participates in the game of "psyching out" each individual instructor in order to give what is wanted at the time and thus pass the program successfully without incorporating the value orientation of the faculty into his own value system.

Once the faculty have identified the desired product and the methodologies by which to enhance the possibilities of success, the next step is the evaluation to determine whether the faculty has, in fact, accomplished what it set out to do. This means a comparison of graduates against the predetermined criteria of a successful practitioner.

By following these steps in her study, M. Epstein's evaluation showed remarkable changes in the graduates of the nursing program. Achievement and autonomy scores rose consistently. There was a gradual decline of scores in intraception and nurturance, but these scores never fell below the scores in achievement or autonomy. There was also a steady decline in abasement. These changes coincided with marked behavioral changes. Once the faculty had identified desirable behaviors and attitudes explicitly among themselves and explored their own philosophies, they were able to arrive at a more consistent approach to the educational process. Instead of a covert, haphazard, individually defined approach to nursing, they were consistently able to encourage those qualities they felt important to bring about a group of more articulate, independent, and self-motivated graduates. Changes were brought about which both faculty and students were able to identify.

A related observation was made by Davis and Oleson[4] in a study dealing with changes of images of nursing. The authors noted that changes in attitudes between first year and graduating nursing students were conditioned by the emphasis of the faculty on specific themes established during the first year and forcefully sustained over the succeeding two years.

In each of the studies cited, certain similarities stand out. One is that students are very sensitive to faculty values, as these are usually the first role models of the profession to which they aspire. Therefore a consistent faculty emphasis and approach can do much to encourage the development of the type of practitioner desired. Second, the values of the individuals selecting the students hold the key to the type of student who will become the practitioner of tomorrow, and I believe they should reflect the explicit philosophy and value systems identified by the faculty. Third, as the relative weight of the interview in the selection process has increased, it becomes increasingly important that desirable characteristics be delineated and agreed upon by faculty. Admission committees should evaluate the extent to which they apply specified criteria to the selection of candidates. Dr. Wellington points out that, despite the emphasis on personality characteristics, committee members put greater emphasis on academic achievement than even they realized. Fourth, and perhaps most important, these studies highlight the incongruity between what we say we are producing, what society wants us to produce, and what we actually do produce. Any change in our system must be preceded by a basic dissatisfaction with our present system and a conviction that we can do better.

It is important that we be clear in our goals for education and that there be unity of purpose between participants in the educational enterprise if we are to shape the direction of our professions.

ACKNOWLEDGMENT

I would like to acknowledge the contributions of Rhoda Epstein to this paper. Many of my comments are the result of our joint discussions concerning Dr. Wellington's paper.

REFERENCES

1. Gottheil E, et al.: Students' perceptions of medicine and their attitudes towards patients. Br J Med Educ 3:355–358, 1969.
2. Kibrick AK: Dropouts in schools of nursing: the effect of self and role perception. Nurs Res 12:140–149, 1963.
3. Epstein R: Transmission of Values and Attitudes via Higher Education. Unpublished doctoral thesis, Boston College, 1973.
4. Davis F, Oleson V: Baccalaureate students images of nursing. Nurs Res 15:151–158, 1966.

CLIFTON O. DUMMETT, D.D.S.

Professor and Chairman, Department of Community Dentistry, University of Southern California

Commentary

I would like to congratulate Dr. Wellington on his presentation of an important and timely topic. The selection of the most suitable students for the health professions is a necessary but thankless procedure that has increased in difficulty in proportion to the numbers of persons interested in becoming bona fide members of those professions.

Dr. Wellington has described his experiences with one school of medicine's admissions committee, but there are elements in these experiences that are quite familiar to those who have worked with similar committees of other medical and health-related schools. It has taken much time and heartache to reach the conclusion that, in today's scheme of events, admission to health professional education institutions is tantamount to entry into the professions. A great deal has been made of the economic waste, not to mention the disruptive interpersonal relationships that result when a student has to be eliminated from his medical class.

Early efforts at selecting students for the health professions were arbitrary and could very well have been responsible for the rejection of capable, ambitious, and desirable young people who might not have quite fitted the then conceptions of "professionalism." By the same token, willful action could just as easily have resulted in the selection of pseudo-professional persons who might have been unconcerned, disinterested, and incapable of responding to the public's legitimate demands for dignified health care.

191

Even though the use of psychological and personal criteria has helped in the selection of an improved caliber of medical student, present selection methods are still not perfect. And so we keep on searching for one way, for *the* method, for *a single* means to accomplish complicated tasks.

Nothing is more complex than human beings choosing and making judgments of other human beings. Insofar as admissions committees are concerned, not every member can be adjudged "well adjusted," and judgments are usually no better than the judges themselves. Consequently, in our continuing searches and efforts to gain further information about the admissions process, we must re-emphasize the need for studies of selection committees and their individual members.

The multistage procedure that Dr. Wellington has described assures due process, fairness, and a degree of public support for an institution's methods of selecting its students for entry into the medical profession. One of the invaluable contributions of the multistage process is that it creates a reservoir of potential applicants from which sensitive admissions committees can more easily select the most able persons who can, in turn, fulfill the demanding requirements of modern health professions.

Dr. Wellington's discussion of the structure of the admissions committee with its subcommittees was illuminating. As a result of society's changing values, I would endorse the need for an increased diversification of the human input in the medical and health professions. Representation from special groups is a key ingredient for change. We have noted that on the part of responsible officials in professional schools, there has been some lessening of discrimination in the acceptance of certain groups for formerly restricted occupations. The increase in the numbers of women, socioeconomically disadvantaged persons, and ethnic minority students in medical schools of the nation is a heartening development. It is quite possible that the expanded memberships on the admissions committees to include representatives of these special groups may have contributed to this increase. With the knowledge and experiences gained by these committees, it should be anticipated that in the future there will be even more spectacular developments in the nation's medical, dental, and other health institutions.

One of the most difficult problems that admissions committees of health professional institutions might be called upon to face in the very near future is the acceptance of students with known homosexual and lesbian tendencies. For such a task, there may be contributions that these human beings can make if they were included on admissions committees. Many of these persons have all of the humane and intellectual qualities for which admissions committees are searching.

The fact is that many of the characteristics and qualities that we are now finding most desirable to inculcate in our health professions are to be found in these persons, as well as in white, Anglo-Saxon, heterosexual males. The ideals and philosophies to which the health professions are dedicated suggest the need to tackle with toughmindedness and flexibility many inelegant problems that, until recently, were refused enlightened consideration.

Nineteenth century conservatism in the selection of medical students has been imitated by the dental profession in the selection of dental students. The legendary emphasis on a "good pair of hands" as the *sine qua non* for the selection of dental students has been so exploited as to have popularized the myth of indubitable digital dexterity even to the exclusion of an intellectual capability. And the cultural lag still exists! It is most probably responsible for an incomprehensible resistance to change that at times the profession has demonstrated regarding efforts to update dental school acceptance requirements.

The acceptability of some current innovations can be attributed to the persistence of a few determined dental educators, the resourcefulness of the Council on Dental Education of the American Dental Association, and the powerful influence of the American Association of Dental Schools. To these groups and individuals are due much of the credit for the fact that admissions committees of the nation's dental schools have begun to recognize the need to increase each school's flexibility both in terms of its curriculum and its admissions policies.

The need for a broader spectrum of students to attend schools of dentistry has been recognized, and committees are making substantive efforts to meet this need. Many committees, for instance, have de-emphasized the absolute essentiality of a strong science background in those who apply to dental schools. There has been discussion about seeking students with degrees in sociology and psychology, and even in music and drama. There has been further talk about reversing a discriminatory tendency toward females, and even taking advantage of the tremendous reservoirs of talent and performance that are available in the chronologically mature female. Most important of the newly found revelations is the admissions committees' search for candidates with honest feelings for their fellowmen.

Some purpose may be served by recounting a few experiences with policies and practices of the admissions committee at a California dental school.

In a study completed by the recently appointed Director of Dental Admissions at the University of Southern California, efforts were directed at developing a profile for every student who was accepted into the school of dentistry from the 1953 entering class to that of 1972.

The typical entering dental student for the last 20 years has been a 22-year-old white male, single, without a college degree, and most likely from a nonprofessional family.

The data indicated that USC's School of Dentistry traditionally has taken the "best" students in the country with respect to their manual dexterity scores on the Dental Aptitude Test (DAT). (Parenthetically, the data indicate that the best students accepted at USC were actually only good students with respect to general academic competence as portrayed by academic averages on the GPA and the DAT.) On the latter test, academic average is a composite score derived from eleven subtest scores. The score measures a student's general intelligence, his ability to read and comprehend scientific writing, and his knowledge of scientific information in the fields of biology and chemistry.

During the past two years, classes with a greater diversity of students have been admitted. Students have been classified as being "well rounded" from both academic and social viewpoints. This designation was arrived at by virtue of the fact that the accepted students had pre-dental grade point averages that had increased, but academic and manual averages on the DAT that had decreased.

In 1973, the admissions committee reported receipt of more than 2,000 applications for the 120 available places in the first-year dental class. The applications were from what were considered highly qualified persons with GPAs higher than 3.0. Current policies of the admissions committee are to procure a comprehensive picture of the applicant's personality by using the grade point average and evaluating the applicant's qualities as evidenced from personal interviews, letters of recommendation, and accounts of extracurricular activities.

From the standpoint of the University of Southern California's dental admissions committee, academic capability and personal qualities as obtained from the personal interview represent characteristics that are now stressed in the selection process.

There have been a number of innovative procedures aimed at convincing applicants of the admissions committee's efforts to be as sensitive as possible in processes that would channel to the committee a number of excellent prospects. In 1972 the director of the admissions office allowed unsuccessful applicants the privilege of discussing their individual cases with him. Dental applicants were also encouraged to take advantage of a number of counseling services.

Dental admissions committees will endorse the need for continuing research into the personality qualities of persons interested in studying for the health professions.

Dr. Wellington has indicated that at least in one institution, traditional values held by the medical profession as they relate to scientific competence and responsibility may not have changed greatly. Academic capability and personal qualities are still the characteristics most heavily weighted in the selection process.

In dentistry, traditional values as they relate to scientific competence and public accountability have undergone changes, the most notable being a diminution in the excessive emphasis previously placed on manual dexterity. Technical excellence used to be considered an endpoint in itself rather than a means toward helping to preserve patient health through dental care. Clinicians are exhibiting greater concern about consumer satisfaction and patient sensitivity, and these changes are being reflected in the dental curriculum and in the type of person selected to study for the profession.

Creating a dentist to fulfill society's needs is as dependent on the development of different scholastic programs as it is on the types of person that admissions committees select. There is a growing demand for dentists to be oral physicians rather than merely dental technicians. This metamorphosis has to begin with the incoming dental student, and this is another reason why the work of admissions committees is so vital.

I would welcome Dr. Wellington's opinions on the matter of student quotas. It is obvious that the academically deprived student cannot immediately compete on a level with the academically nondeprived. Therefore, if the former is to achieve the goal of a profession, he must gain admittance, despite somewhat lower credentials, and be provided tutorial assistance as needed. It cannot be assumed that his performance scores are completely representative of his potential, inasmuch as these scores reflect the system that brought him to this level as well as his performance within it. Thus, a special place needs to be created for this student in order to give him that extra boost that he has earned through desperate years of second-class, second-rate, and second-best status. It thus becomes apparent that only by setting aside a stipulated number of openings to be available to this category of student can some form of "inequitable equity" be established to begin to compensate in a small way for the long years of neglect. No matter how much one may disagree with a quota system per se, it does serve a useful purpose in allowing disadvantaged students to meet the handicap of academic weakness. It goes without saying, however, that these students must understand from the very beginning that preparation for dentistry is a formidable task and that there are no substitutes for study, industry, concentration, and ethics! Moreover, dentistry should not be expected to lower hard-fought-for standards just to make it "easier" for members of minority groups. The effort should be directed toward trying to attract as many academically qualified persons as possible who are interested in the health professions.

The vehemence of reactions against the steps taken by some of our nation's most illustrious institutions is surprising, but not unpredictable. These schools announced that they would accept persons who were socioeconomically different from the majority of the school population and that such persons would comprise 25 percent of each class. This accommodation was made on the basis that these persons would find it difficult to meet regular acceptance standards of dental and medical schools. In the procedure, qualifying test score requirements were lowered. Many students had grades and test scores that were not as high as normally considered essential in the past. However, many honest dental educators would attest to some lack of correlation between the grades and test scores at the time of entrance and the subsequent performances of the students. Several schools feel it is of utmost importance to interview minority students as an additional aid in considering their test scores and grades. In this way they are better able to evaluate how the students would perform and then weigh the academic considerations in relation to what the committee feels these students could contribute to dentistry, as well as to the communities from which they come.

I believe that, even though they have been slow and deliberate in their progress toward consideration of dental education's urgent issues, our professional schools have started to correct many of the educational ills and long-standing inequities that have plagued the professions. There is still a long way to go, and there is the need to accelerate the pace of consideration, but essentially many of our mature educators are now alert to the issues.

RENÉE C. FOX, Ph.D.

Chairman, Department of Sociology, University of Pennsylvania

Is There A "New" Medical Student?

A COMPARATIVE VIEW OF MEDICAL SOCIALIZATION IN THE 1950s AND THE 1970s

I

Writing about the socialization of physicians in the 1970s is a paradoxical intellectual experience. Due notice is being taken of the dramatic increase in the number of persons applying for admission to medical school. Discussion regarding not only the intellectual and scientific qualifications of the men and women opting for medical careers but also their social backgrounds, life experiences, attitudes, and convictions is rampant. The advantages and drawbacks of actual and potential curriculum changes are being debated by medical educators throughout the country, who are attempting to evaluate the impact of these changes on the competence and outlook of physicians now in training. In many educational and professional circles, and in the public arena, there is great preoccupation with the quality, as well as the distribution and cost, of health care in the society. To what is perhaps an unprecedented degree, this concerned interest has come to include questions about the ethical and existential dimensions of modern medicine along with its scientific and technical aspects. These various developments are accompanied by general recognition that there is a significant relationship between the perceived strengths and weaknesses of the American medical system and the process of socialization for physicianhood that is an integral part of medical training. It could even be said that another

197

characteristic of the present medical historical juncture is heightened
awareness of the professional socialization process. Today's medical
students, house officers, and their teachers seem to be impressed with
the fact that the educational sequences in which they are participating
not only convey knowledge and skills but professionally relevant values,
attitudes, and behavior patterns as well.

One would expect these characteristics of present-day medical educational milieux to generate significant, clinically perceptive, and socially
sensitive research on the process of becoming a physician. But, to our
knowledge, no such major study is being conducted. This stands in
sharp contrast to the late 1950s when a number of important social
scientific inquiries into the process of becoming a physician were undertaken.[1] Why the current paucity of work on medical socialization exists
is a subject for study in and of itself. Its explanation is intricately associated with the stage of development and the collective mood both of
social science and medicine and with more general cultural, economic,
and political trends in the society that affect these disciplines. But
whatever its origins, the lack of research on this subject means that any
discussion of medical socialization in the 1970s is necessarily speculative. This is as regrettable as it is curious. For it occurs at a time when—
for both social scientific and medical educational reasons—it would be
valuable to study the social and cultural changes that seem to be taking
place in the attitudes and values of medical students, the education they
are undergoing, and the profession into which they are graduating. Instead, what is happening is that the many strongly felt but undocu-
mented opinions that are being expressed on these matters are being
presented and accepted as fact and are beginning to influence policy
decisions about present and future medical training.

II

This paper is based on social scientific observations made in various
medical school settings, principally in the 1950s and in the 1970s. One
set of materials on which I draw are my own firsthand research experiences as a member of the Bureau of Applied Social Research–Columbia
University team that undertook studies in the sociology of medical education in the mid-1950s at Cornell University, the University of Pennsylvania, Western Reserve University, and the University of Colorado. I
was the chief fieldworker for the project, and in this capacity spent four
years as a participant observer at Cornell University Medical College,
watching and taking part in the academic, clinical, and interpersonal
events that contributed to the processes of medical education and so-

cialization through which students passed. I also had access to the data that my colleagues obtained from students in the four medical schools under study, through the periodic administration of a panel-type survey questionnaire.[2] As already implied, this was a "golden era" of research on professional socialization. Not only were several studies of psychosocial aspects of becoming a physician en route, but these were characterized by a continual exchange of insights and information between them. Thus, my data from the 1950s include unpublished as well as published observations made available to me by social scientists and physicians associated with the University of Chicago, the University of Kansas, Tulane University, and Harvard University, among others.

As already implied, my data from the late 1960s and early 1970s are more impressionistic. They have not been gathered within the framework of a large, systematic study. Rather, they are the product of my own, more sporadically collected observations and documentation, which several of the roles that I now occupy have made possible. Since 1969, in my capacity as Professor of Sociology in the Department of Psychiatry and the Department of Medicine at the University of Pennsylvania, I have been engaged in teaching medical students and in observing and interviewing them in order to help appraise the consequences of certain curriculum reforms. In addition, I have served both on the admissions and the curriculum committees of the medical school. Beyond those functions, because I have now done research, writing, and teaching in the field of the sociology of medicine for more than 20 years, I am often invited to visit and lecture at other medical schools. These activities have enabled me to have various kinds of contact with medical students and faculty in multiple settings of different medical schools. I have kept a fieldworker's record of these experiences. These notes are the primary source for the account of medical socialization in the 1970s that I shall present.

III

Medical education in the 1950s was more tightly and uniformly organized than it is now. Looking at it from the perspective of the 1970s, the medical school curriculum was arranged in a "lock-step" way, with little room for individual variation or choice. The first two years of training were devoted *en bloc* to lecture hall presentations and laboratory work in the so-called preclinical or basic sciences. Patient contact was minimal, largely confined to the cadaver in the anatomy laboratory, the newly deceased patient in the autopsy room, and to live patients who were briefly presented to the class by an instructor, generally to demonstrate some biological principle or phenomenon. Only toward the end of the second year—in the context of their physical diagnosis course, where students learned to take medical histories and conduct physical examinations—did they have more sustained and clinically oriented exposure to patients. Although students were divided into smaller working groups for some of their laboratory and clinical tasks, assignment to these groups was determined by alphabetical order. Thus, student teams were comprised of those whose family names were alphabetically close. The third year of medical school represented the great crossing over to the clinical phase of training. Third and fourth years were largely made up of a series of clinical clerkships in the various branches of medicine and surgery. The same alphabetical criterion that applied to the first two years ordered the sequence in which students rotated through their clerkships, although there were carefully defined circumstances under which some student preferences in this regard were honored.

The highly patterned, collective, and relatively unvarying nature of each stage of medical school training was reflected in the students' characteristic dress and equipage. For, although they were not expressly required to wear uniforms and were not aware that they did so, the self-presentation of each cohort of students was so similar that one could identify the phase of their training by their costume. First-year students tended to dress in long white laboratory coats, worn over khaki pants and sports shirts. They moved through the corridors of the medical school, arms laden with clipboards, notebooks, and large, atlas-like texts. Toward the end of second year, when they were beginning to see patients in physical diagnosis, students looked more freshly barbered, donned neckties and more formal woolen trousers, and self-consciously carried unmistakably new little black bags wherever they went. During the clinical clerkships of third and fourth years, the long white coats gave way to short, jacket-length ones. Students pinned identifying name tags on their lapels and allowed their stethoscopes to hang conspicuously out of their hospital coat pockets. Some fourth-year students, emulating the interns they would soon become, knotted a rubber tourniquet around one of their belt loops, as if they were perpetually ready to draw blood or start an intravenous infusion.

In certain medical schools (among them, the four that were studied by the Columbia team of sociologists), the 1950s were also a time when various educational innovations were being tried. The most extensive changes were those initiated by the School of Medicine at Western Reserve University, where the traditional curriculum was razed and another progressively put in its place. By and large, the experiments in medical education that were launched during this decade were oriented toward a number of common themes.[3] Organized attempts were made to design opportunities for students to have earlier patient contact. Ways were also devised to introduce students to patients with "normal" health problems, such as those of uncomplicated pregnancy or everyday pediatrics, at the same time that they were being introduced to the more tragic and extraordinary dimensions of medicine through the anatomy laboratory, the autopsy, and their first encounters with chronically ill and dying patients. Various modes of more broadly defining the physician's role and of effectively emphasizing the role of social and psychological factors in the genesis and treatment of illness were tried. These included developing and conveying the concept of "comprehensive care" and teaching, as well as efforts to incorporate more behavioral science into the medical curriculum. They also entailed trying to upgrade the importance of experience in outpatient clinics, based on the conviction that providing students with continuing responsibility for ambulatory patient care would train them in a more inclusive approach to medicine. Finally, there were some endeavors to increase the amount of free or elective time in medical students' programs. As the foregoing suggests, although these modifications in the curriculum were oriented to greater "liberalization" of medical training in several senses, they were as structured as the aspects of the traditional curriculum that they sought to modify.

The medical curriculum of the 1950s was not only highly organized, it was also characterized by a remarkable degree of internal logic. The learning sequences that it embodied unfolded in a systematic way, with each new step building on the ones that preceded it. This kind of order was a distinguishing feature of the attitude, as well as the cognitive, learning that took place in medical school. Students were as progressively trained in certain values, attitudes, and norms as they were in biomedical knowledge and skills. This is all the more impressive because, by and large, these psychosocial aspects of learning built into the curriculum were not planned as such by medical educators. To a significant degree, they were unanticipated and unrecognized consequences of the more deliberately arranged scientific and clinical training that students received and of the kinds of relationships with faculty, patients, and each other that students typically developed in medical school. In fact, one of the primary tasks that the social scientists involved in the socialization studies of the 1950s performed for medical educators was to identify the formal and informal medical school contexts in which professionally relevant attitude learning inadvertently occurred.

The nonrandom nature and the psychosociology of attitude learning in medical schools of the 1950s can be illustrated by several examples drawn from my own observations. Two such learning sequences in which I became particularly interested were what I came to call training for uncertainty and training for detached concern.[4]

Training for uncertainty consisted of the flow of medical school experiences that progressively taught students to perceive the uncertainties of medicine, to acknowledge some of their implications for the role of physician and the welfare of patients, and to cope with them. Students were confronted with three basic types of uncertainty as they advanced from one phase of the curriculum to another: (1) uncertainties that stem from the incomplete mastery of the vast and growing body of medical concepts, information, and skills; (2) those that come from limitations in current medical knowledge and techniques; and (3) the uncertainties that grow out of difficulties in distinguishing between personal ignorance or ineptitude and the open-ended, imperfect state of medical science, technology, and art.

In the preclinical years, gross anatomy, the first and most massive course that students experienced, played an important role in confronting them with the realization that no matter how well informed or skilled they might become, their mastery of all that is known in medicine would never be complete. For, over the centuries, this field has gradually traced out what students described as nothing less than the "blueprint of the body." The "huge body of [anatomical] facts" symbolized for students the "enormity" of medicine and the impossibility of commanding it all. Pharmacology, which came later in the preclinical curriculum, significantly contributed to acquainting students with uncertainties that result from limitations in the current state of medical knowledge, rather than from their own inadequacies. The lack of a general theory of drug action that characterizes this science, along with the associated difficulties of predicting how individuals will respond to any given drug, dramatized for students the fact that "there are so many voids" in medical knowledge that the practice of medicine sometimes seems largely "a matter of conjuring . . . possibilities and probabilities."

The third kind of uncertainty, that of determining where personal limitations leave off and those of medical science and technique begin, became more salient for medical students at the end of their preclinical years in physical diagnosis. Here, as they learned examination, observational, and history-taking methods relevant to defining the nature of the patient's problem, students were acutely faced with difficulties in ascertaining how much of their "trouble . . . hearing, feeling or seeing [was] personal," and how much of it had to do with "factors outside of themselves," with "the fault of the field, so to speak."

The range of course-related experiences bearing upon students' training for uncertainty was as broad as it was systematic. Throughout the curriculum, students were recurrently exposed to experiences that contributed to this aspect of the attitude learning they underwent. In the clinical years, for example, the several forms of medical uncertainty to which they were subject were compounded for them by their contact with patients and by their developing sense of professional responsibility. As students' awareness of the imminence of their doctorhood grew, their obligation to "know enough to do justice to [their] patients" also increased. And they came to regard "gaps in their knowledge" or "unsureness" on their part as more serious than in earlier stages of their training.

One of the cardinal experiences that linked students' training for uncertainty in the preclinical and clinical years were the various contexts and guises in which they faced death. These included dissecting a human cadaver in anatomy, witnessing and contributing to the death of some of the laboratory animals on which students worked in their basic science courses, observing the conduct of autopsies, and meeting terminally ill and dying patients. Students were astonished and disquieted to learn that although death is an ultimate and finite certainty for human beings as for all living creatures, it is also more ambiguous and more mysterious than they had supposed. Whether death will occur in a given case, when it will come to pass, what causes it, and why it happens, students discovered, are all questions that in many instances cannot be easily or categorically answered. Furthermore, they began to see that the relationship between the physician's knowledgeable and skillful intervention in a patient's condition and his ability to forestall or prevent that patient's death is more tenuous than they had assumed.

There was a structured discontinuity in students' experiences during the preclinical and clinical years that also significantly contributed to their training for uncertainty. The ethos created by their instructors in the first two years of medical school were what students described as an "experimental" and "philosophy of doubting" point of view. Pervading the basic science teaching that they received was the "message" that an irreducible minimum of uncertainty is inherent in medicine, that uncertainty is "legitimate," as well as "inevitable," that it can be conducive to medical scientific creativity and progress, and that, in any case, it is best handled by openly facing up to it. In the clinical years, this systematic doubting continued. But, from their clinical instructors and from their patients, students now began to learn about some of the undesirable consequences of "doubting too much." However exquisitely aware the physician may be of the ambiguous and indeterminate aspects

of a case, students were made to realize, he (she) nonetheless must sufficiently commit himself to some tentative diagnostic and therapeutic
judgments so that he can act on behalf of his patient. And although patients may welcome the physician's willingness to admit his uncertainty
and that of the field, too great a display of unsureness may alarm them
or undermine their confidence and trust. These insights were gradually
assimilated and applied by students in their third and fourth years of
medical school so that, by the time they reached graduation, most had
achieved some balance between Hamlet-like doubting and its opposite
extreme, supercertitude.

The training for the detached concern dimension of students' attitude
learning unfolded with an equally impressive orderliness. What it entailed was progressively acquiring the ability to bring the objectivity and
empathy, the equanimity and compassion expected of physicians into a
supple balance with one another so that the care they rendered was at
once competent, clear-sighted, and humane. Over the course of the four
medical school years, students were recurrently involved in experiences
that had powerful implications for their training in detachment, concern, and the dynamic equilibrium between them. As with all medical
school sequences, it began in the anatomy laboratory, where students
were introduced simultaneously to the cadaver, death, nudity, anonymity,
and to both the obligation and prerogative to cut and explore the human
body. However potentially stressful these encounters were, as students
put it, the "very dead" appearance and texture of the cadaver helped to
shield them against the full emotional realization that the body on
which they were working was once a human being. Only when they dis-
sected the hands, face, and genitalia did the "humanness" of the cadaver
become acutely problematic for them. Students' scientific involvement
in learning anatomy and in performing well in the laboratory, their
teamwork, and the gallows humor in which they mutually engaged were
their chief ways of coping with the evocative aspects of dissecting a
cadaver.

From anatomy, students moved on to work with live laboratory animals in various of their preclinical courses. Both because students were
no longer working on the human form and because the anatomy laboratory had given them some emotional as well as technical preparation for
manipulating and cutting into a body, this set of experiences was not as
disturbing in certain regards as contact with the cadaver. At the same
time, students testified, the new experience that challenged their equanimity somewhat was the fact that, unlike the cadaver, these animals
were alive, moved, and bled and, as the euphemistic expression went,

were "sacrificed" as part of the process of training doctors. It is interesting that, in this sequence of laboratory exercises, students worked on cats before they carried out procedures on dogs. By and large, they found it emotionally more difficult to practice on dogs, attributing their sentiments to the fact that more of them had dogs than cats as pets to whom they had been attached. Although this arrangement made a great deal of socialization sense, its latent consequences were neither anticipated nor recognized by medical educators. The cats-before-dogs progression was an inadvertent by-product of purely technical, didactic decisions made by preclinical faculty.

In their second year of medical school, students underwent a major rite of passage experience that had great import for their training in detached concern. This was their first autopsy in their pathology course.[5] In many ways, students reported, the autopsy reminded them of the anatomy laboratory. But now, they found themselves simultaneously confronted with death as "recent life," as an ultimate certainty and an irreducible mystery, and with the chastening realization, as one of them put it, that "on the wards of learning" and throughout our professional careers "some of our patients will die." Despite the anticipatory socialization that they received through their prior work on the human cadaver and on live laboratory animals, students were profoundly affected by the autopsy. Once again, engrossment in the scientific, technical, and learning tasks at hand helped them to handle their feelings, along with their strong motivation to "do well" and "act professional." But in this setting, by tacit agreement ("unwritten law"), they dealt with their deepest emotions in mutual silence. ("You don't bare your heart about the autopsy. . . . You sort of sit on the lid of your feelings. . . .") This stood in sharp contrast to the easy verbalizing and vigorous discussing that generally characterized the student group and, particularly, to the counterphobic black humor that they used to cope with death in the anatomy laboratory.

Still later in the second year, in anticipation of the approaching clinical phase of their training, students began to try certain procedures on themselves and on their classmates. In some of their basic science courses and in physical diagnosis, for example, they became the subjects of urinalyses, glucose tolerance tests, capillary punctures, venipunctures, auscultation, percussion, blood pressure determinations, nose and throat swabs, fluoroscopy of the gastrointestinal tract, typhoid vaccinations, and of personal and psychiatric case histories. This phase of their experience and development was notable for the collective state of hypochondriasis that it elicited. The sociodynamics of this reaction were incisively analyzed by one student who explained, "We are now in the process of contracting the diseases we are studying, in order to develop emotional immunity to them."

The ultimate focus and raison d'être of the training in detached concern that students received was their relationship with patients. In a sense, the cadaver, the laboratory animals, the deceased person on the autopsy table, and the classmates on whom students worked were all "prepatients." It was not until the end of the second year, chiefly in physical diagnosis, that students began to have face-to-face contact with "real" patients. The process was very gradual, beginning with short, task-delimited, group visits to hospitalized patients, chaperoned by instructors. Gradually, these patient contacts were lengthened, came to include more interaction and responsibility, and were no longer flanked by supporting clusters of classmates and faculty supervisors. Finally, the day arrived when the medical student "soloed," taking a patient's entire medical history and carrying out a complete physical examination without the presence or aid of anyone else.

Certain aspects of the history and physical were particularly embarassing and emotion-laden experiences for students: for example taking a sexual history; examining a woman's breasts; doing a vaginal or pelvic examination; palpating a man's testicles or a person's abdomen; carrying out a rectal examination. These intimate and potentially erotic aspects of the clinical tasks they were learning to perform, along with "any very emotional reaction" by a patient were likely to be disturbing to students. For, at this point in their training, most students were struggling to manage their own overabundance of concerned feelings and to achieve greater detachment as they undertook their still very new, physician-like role.

The third and fourth years of medical school, the clinical phase, were organized around interviewing and examining patients. Although, with experience, students gained more skill and poise in these functions, particular kinds of patients were likely to make them feel anxious, frustrated, or sad. Sick children, psychiatric patients, alcoholics, hostile, "uncooperative" patients, the elderly, and dying patients confronted students with problems of suffering, vulnerability, competence, adequacy, mortality, and of meaning that challenged their equilibrium and control.

Somewhere in the course of the third year, students' difficulties in relating to patients shifted from what they had previously experienced as too much concern to that of too much detachment. They were no longer so preoccupied with how to manage superfluous emotion as they were troubled about what had happened to their former capacity to respond feelingly to patients and their predicaments. This was a period that students apprehensively described as a time of "emotional numbness." In part, they were taking note of a degree of overdeterminism in the greater capacity for detachment that their medical training seemed to have instilled in them. But this was a temporary socialization phase. By the time students reached their senior year, they had progressed beyond this hyperdetachment to a new level of integration that enabled them to more effectively blend objectivity and equipoise with compassionate concern.

IV

There were at least three fundamental differences in the studies of medical socialization conducted in the 1950s. Some of the inquiries were more psychodynamically than sociologically oriented, emphasizing the personal development of medical students, the impact of their medical school experiences on them as individuals, and the inner or unconscious meaning of those experiences.[6] A second major difference in the studies of the 1950s has been the subject of commentary and debate in the social science literature. Whereas Columbia University sociologists viewed the medical school as training "student-physicians," University of Chicago sociologists saw it as training "boys in white." The Columbia group was impressed with the extent to which the medical school curriculum provided both latent and manifest forms of "anticipatory socialization" for values, attitudes, and behavior patterns relevant to the role of physician. In their view, medical school courses and experiences made up an ordered continuum that progressively moved students toward physicianhood, attitudinally, as well as intellectually and technically. In contrast, the Chicago group saw whatever socialization medical school effects as much more dissociated from becoming a physician and assuming the physicianly role. Rather, it seemed to them that the greater part of the training that students underwent in this respect entailed learning to adroitly play the *student* ("boy") role, so as to excel academically in ways that would enable them to master the vast amount of knowledge and technique they had to assimilate, earn them high grades, curry favor with their teachers, and make them eligible for the professionally critical reward of a "good internship." According to this perspective, becoming a physician in deeper, less expedient senses was almost a luxury that had to be postponed until the hurdle of medical school was successfully passed. And students neither were granted nor took the kind of

responsibility that made them feel successively more like physicians. As
the foregoing implies, unlike their Columbia colleagues, the Chicago
group was disinclined to argue that, below the surface of the students'
manifest learning experiences, a process of latent learning was shaping
their future attitudes and behavior as physicians. The utilitarian, achieve-
ment-oriented, competitive outlook and actions of the medical students
reported by the Chicago sociologists would have been interpreted by
the Columbia group as socialization for physicianhood and not just for
"studentry."

Whether the disparities in the Chicago and Columbia studies were
more a reflection of the divergent assumptions that the two groups
brought to their research or of the differences in the milieux of the
medical schools where they did their respective fieldwork has never been
resolved. Probably both sets of factors contributed to the "student-
physician" versus "boys-in-white" pictures of socialization that emerged
from their inquiries. The University of Kansas School of Medicine studied
by Chicago is a state-supported, midwestern institution that in the
1950s had a curriculum and an educational philosophy that were relatively traditional. Cornell University Medical College, where the major
part of the fieldwork for the Columbia study was conducted, is a private, ivy league school with a greater commitment than Kansas to educational experimentation and innovation. In addition, however, it could
be said that the implicit "world views" of the Chicago and Columbia
schools of sociology varied sufficiently to account for some of the differences in the ways that they perceived and reported the medical socialization process. This is made apparent by a third basic distinction
between the 1950s studies. The Chicago group, renowned for its firsthand work on the sociology of deviance and for its insights into "cool-
ing the mark" attitudes and behaviors, found evidence of these phenomena in the subculture of the medical students that they observed,
while the Columbia group did not. Furthermore, the Columbia study
described the self-regulating "little society" of medical students as a
straightforward, informal organization of peers that openly supported
and reinforced values and norms espoused by faculty as well as themselves. According to the Columbia observations, they had no "under-
cover" aspect to their group such as portrayed by the Chicago sociologists, who reported that the medical student world that they came to
know was one that presented a conformist public face to the faculty,
while, in private, students collectively believed in deviating from some
of the rigorous standards of excellence and etiquette that the faculty
expected them to meet.

V

These differences notwithstanding, the medical socialization studies of the 1950s were significantly alike in ways that reflected the perspective on becoming and being a doctor that medical educators, social scientists, and medical students shared in that decade. Attention was focused on students' interaction with their teachers, with patients, and with each other. Although their relationships with nonphysician members of the medical team were not ignored, they were subordinated to other aspects of students' role set. There was consensus that medical students formed a subculture that importantly influenced the direction and content of socialization. Peer relations were thus acknowledged as critical to nascent physicianhood and, by implication, to the practice of medicine by mature physicians. Teachers were viewed more as positive than as negative role models. But the sacred center and ultimate goal of medical education and socialization was taken to be the relationship that medical students learned to develop with patients. Ideally, it was supposed to combine high competence in the most advanced, specialized, and vigorous medical scientific treatment of the patient's problems with a comprehensive, humanistic approach to what was sloganistically called "the patient as a whole person." Medical practice was implicitly depicted as a chain of dyadic relationships between individual physicians and their individual patients. Teamwork with fellow physicians, nurses, social workers, and other medical and paramedical professionals was invoked, but there was virtually no reference to the medical care system as system, or as more than the sum of its interpersonal parts. The medical school was studied as a microcosm. Outside its doors lay the larger medical profession that it was training students to enter. Yet physicians, patients, and medical professionals whose trajectories extended beyond the medical school and university medical center were rarely seen, or merely glimpsed in passing. The organization of the medical profession was only occasionally mentioned. And even the social system of the medical school was examined in a selective way. Its academic structure was thoroughly explored, but its economic and political dimensions and their potential impact on the educational and socialization process were hardly considered.

The 1950s studies concentrated on certain attitude-learning sequences to which the medical school seemed to contribute. Training for uncertainty and limitation, training in detached concern, and training in teamwork have already been mentioned. In addition, training in the allocation and management of scare time was studied, not only for its own sake, but also as indicative of both the values and skills that students were acquiring. The so-called "fate of idealism"[7] was followed through medical school: that is, the process by which students came to temper their Olympian medical standards, their sense of calling, and their high commitment to the profession with "reality-situation" factors of which they progressively became aware. There was considerable interest in how students learned to deal with the competitive, achievement-and-success-oriented aspects of their medical school experiences, and with how they reconciled these self-interested aspects of their role with the disinterested professional obligation to be primarily concerned with the welfare of patients. Students' training for responsibility and their training in medical morality, rather specifically conceived, were other foci of attention.

An interesting common pattern that emerged from the 1950s studies was that a good deal of the socialization that took place in medical school seemed to entail the blending of counterattitudes: uncertainty with certainty, detachment with concern, idealism with realism, self- with other-orientation, and active responsibility and meliorism with humility and the ability to desist. Furthermore, each of the attitude-learning sequences traced out was characterized by a phase that generally occurred midway in the curriculum, when students seemed to have temporarily *over*learned one of a set of counterattitudes. Thus, at a certain point in their third year of medical school, for example, students were inclined to behave with exaggerated "certitude," often complained of feeling "emotionally numb," and appeared to be more "cynical" than "idealistic." Yet by the end of their fourth year these attitudes seemed to be more equitably balanced in what we earlier described as a dynamic equilibrium. It has not been determined whether this attitude-learning pattern is distinctive to medical education, or whether it is applicable to professional and adult socialization in other contexts as well. This is a question of potential basic and applied significance that merits further attention.

VI

Medical education and socialization in the 1970s are proceeding under circumstances that are markedly different from those of the 1950s. To begin with, as already stated, an unprecedented number of young men and women are now aspiring to the career of physician. Although the 1950s were marked by a post-World War II increase in applicants to medical school, what was then considered a "boom" period in this regard did not approach the ratio of at least three applicants for every one medical school place that characterizes the 1970s. At present, this tendency continues unabated and even appears to be gaining momentum. The attraction of so many young people to medicine is occurring at the same time that law schools are experiencing a comparable increase in applicants. This suggests that a more generalized movement toward the liberal professions may be taking place. Why this is happening, what attributes of medicine and law are motivating college students to try to gain entrance to a professional school, from what social backgrounds are these students being drawn are all questions that have not yet been systematically investigated.

There is a great deal of speculation among medical educators about whether the men and women now enrolled in a medical school or hoping to be accepted by one constitute a "new" type of medical student with different conceptions of the profession and their future roles in it than those of their predecessors. Those who contend that there is, indeed, a new medical student say that he (she) is socially concerned, critical of the way that health care is organized and delivered in American society (particularly to the disadvantaged), determined to practice a more equitable, feeling, and less driven medicine than his elders, and committed to actively reforming medicine in ways that he hopes will be ramified in nonmedical sectors of the society. Those who argue that the present generation of medical students is not really new in these or other respects tend to regard the social criticism and social commitment statements made by students as "rhetoric"—"ideology" that, however sincere, is ephemerally idealistic. What is more, these skeptical observers maintain, the students who articulate these new values are not representative of the present generation of medical students. They come from privileged backgrounds and attend certain elite eastern medical schools where they constitute a vociferous minority of the student body. Once again, the data needed to resolve the question, "Is there a 'new' medical student?" are lacking.[8] But those who believe and those who disbelieve in the existence and importance of the new medical student are reacting to the same phenomena of which they have mutually taken note. And it seems to us that medical students of the 1970s must be sufficiently different from those to whom medical educators were previously accustomed to have elicited all this discussion and controversy about them.

In addition to the fact that many more students are now applying to medical school than in the past and that numbers of those who are admitted begin their study of medicine with a "new" socially conscious and critical ideology, medical curricula have changed in ways that distinguish them from the programs of the 1950s.[9] Organized attempts have been taken to loosen and diversify the "lock-step" curriculum.

Both elective and free time have been expanded. Multiple "tracks" have been created so that there now exist a number of patterns in which students can proceed through medical school in accordance with their present interests and future career plans. Combined M.D.-Ph.D. programs have been created that allow students to broaden, intensify, and accelerate their competence in a variety of medically related fields. The course of studies is no longer sharply dichotomized into preclinical and clinical years. Rather, a required "core curriculum" has been instituted, which from the first medical school year on tries to integrate the various basic sciences with each other and with clinical training. Numerous medical schools have been experimenting with ways to shorten the duration of professional training. Chiefly, these take the form of selectively granting students early admission or advanced placement, making it possible for them to complete the medical curriculum in three years, and eliminating required internships in some fields. Medical school departments and programs of community medicine, social medicine, preventive medicine, and family medicine have been created. Students have been given opportunities for fieldwork and practicum experiences outside the walls of academic medical centers. The aim here has been to acquaint them with more than "ivory tower" medicine, to familiarize them with the health and medical care delivery problems of disadvantaged groups in the society, and to develop their general ability to think of health, illness, and care in a social system framework. (It is interesting to note that some of these extramural experiences were originally sought out or created by students and subsequently accepted for credit by faculty.) Greater emphasis has been placed on the relevance of behavioral science training to physicians' collective ability to improve the health care system, as well as to their development as humanely competent individual practitioners. Courses and even programs in medical ethics have been launched by medical schools throughout the country. These courses go beyond the "do's and don'ts of doctorhood" to consider the ethical component in medical decision making and to ponder such questions as "death and dying" and the moral and metaphysical implications of particular biomedical advances. Along with all these other changes, many medical schools have replaced their traditional "A through F" grading systems with a "pass–fail"-type of evaluation. And an increasing number of medical schools have been making concerted efforts both to recruit and admit more minority group students (especially nonwhite, nonaffluent, and women students) to training for physicianhood.

These sorts of modification of the curriculum and ethos of medical schools have all come about in the past decade. They constitute a set of educational arrangements and perspectives that grow largely out of the

criticism and self-criticism to which the American medical profession
and health care system have been subject in recent years. In turn, these
alterations and the inner and outer pressures that have helped to produce
them are part of a much broader process of social and cultural change
that surfaced in the 1960s and continues to the present. During this
period, medical schools, like many other institutions, have been questioned, challenged, and reproached. Various medical, professional, student, government, patient, and community groups have held them responsible for the fact that many of the physicians they have trained have
practiced medicine in ways that have contributed to the keenly felt problems with which the American medical system is currently faced. The
innovations in medical school curricula already described represent *ad
hoc* organized attempts to meet this criticism. Medical educators have
introduced these changes on the assumption that they may influence
physicians-in-becoming to participate actively in the development of a
high quality, reasonably priced national system of health care that is
more equitably distributed, accessible, universalistic, socially aware, and
humane.

More explicitly than in the 1950s, then, the new curriculum is premised on the notion that medical education not only affects the outlook
and comportment of individual physicians but also the attributes of the
profession and the contours of the larger medical system of which doctors are unitary parts. In this respect, the present generation of medical
educators has high "socialization consciousness." Yet, there are several
anomalous features that characterize their view of professional socialization that would seem to belie such an allegation. As mentioned earlier,
by and large the evaluations of what impact curriculum changes have
had on students that medical schools are now conducting do not include
attempts systematically to appraise attitude learning. Rather, the tendency is to measure the amount and quality of cognitive learning that is
taking place, chiefly in the form of National Board Examination scores,
and to ascertain what aspects of particular courses students and faculty
like and dislike. They are not exploring the following sorts of questions.
Does the supposedly less invidious pass–fail grading system actually
quell acquisitively competitive tendencies in students? What effect does
it have on students to be alternately dissecting a cadaver in the anatomy
laboratory and seeing gravely ill patients in the hospital during their first
medical school year, instead of having these two sets of experiences
separated in time from one another as they were in the traditional curriculum? Does the increased contact with poor and deprived patients
now provided strengthen students' belief that, as physicians, they
should and can do something to improve such persons' health and the

medical care they receive, or does it discourage and dissuade them from this conviction? Does the core curriculum–multitrack educational sequence result in as coherent and cumulative a socialization process as the one that existed in the 1950s? Are there any discernible subpatterns in the more diversified effects that the curriculum can be expected to have on students now that it is not as monolithic as it was formerly? Does the increased individuation of course work and medical school experiences that is permitted and fostered by the curriculum reduce the socialization role played by the corporate student peer group? If so, what are the intellectual and psychosocial consequences of such a change in students' role set?

Along with their failure to inquire into such matters, medical educators seem more reluctant than they were in the past to verbally admit that what they teach significantly shapes attitudes as well as conveys knowledge and that these attitudes may have long-range implications for how students will enact the role of physician. Medical educators proceed on this supposition in their daily rounds and in their curriculum planning as we have seen. But they are inclined to disavow that they really believe this when they are called on to discuss their sentiments and convictions about professional education.[10] The source of such faculty ambivalence about the socialization dimension of the medical educational process is not easy to identify. It is almost as if medical faculty members were protecting themselves against being held too accountable for whatever the beliefs, attitudes, and conduct of the new generation of physicians may turn out to be. This stance may be a defense mechanism to which medical (and other) educators have resorted in an era when they have been continuously subject to criticism concerning the social attitudes that they do and do not successfully convey. It may also be a way of implicitly acknowledging that a perplexing "generation gap" exists between them and their students for which they cannot thoroughly account and do not wish to be held largely responsible.

Medical students' attitudes toward their own professional socialization seems more ambivalent than those of their instructors. Many students begin their medical school training with the determined hope that it will not transform them into the kinds of persons and physicians that they are trying not to become. As compared with their counterparts in the 1950s, students now tend to view their teachers as negative role models, not necessarily with rancor or disesteem but more as a symbolic expression of their resolve to be "different," "better," more socially responsible physicians than the medical "establishment" with which they identify their instructors. From the outset, however, students are convinced that "The System" the medical school both represents and comprises is seductive and powerful. In their eyes, it has the insidious capacity to change them into what they are resolved not to be. When asked to predict what effect they think their medical education will ultimately have on them, they are inclined to the opinion that, both because of the forcefulness of the system and their own potential pliancy in the face of it, they are likely to end up replicating the past generation's professional attitudes, behavior, and even their personal style of life.[11]

Thus, in the medical school climate of the 1970s, change-oriented students, who are persuaded that the latent socializing impact of their professional education is subtly but irresistibly converting them to the status quo, meet faculty members who deny that medical education per se has potent socializing effects but who have nonetheless altered the traditional curriculum in order to better train young physicians, attitudinally as well as intellectually, to tackle the health care and medical services delivery problems now facing the profession and the society. Complicating the socialization picture further are the attitudes expressed by some of the social scientists with whom medical faculty and students have conferred about the present and future education of physicians. As already noted, no studies of medical socialization of the magnitude of "boys in white" and "student-physician" are currently in progress. In our opinion, this is as much a consequence of social scientists' brand of ambivalence toward the socialization process as it is a question of medical schools' receptivity to such undertakings or availability of funds to carry them out. In recent years, for example, several prominent sociologists of medicine have become critical of the importance that they and their colleagues formerly attached to medical education and socialization. They now contend that the physician's "immediate work environment,"[12] the "exigencies. . .and realities of practice,"[13] are more significant determinants of the way a man or woman performs in the physician's role than the anticipatory socialization that medical schools supposedly provide. Partly for this reason, they are not enthusiastic about launching studies of becoming a physician in the 1970s and are even less disposed to cast them in the conceptual framework of the 1950s. Insofar as they would be at all willing to conduct research in medical school rather than in medical practice settings, these sociologists would lay greater stress on studying the faculty, the social organization of the medical school, and especially its organization of power than on inquiring into student attitudes, experiences, and culture.[14] They seem to be more interested in political and economic facets of the medical school than sociologists were in the 1950s and more intent on doing research that will have policy implications. One detects in their orientation a certain undercurrent of disappointment over the fact that the sociology of medical school inquiries carried out 20 years ago did not lead to reforms in the educational process that significantly improved the way that medicine is organized and practiced in our society. These activist yearnings and regrets on the part of sociologists, along with their increased social structural determinism, are not conducive to their undertaking studies of medical socialization in the 1970s.[15]

Meanwhile, a new generation of students is passing through a greatly changed medical school en route to becoming physicians. We know remarkably little about these students, or about the impress that their medical education is making on them. Yet, at present, a number of medical schools are considering "rolling back" certain of the curriculum reforms of the 1960s on the grounds that they have already had some undesirable consequences for the intellectual and attitude learning of medical students.[16] Is this an accurate diagnosis and an appropriate set of responses to it? Will such revisions become widespread and, if so, will they usher in a state of retrenchment in the medical profession and the process of being educated and socialized for it? There is little data on such matters either available or being collected.

VII

By way of conclusion, I would like to essay a portrait of the "new" medical student based on my observations and constructed out of my field notes.[17] Whether such students exist in significant numbers, what role the medical school relative to other institutions is playing in their development, and what effect their graduation into physicianhood will have on the medical profession are questions to which there are as yet no valid or reliable answers.

Despite the efforts being made to recruit young persons into medical school from minority groups and nonprivileged social class backgrounds, the new medical student is still likely to be a white, middle-class man. He arrives in medical school garbed as he was in college, in blue jeans or modishly colored sports slacks and tieless shirt. His hair is long, though usually not unkempt, and he may have grown a moderate beard. When he begins to see patients, he often starts wearing a tie and sometimes a jacket. He may also cut his hair on the short side of long and shave more closely.

Although he is fiercely intent on being accepted by a medical school, unlike his counterparts in the 1950s, the new medical student is generally a "late decider." It is not uncommon for him to have committed himself to becoming a doctor in the second half of his college career. Because of his "delayed" decision, he may have had to take his premedical courses in summer school or in a concentrated postundergraduate year. In any case, he worked hard and competitively as a college student in order to earn the very high grade point average that made him eligible for admission to medical school. Although aggressively achievement oriented, he deplores it in himself, his classmates, his teachers, the medical profession, his parents, and in American society more generally. As engaged as he is by medicine, he wonders continually whether it is really his "vocation." The "on-call 24 hours a day" demands associated with the traditions and responsibilities of many branches of medicine contribute to these doubts. For he is concerned about what this kind of relentlessness may do to his person, his relationships to patients and colleagues, his family life, and to his capacity to participate in cultural, civic, and recreational activities that he considers healthy and humanizing, as well as pleasurable.

Such a student is likely to have come to medical school with declared interests in fields like community medicine, public health, family medicine, psychiatry, and pediatrics (pediatrics, he feels obliged to explain, because it is "holistic" medicine and entails caring for "new and future generations"). In the end, these may not be the fields that he will actually enter. But they express the interpersonal, moral, and societal perspective on physicianhood that he brings with him from college. He is actively committed to such humane and social goals as peace, the furtherance of civil rights, the reduction of poverty, the protection of the environment, population control, and improvement in the "quality of life" for all. He extends the principles that underlie these commitments to medicine and the role of doctor. In his view, health and health care are fundamental rights that ought to be as equitably distributed as possible. For this reason, as he sees it, the physician should care for the psychological and social, as well as physical, aspects of his patient's illness. He should have a "genuine concern for the total health of mankind." He should take initiative in dealing with some of the factors at work in the society that adversely affect health and keep the medical care system from functioning optimally to maintain and restore it. Although the doctor's social dedication should be universalistic, the new student believes, he has special obligations to those who are disadvantaged or deprived.

The new medical student is also staunchly egalitarian in his conception of the doctor, the doctor's relationship to patients, and to nonphysician members of the medical team. The student disapproves of "all-knowing" or "omnipotent" attitudes and behavior on the part of physicians. ("The doctor is not a king. . .a high priest. . .or a technological master who can control or dominate all.") He maintains that physicians should approach patients "as human beings" with "respect for their feelings and opinions," rather than as "diseased specimens," or persons incapable of understanding their own medical condition and the treatment prescribed for it. Ideally, a collegial, "nonauthoritarian" relationship with patients ought to be developed, one that is "honest," "open," and nonmanipulative. ("The physician should reach people through conversation that is not like that of a salesman. . . . He should have open communication with patients. . .and hide as little as possible from them.") "Integrity" that is emotional and moral, as well as intellectual, is basic to this relationship too. It entails more than being honest and consistent in what one says and does. It is actively critical and self-critical, involving the "questioning of self, colleagues, teachers, physicians and the intentions of the institution."

A "detached concern" model of relating to patients is not one that the new medical student admires or would like to exemplify. Rather, he places the highest value on feeling with the patient. Although he recognizes the need for maintaining some objectivity in this relationship, he does so with regret. For him, to feel is to be human and compassionate; it dignifies and heals; and the more one feels, the better. However scientifically and intellectually inclined he may be, the student believes that it is all too easy to distance one's self from patients (and from one's own humanity) by approaching the problems for which they seek the doctor's aid in an overly conceptual and technical way. He considers "direct experience," or what one student calls "phenomenological contact," to be the method *par excellence* by which the physician should learn and come to understand. It allows him to maintain close contact with patients and "reality," and also to seek knowledge and truth that go beyond the passive acceptance and mastery of what is handed down to him by past generations. ("We are experiencing physical diagnosis in relative virginity. . . .We still don't know the 'rules of the game' and are therefore likely to violate them in worthwhile ways.")

Finally, although the new medical student would not downgrade the importance of training, knowledge, skill, and experience for competent physicianhood, he also insists that the doctor's values, beliefs, and commitments are a critical part of his ability to help patients, reform the health care system and "improve society." ("Ethical, moral and social issues are a base on which a superstructure of scientific knowledge should be built, rather than the over-Flexnerian tradition in which scientific schema formed the base. . . .") And so, the physician must be more than just a "good human being." He must also concern himself with the "philosophical" problems of life and death, suffering and evil, justice and equity, human solidarity and ultimate meaning in which his chosen profession and the human condition are grounded.[18]

This is the simultaneously critical, activist, and meditative ideology or world view that the new student brings to medical school. How predominant it is, whether it will prevail, and whether in interaction with the medical school environment and the social climate of the seventies it will produce a new type of physician will be revealed in time, the professional socialization process, and, perhaps, studies of it.

REFERENCES AND NOTES

1. Major publications based on these studies include Becker HS, Geer B, Hughes EC, Strauss AL: Boys in White: Student Culture in Medical School. Chicago, University of Chicago Press, 1961; Hammond KR, Kern F, Jr: Teaching Comprehensive Medical Care. Cambridge, Harvard University Press, for the Commonwealth Fund, 1959; Horowitz MJ: Educating Tomorrow's Doctors. New York, Appleton-Century-Crofts, 1964; Merton RK, Reader G, Kendall PL (ed): The Student–Physician: Introductory Studies in the Sociology of Medical Education. Cambridge, Harvard University Press, for the Commonwealth Fund, 1957; Miller GE: Teaching and Learning in Medical School. Cambridge, Harvard University Press, for the Commonwealth Fund, 1961. In addition, at least two major books on the house officership phase of medical training came out of that period: Miller SJ: Prescription for Leadership: Training for the Medical Elite. Chicago, Aldine Publishing Co., 1970; Mumford E: Interns: From Students to Physicians. Cambridge, Harvard University Press, for the Commonwealth Fund, 1970. For a state of the field review of these and other sociology of medical education studies, see Bloom SW: The sociology of medical education: some comments on the state of the field. Milbank Mem Fund Q 43(2):143–184, 1965.
2. For a sample of the questionnaire and a discussion of how it was developed and administered, see Merton RK, et al. (ed): *op. cit.*, Appendix D, pp 307–351.
3. As the citations listed under note 1 suggest, many of these experiments in medical education, and the studies that described, analyzed, and attempted to evaluate them, were sponsored by the Commonwealth Fund.
4. See Fox RC: Training for uncertainty, in RK Merton, et al. (ed): *op. cit.*, pp 207–241; Lief HI, Fox RC: The medical student's training for "detached concern," The Psychological Basis of Medical Practice. Edited by HI Lief, VF Lief, NR Lief. New York, Harper & Row, 1963, pp 12–35.
5. See Fox RC: The autopsy: its place in the attitude-learning of second-year medical students. Although this paper, written in 1958, has never been published, it has had wide, informal circulation; available from author.
6. Notable among these are the studies carried out by Daniel H. Funkenstein and Harold I. Lief, as well as Milton J. Horowitz's *Educating Tomorrow's Doctors* already mentioned. See, for example, Funkenstein DH: Medical students, medical schools, and society during three eras, Psychosocial Aspects of Medical Training. Edited by RH Coombs, CE Vincent. Springfield, Ill., Charles C Thomas, 1971, pp 229–281; Funkenstein DH: The learning and personal development of medical students: reconsidered. New Phys 19: 740–755, 1970; Lief HI, et al.: A psychodynamic study of medical students and their adaptional problems: preliminary report. J Med Educ 35:696–704, 1960.
7. Becker HS: The fate of idealism in medical school. Am Sociolog Rev 23:50–56, 1958.

8. Daniel H. Funkenstein is virtually singular in providing data supporting the contention that a "new breed" of what he calls "community era" medical students has emerged, and "first became the majority of an entering class in the Harvard Medical School in 1968." See Funkenstein DH: Medical students, medical schools, and society during three eras, Psychosocial Aspects of Medical Training. Edited by RH Coombs, CE Vincent. Springfield, Ill., Charles C Thomas, 1971, pp 229–281.

9. For a useful summary of the major characteristics of these curriculum changes, and also some speculative comments on the new medical student, see Thorne B: Professional education in medicine, Education for the Professions of Medicine, Law, Theology, and Social Welfare. Edited by EC Hughes, B Thorne, AM DeBaggis, A Gurin, D Williams. A report prepared for The Carnegie Commission on Higher Education. New York, McGraw-Hill, 1973, pp 17–99.

10. In the way of an illustrative anecdote, at a recent dinner discussion meeting about premedical and medical education at the University of Pennsylvania, all the medical faculty members present heartily agreed with a professor of religion who affirmed that it was "too messianic to believe that education forms moral character."

11. It would be interesting to explore the psychodynamic as well as social reasons for which this generation of medical students feels so malleable in the face of what they conceive to be "the system." This is the kind of question that lends itself to an Erik Erikson type analysis.

12. See, for example, Freidson E: The Profession of Medicine. New York, Dodd, Mead & Company, 1970, p 89.

13. Freidson E: Professional Dominance: The Social Structure of Medical Care. New York, Aldine-Atherton Press, 1970, pp 17–18.

14. These sentiments were forcefully and recurrently expressed by the social scientists who participated in a 2-day meeting on medical education research convened by the National Center for Health Services Research and Development, of the Department of Health, Education, and Welfare, and held on November 22 and 23, 1971, in Rockville, Maryland. A verbatim transcript of these sessions exists. All of us who participated in these meetings are particularly indebted to Drs. Arthur J. Barsky III, Ralph B. Freidin, and David M. Levine who organized them.

15. Perhaps a personal announcement is not inappropriate here. Diana Crane and Frank Furstenberg, members of the Department of Sociology at the University of Pennsylvania, and I are currently working on a proposal to study the process of becoming a physician in the 1970s (which is cross-cultural as well as comparative with training for the law), and that we will prove an exception to this regrettable trend.

16. See, Goldhaber SZ: Medical education: Harvard reverts to tradition. Science 181: 1027–1032, 1973. Although this article somewhat simplifies and exaggerates the "strong trend toward retrenchment and reinstating the traditional educational system" at Yale as well as Harvard, it is nevertheless a significant and perhaps even a premonitory piece.

17. All the quotations in the "portrait" that follows are taken from verbatim spoken or written comments made by medical students.

18. Parsons T, Fox RC, Lidz VM: The "gift of life" and its reciprocation. Soc Res 39(3):405–410, 1972.

ROGER J. BULGER, M.D.
Executive Officer, Institute of Medicine

Commentary

It is, of course, to some degree presumptuous for a physician to be commenting on a distinguished sociologist's analysis of the socialization of student-physicians as they proceed through medical school. As one of those students who had the medical school experience in the 1950s, I was intrigued by Professor Fox's summarization of her own and others' studies of that era. I found particularly illuminating and insightful Professor Fox's discussions of those learning sequences she calls "training for uncertainty" and "training for detached concern." My only difficulty is in being able to accept wholeheartedly what I take to be her conclusions that, in each of these two particular instances, students generally came out very well:

- [In training for uncertainty,] insights were gradually assimilated and applied by students in their third and fourth years of medical schools, so that by the time they reached graduation, most had achieved some balance between Hamlet-like doubting and its opposite extreme, supercertitude.
- The training for the detached concern dimension of students' attitude learning unfolded with an equally impressive orderliness. What it entailed was progressively acquiring the ability to bring the objectivity and empathy, the equanimity and compassion expected of physicians into a supple balance with one another so that the care they rendered was at once competent, clear-sighted, and humane.

221

Since my doubts on these points are subjective, I bow to Professor Fox
who has wide experience and data to support her views, but I cannot
do so without expressing the fear that, in jettisoning the curriculum of
the 1950s that could accomplish such excellent attitude learning, we
may have thrown at least a part of the baby out with the bath water.

As Professor Fox points out, analyses of medical education of the
1970s with regard to attitude learning are, of necessity, highly subjective
and speculative because of the unfortunate dearth of proper evaluative
studies. Therefore, I feel a little freer to speculate with her about these
matters. As I see it, there are several major elements to the confusing
picture we see in this country at this time.

First, very few faculties of medical schools have defined what attitudes
they would like to teach, much less to consider how best to teach them.
Second, curricula are so varied from school to school that studies carried
out in one institution are likely to be of dubious relevance in most
others. Third, the nature of the faculty of the 1970s is probably quite
different from that of the 1950s and is quite at variance with the value
sets likely to be seen as desirable for service-oriented practitioners.
Fourth, similar comments can be made about some medical school administrative practices and organization. Fifth, the curriculum pressures force
college and medical students into an intensive competition for competence
and achievement in the biomedical sciences.

The problem of explicit articulation of behavior and attitude objectives is a complex one, and the implication I would least like to leave behind is that I think it is possible at this time to delineate a detailed set of
such objectives that would find universal acceptance in schools across the
country. Quite to the contrary, I believe that each school should try to
establish its own set of objectives in this area and that the likely outcome
of such a universal effort would be an extraordinary variety of content.
The only requisites in my view are that each institution should try it and
that significant consideration be given in the effort to lay opinion.

For example, one can envisage some statements based on the Hippocratic Oath that speak to attitudes toward learning and human values
that might be appropriately fostered by more free time, flexibility, and
multitrack curricula. One can imagine that other institutions might focus
on meeting certain manpower needs, such as more primary physicians.
Still other institutions, like the Abraham Lincoln School of Medicine in
Chicago, might undertake a rather impressive and comprehensive delinea-
tion of habits and attributes it deems desirable in its graduates.[1] Finally,
the likes of Ed Pellegrino,[2] George Engel,[3] Kerr White,[4] and Richard
Magraw[5] would most likely prefer a more searching analysis and understanding of the patient–physician transaction, including, of course, an

assumption that transaction in and of itself has great therapeutic possibilities on the one hand and significant counterproductive potential on the other. Such people would emphasize, I believe, that the physician must be a continuing, life-long expert in and student of the nature and ethics of that transaction.

In other settings, statements of objectives might pattern themselves after the structuring presented earlier by Jonson and Hellegers, addressing the virtues, duties, and societal responsibilities of the physician. Dr. Redlich[6] last year presented an interesting list of virtues for an ideal physician; these included (1) knowledge and competence, (2) helpfulness, (3) professional empathy, (4) cleanliness, (5) parsimony, (6) responsibility, punctuality, and reliability, and (7) courage. (I presume he assumed honesty.) It is of interest in this regard to consider what William Osler,[7] in many ways the father of modern American medicine, said some 70 years ago:

In these days of aggressive self-assertion, when the stress of competition is so keen and the desire to make the most of oneself so universal, I may seem a little old-fashioned to preach the necessity of humility; but I insist for its own sake and for the sake of what it brings, that *due humility* should take the place of honor in the list. For its own sake, since with it comes not only a reverence for truth, but also a proper estimation of the difficulties encountered in our search for it. More perhaps than any other professional person, the doctor has a curious, shall I say morbid? sensitiveness to (what he regards) personal error. In a way this is right; but it is too often accompanied by a cocksuredness of opinion which, if encouraged, leads him to so lively a conceit that the mere suggestion of a mistake under any circumstances is regarded as a reflection on his honor, a reflection equally resented, whether of lay or professional origin. Start out with the conviction that absolute truth is hard to reach in matters relating to our fellow creatures, healthy or diseased, that slips in observation are inevitable, even with the best trained faculties, that errors in judgment must occur in the practice of an art which consists largely in balancing possibilities—start, I say, with this in mind, and mistakes will be acknowledged and regretted; but instead of a slow process of self-deception, with ever increasing inability to recognize truth, you will draw from your errors the very lessons which will enable you to avoid their repetition.

Lastly, in some institutions, an attempt might be made to delineate some differences in socialization objectives among groups of physicians, e.g., primary care physicians, medical specialists, clinical investigators, and basic biomedical scientists.

Whatever the ultimate shape and content of a given institution's "socialization" objectives, such an effort must be subject to constant scrutiny and review. It is only through this effort at stating objectives that a school can attempt to bring its students' values into more appro-

priate consonance with those of society. Thus, the faculty must come
to understand that its curriculum's objectives should and will be affected
by societal shifts in attitudes or values; the faculty will need to appreci-
ate such shifts and their impact on the appropriateness and relevance for
the future of any given stated socialization objective. In a more ideal
world, then, the schools will be good at understanding what is going on
around them.

The problem of curriculum variability from school to school will, I
believe, be a major stumbling block to any evaluation of the socialization
process. It may be fairly easy to determine that a new curriculum has
changed the learning sequences in certain specific ways from that of the
1950s; but it will not be so easy to determine from the outside which
curricula are attempts at repackaging the old product in new wrappers
versus those that are truly innovative and creative. In one school, for
the past five years, the first-year students have had all their mornings
entirely free of required courses in order to encourage them to participate more fully in the intellectual life of the rest of the university. A
symbolic bridge exists across the road that separates the health sciences
from the rest of the university campus. Despite this, however, only four
students from the medical school crossed that bridge to sign up for a
grand total of five courses during the five-year period; the remainder of
the students spent their elective time at the medical school trying to
pick up, according to individual needs, some of the material that had
been excised from the old required curriculum. How can one compare
this kind of curricular approach to the one, for example, at Penn State
where a department of the humanities has been created that participates
fully in the curriculum and in the life of the school generally?

Another sort of difficulty for the evaluating sociologist can be exem-
plified by the family practice phenomenon. It has been legislated in
many states that there be created departments of family practice, and,
in response to such legislation, it is hardly an understatement to indicate
that compliance was obtained with differing degrees of institutional enthusiasm. Some schools' responses seem analagous to the man Abraham
Lincoln used to tell about who was to be tarred and feathered and run
out of town on a rail, and said, "Folks, if it weren't for the honor of the
thing I'd just as soon pass up this affair." Thus in some institutions the
letter of the law has been adhered to but perhaps not the spirit, and it
would be of interest to identify such schools and the outcomes of their
programs. In others, rather major and sweeping curricular and administrative changes have been made to pave the way for a more wholehearted
institutional effort at developing a family practice program.

At one such place with which I am familiar, the administration took the leadership in designing, building, organizing, and staffing a clinic within the university hospital especially geared to the teaching of primary care. Special efforts were made to cultivate and sensitize department chairmen and other faculty so that, when the time came for the program to begin, admission of family practice patients to the university hospital, surgical, orthopedic, and obstetrical prerogatives were all worked out relatively easily. In every way possible the family practice faculty became equal and respected partners in the school's machinery. The curriculum tracks were established to include one in family practice. The results over the past five years indicate that from 35 to 40 percent of students are going into primary care and that this group includes many of the students with the best academic records. There is an impression, but no data, that the existence of a respected faculty and a group of happy, competent family practice students and residents within the medical school structure is serving to have its own "socializing" effects on the others. These things it seems to me need to be studied.

The nature of the medical faculty of the 1970s is surely different from that of the antecedent generation. Although it is reassuring to have Professor Fox indicate that we are more sensitive now to the fact that socialization occurs through medical education, it seems quite likely that the attitude profiles of the modern faculty will be at variance with what the students want to become on the one hand and what the public might want the students to become on the other. My speculation is that studies would show that the faculty of the 1970s is full-time and predominantly research oriented, having grown up in a tertiary care, specialist-dominated, intellectual elite setting. Further, I believe that such studies would show that the successful, modern faculty member is by nature entrepreneurial, competitive, "cure" rather than "care" oriented, and would tend not to understand, believe in, or give much weight to such concepts as the following: (1) the patient–physician interaction as a therapeutic device in and of itself; (2) the faculty role model function; and (3) the analogy that, in my experience, seems not to escape the students that the faculty-student relationship has aspects that are transferable or are transferred to the physician–patient relationship.

None of this is said in a critical or pejorative sense, nor should it imply that the faculties must be by-passed or dismissed à la Chairman Mao and his cultural revolution in attempting to achieve socialization objectives. Rather, I think it underscores the need for studies of their characteristics and for overt attempts to establish socialization objectives, so that faculties can begin to review their behavior in light of new information about themselves and what they want at least some of their students to be.

Finally, there is the effect of the growing number of qualified, clamor-

ing candidates for entrance to medical school and the forces calling for
a decrease in the length of the training period, an increase in curricular
flexibility and free elective time, while at the same time a maintenance
of high quality and an active exploration of new, quite untried curricular
forms. There seems little question that all this puts enormous pressure on
college and medical students to spend every available moment developing
their scientific and technical competencies with the tendency always to
leave other interests for another time. I think the data support the view
that over the last decade there has been no increase in the small minority
of college students concentrating in the liberal arts who gain admittance
to medical school. Without belaboring this issue, it seems highly likely to
me that there would be an obvious, serious dysjunction between what
socialization objectives might be for a service-oriented primary care physician and the pressures and values inherent in the educational obstacle
courses students are made to negotiate on the road to their license to
practice.

One final comment concerning the excellent section on the modern
student by Professor Fox. After reading it, one's first reaction is that the
world will be in good hands at last. I, however, believe there is still something for such students to reflect upon. The question is raised by another
sociologist, David Riesman,[8] in discussing the modern Harvard College
undergraduate:

They want to be of use, they want to be needed. I think that's a general proposition
about people. But at its most extreme, service to mankind is paradoxical—you know,
love mankind, but hate patients. They want to be concerned with the distribution of
medical care, but daily patient care? That's a less attractive prospect.

In summary, I would like to support wholeheartedly Professor Fox's
call for intense evaluation of the effect of the medical school curriculum
of the 1970s on the behavior patterns and attitudes of the students. I
believe, however, that such an evaluation will be most useful if the effort
coincides with an attempt to establish in each school explicit behavioral
and attitudinal objectives for the curriculum. Furthermore, it seems that
studies of curriculum effect on attitude learning will be incomplete if
not accompanied by and correlated to intensive investigation into faculty
attitudes and behavior. Studies structured similarly to those of the 1950s
will yield most interesting comparative data, but I believe the sociological
evaluation can gain additional relevance if this is done in the context of
explicit institutional goals, which for most schools remain to be developed.
It seems high time that medical educators formally recognized that the
curriculum design and its implementation have as major an impact on
the socialization of the student as they have on the cognitive elements he

or she absorbs. Until carefully considered, socialization objectives are articulated for the curriculum, and unless attempts are made to modify the curriculum, as well as faculty and administrative behavior in order to better support these objectives, the educational process will be mindlessly and almost randomly determining the outcome, at least in this major area of professional education. We are not likely to see this kind of activity develop on a universal basis until school accrediting agencies make such socialization curricular objectives a part of the accrediting guidelines.

REFERENCES

1. Curriculum of the Abraham Lincoln School of Medicine of the Illinois College of Medicine. Chicago, University of Illinois College of Medicine, 1972, pp 22-25.
2. Pellegrino ED: comments on Government Decision Making and the Preciousness of Life by K Arrow, this volume.
3. Engel GL: The best and the brightest. The missing dimension in medical education. Pharos, Oct 1973, pp 129-133.
4. White KL: Life and death and medicine. Sci Am 229:22-33, 1973.
5. Magraw RM: Social and medical contracts: explicit and implicit. What is medical care?, Hippocrates Revisited. Edited by R Bulger. New York, Medcom Press, 1973, pp 148-157.
6. Redlich F: Talk presented at Institute of Medicine Spring Meeting, Washington, D.C., May 10, 1973.
7. Osler W: Teacher and student, Aequanimitas. Philadelphia, P. Blakiston's Son & Co., 1932, p 38.
8. Reisman D: Quoted in What's happened to Harvard, by S Isaacs, Wash Post, Nov 25, 1973, pp C1-C4.

V

Care Settings
and Values

The fee-for-service setting and organizational programs such as the Health Maintenance Organization have their own underlying values in terms of the quality of care that is provided and the amount of choice that is given to the consumer of health services. The papers in this section examine these underlying values from the standpoint of which settings would be more desirable ethically for both the provider and consumer of medical care.

MICHAEL J. HALBERSTAM, M.D.
Internist, Washington, D.C.

Professionalism and Health Care

Healing, like any form of personal service, requires that the servor be compensated. In the beginning this was achieved through fee for service. Fee for service, of course, did not originate in the healing arts, but more probably as an extension of bartered food exchange. By the time currency of some sort had replaced barter in the ancient world, men were hiring each other's time, skill, and strength in tasks such as farming, home building, and transportation. A task was desired, a fee set, and the bargain completed.

The simplicity of fee for service made it the natural method of compensation when a specialized class of healers began to develop. Indeed, this near-universality makes it difficult to trace development of physician payment, since most chroniclers and historians have taken a direct healer's fee for granted. Writing of the earliest Greek physicians, Bullough[1] says, "They [the priestly physicians] probably treated people of high status and left the more empirical practitioners to deal with the poor." He does not mention how these practitioners were paid because it is assumed that it was by fee. The Code of Hammurabi (?1704–1662 B.C.) contains the earliest written healing ethic. Among other things, it specifies a fee schedule based on what later came to be known as the "Robin Hood" principle:

If the doctor has cured the shattered limb of a gentlemen or has cured the diseased bowel, the patient shall give five shekels of silver to the doctor.

231

If he be the son of a poor man, he shall give three shekels of silver.

If a gentleman's servant, the master of the slave shall give two shekels of silver to the doctor.

This kind of direct fee system is implied in the history of healing in most ancient or preliterature cultures, including the Chinese, Hindu, and American Indian.[2] When other payment arrangements existed, they were unusual enough to warrant special mention. Bullough[3] quotes the Greek historian Diodorus Siculus (first century B.C.) to the effect that among the Egyptians:

...in expeditions and journeys from the country all the sick are taken care of without giving pay privately. For the physicians receive support from the community and they provide their services according to a written law compiled by many famous physicians of ancient times.

This kind of community arrangement for personal healing appears to have been extremely rare in the past, although in the Middle Ages and later, many cities developed the prototype of what would be called the "city physician" or "the community health officer." A more common kind of contractual healing arrangement in the past existed among the rich or noble, who had personal physicians. The type of contract varied from nation to nation and from one era to another; generally, however, the personal or court physician was retained on a yearly or lifelong basis by a powerful family. While the physician was in essence salaried, he often received a bonus if his work was unusually skillful and was subject to dismissal if he lost favor. It is probably this kind of contract that gave rise to the notion that the Chinese paid their physicians to keep them well and received money back if they became ill. While this may have been true in court circles, there is no evidence to suggest that the millions of villagers received care on any but a fee-for-service or barter agreement.

One tradition in healing ran strongly against fee for service. Of all occupations, the priesthood was most isolated from simple commerce and most intimately linked to medicine. The separation of natural from supernatural healing was not nearly so evident to past societies as it appears to be to ours, and in many cultures the evolution of healers as distinct from priests was a very slow process (indeed, the process is by no means complete today). Payment to the priesthood occasionally takes the form of fee for service (as in the Navajo tradition, where a "singer" is paid so many sheep for a healing chant, or the Episcopal, where the parish salary is supplemented by gifts for special services such as marriage), but community subsidy has long been dominant. As healing evolved as a separate discipline, the priesthood showed some conflict. The emergence of Jewish physicians during the Middle Ages stemmed in part from rabbis who, possessing a knowledge of both the Torah and botany, felt it improper to earn a living through the former. Medicine became a favorite alternative livelihood.

The connection between theology and medicine continued on to colonial New England, where many of the great Puritan ministers were also schooled in alchemy and botany. There, however, the situation was somewhat the reverse of the medieval rabbis, for physicians were poorly paid and often had to go to court to collect their fees, while ministers were well rewarded. Giles Firmin of Ipswich complained in 1638 that he was "strongly set upon to study divinity. My studies else must be lost, for Physick is but a mean help."[4] Out of this matrix grew a tradition of ministers (and/or their wives) who provided rudimentary healing services to frontier communities. As a mode of medical practice in the new nation, it was soon overshadowed by physicians trained in the English model, practicing on a fee-for-service basis.[5]

Before the Industrial Revolution and urbanization, a large number of other occupations that today are salaried existed on a fee basis. Like so many night club comedians, university professors once lived directly on the fees paid by individual students to attend their lectures. Firemen put out—or attempted to put out—fires on the basis of combined fee for service and insurance. Similarly, circuit-riding judges got so much per case.

Fee for service became so inseparably tied to the practice of medicine that it gave rise to a whole literature of epigrams, doggerel, and witticism. The literature was for the most part mordant, its cynicism directed equally toward patients ("The doctor is one on whom we set our hopes when ill, our dogs when well") and physician ("To give a surgeon a pecuniary interest in cutting off your leg is enough to make one despair of political humanity").[6] What is striking about these comments is their transcultural, international origin. They come from every era, every continent. The physician and his fee seemed an inseparable combination.

With the Industrial Revolution, however, a new model for providing health services appeared. Increasing numbers of men, women, and children labored for fixed cash salaries instead of subsisting in marginal agriculture. As the single factory then gradually gave way to the large corporation, an expanding managerial class made decisions for industries in which they, unlike the original factory owners, had little personal stake. Managers developed special skills that were interchangeable—work done for Standard Oil was the same as that done for Shell—and managers advanced their careers by switching corporations instead of waiting patiently for promotion. The success of this production system impressed health planners.

Within medicine itself organic changes occurred that suggested a new organizational form might be better than the traditional one. Specialization made it difficult for a single physician to give all the service that medicine could now offer. Groups of physicians began to practice together in hospitals, clinics, or groups.

During the nineteenth and twentieth centuries a strong nation-state replaced the loose confederacy of principalities that had previously marked most of Western Europe. As the nation-state prospered, it took increasing responsibility for the social welfare of its citizens. No longer did people look to charities or the church for housing, food, or pensions. The state assumed responsibility for these and other social services. Among the other social services, medical care became increasingly important.

The changes in production, medicine, and the social obligations of the state combined to give a new view of medical care. An ethic grew that saw medical care as a right, subsidized by the state if otherwise unavailable, as an expense that should be shared among the community at large, and as a service that could be organized rationally along the lines of an industrial process. This brought inevitable conflict with an equally important concept of the industrial society, the ideal of professionalism.

PROFESSIONALISM

The development of the professions is one of the characteristics of modern Western society. "The professions are as characteristic of the modern world as the crafts were of the ancient," according to Graubard,[7] and few would argue with Bullough[8] that "The striving to be identified as a professional is one of the motivating factors in modern life." Goode states, "An industrializing society is a professionalizing society." At times it appears that the desire to be identified as a professional outweighs in some aspirants the desire to practice their profession in the first place, and the vigorous attempts to make such disparate occupations as accounting, psychology, and chiropractic recognized as professions has often led to intensive lobbying and political campaigning.

It could be said that everyone wants to be a professional, but no one knows what a profession is. Experts from Alfred North Whitehead to Abraham Flexner have tried to put ropes around the concept, with varying degrees of success. Flexner[9] noted six criteria: (1) intellectual operations coupled with large individual responsibilities, (2) raw materials drawn from science and learning, (3) practical application, (4) an educationally communicable technique, (5) tendency toward self-organization, and (6) increasingly altruistic motivation. Additions and modifications of these criteria are many and include Cogan's[10] that, "The profession, serving the vital needs of man, considers its first ethical imperative to be altruistic service to the client."

A profession differs from a craft such as woodworking, for example, in its dependence on a large body of theoretical information and its tendency toward innovation rather than tradition. It differs from occupations such as business and advertising in its stated emphasis on community service and altruism. On a practical level, therefore, professionals do not advertise, while businessmen do not have to apologize for seeking to maximize profit, even if it means moving a factory at the expense of many local jobs.

The combination of theory with practical application is essential to professionalism. The professor of romance languages is a scholar, not a professional, for we may assume that the public at large does not demand a knowledge of the consonant shift in Old English. Scholars may form professional organizations, but their essential loyalty is to their discipline and to the ideals of scholarship, not to the public at large or even to the institution that may employ them.

Since, in addition to social status, the professions gain certain practical advantages, including a degree of self-regulation and higher fees, it is not surprising that many people consider themselves professionals who are not so regarded by the world at large. The definitions of professionalism are not hard and fast, nor are they embodied in statutes. There are many occupations in a kind of twilight zone, and many members of accepted professions do not always function as true professionals. Thus, as Paul Goodman[11] points out, "From medieval times, a professional—typically, physician or lawyer—was an artist in that he dealt with individual cases, each one unique. A physician treats a patient, not a pathology or a syndrome. He himself is engaged as a person, not merely as a scientist." Goodman contrasts this traditional role of the physician with that of the social worker, nurse, or engineer who is not employed directly by his client, but instead by an organization (a city department, hospital, or conglomerate) that itself limits the professional's autonomy: "It is the organization, not the professional, that has final responsibility."

Although medicine has usually functioned as an independent profession, it is nowhere writ that this cannot change. This was implied by H. L. Mencken[12] when he wrote,

The essence of a professional man is that he is answerable for his professional conduct only to his professional peers. A physician cannot be fired by anyone, save when he has voluntarily converted himself into a jobholder; he is secure in his livelihood so long as he keeps his health, and can render service, or what they regard as service, to his patients.

Mencken's point is that a physician who, for example, becomes a full-time employee of a university health service is a "jobholder" and therefore no longer a professional. Many physicians in full-time institutional practice would dispute this, and yet there is little doubt that professional independence must be compromised to meet the requirements of the employer. At times the compromise may be untenable, leading either to resignation or the kind of public protest that municipal physicians in New York employed over inadequate equipment in public hospitals. More often, an accommodation is reached, so that the physician reconciles his professional image with what is required of him as a jobholder. The physician for a steel company, for example, believes that by stressing on-the-job safety, treating industrial accidents, and counseling workers about alcoholism he is doing socially valuable work. Indeed, he probably is; but when certain loyalties conflict, it is apparent that his obligation is not the physician's traditional one to the patient, but is directly to his employer, the company.

So long as everyone involved recognizes the dynamics of such a situation, no immediate harm is done. During the 1973 World Series, for example, the unfortunate Mike Andrews committed several horrendous errors at second base for the Oakland Athletics. Sportswriter Shirley Povich wrote that "an angry Charlie Finley [the Oakland owner] fired Andrews clear out of the Series, in the guise of a medical discharge obtained through a friendly neighborhood team doctor who works for Finley."[13] A more sinister side of the same practice was revealed in 1973, when the team physician of the San Diego football team admitted regularly supplying the players with large amounts of dangerous amphetamines and steroids.

Physicians employed directly by companies, teams, or government agencies are rightly considered by their patients to be "company doctors" or "team doctors" or "agency doctors." Although it is never stated in so many words, and while it may be ignored in certain cases, the employer's interests supersede those of the patient. The physician himself has become an agent of the employer—i.e., "personnel" in the definition supplied by Goodman, meaning "the body of persons employed in a public service, as the army or navy, as opposed to the materiel."

We need not assume that physicians so employed are venal or permit harm to come to patients so long as the employer is well served. The decisions that such physicians are required to make often involve equities on both sides. The company physician, for example, may discover evidence of alcoholism in an employee who has been frequently absent. Though it might be more enlightened to keep the man employed while enrolling him in an alcoholic rehabilitation program, the employer has no obligation to keep on an unreliable worker. The company physician's advice and consent in such a conflict is needed, and it is clear that his obligation to the employer is certainly as great as to his "semipatient."

Workingmen, athletes, college students, and government employees are often cynical about the function of their agency's physician. They are aware that the agency, while it may in fact have a genuine and benign desire to keep its workers healthy, must in the end decide in favor of what is best for the institution, not for the individual patient. Therefore, it is common for a military officer who notices symptoms of chest pain to consult an "outside" physician, because he knows that the company physician will make higher echelons aware of a complaint that might hurt promotion.

Since the employee in such circumstances enters into the relationship with the company doctor knowingly, not much individual harm is done. I suggest, however, that the proliferation of team, company, college, and agency doctors, however well intentioned, has had an erosive effect on the profession of medicine. From the outset one of the basic Hippocratic concepts is violated, for the physician transmits what he learns in the course of his practice to another person—the employer (or dean or coach). Of course, the "patient" signs in advance a statement waiving confidentiality, but often this is done with the patient caught in a no-win game: He can't get the position without having a medical exam by the employer's doctor, and he can't have the medical exam without waiving confidentiality. Sometimes the pressure to consult the company doctor will be more subtle, but it exists nonetheless.

One result of all this is a blurring of people's faith in doctors. They are aware that many physicians are no longer paladins, single-mindedly devoted to their patient's welfare in return for a fee, but agents of society. The physician's own sense of responsibility becomes unfocused when so many social agencies request his services and he becomes increasingly used to working, not for the patient, but for someone who has hired him to examine the patient.

Just as invidiously there has blossomed the notion that the profession of medicine is the final arbiter about what people can or cannot do. If you run a college or a summer camp or a sports program and you're worried about lawsuits, you get a physician to certify the health of your enrollees in advance. If you don't want to stand trial or do jury duty or travel second class, society asks you to get a physician's certificate as to your infirmity. If you want to drive a car or fly a plane or do scuba diving or get life insurance, society requires that a physician testify to your wellness. Increasingly, the doctor has become the gatekeeper to a vast number of activities. Institutions and organizations hire physicians to do the dirty work they are reluctant to assume themselves.

Consider this actual example. A government agency is created to send idealistic volunteers, most of them young, into poverty areas for a period of two years. The government agency is naturally concerned that these volunteers be physically and emotionally stable. If fears that illness, particularly mental illness, will not only reflect on the validity of the entire program but that it may cause damage to the agency's clients and involve the government in lawsuits. Accordingly, the agency hires a physician to help screen the volunteers. The physician requests applicants to fill out a form listing any previous medical treatment. If significant illness is noted, the government physician then requests the previous physician to give details of treatment. Often the previous physician himself may have been hired by a college to care for its students and, especially if the treatment was psychiatric, may be reluctant to release details of treatment, even with the patient's consent. The government doctor feels that he must act to prevent his agency from taking on a host of neurotic, counterproductive misfits. The university psychiatrist feels that he must protect the integrity of his program, refusing to give out records of treatment even with the patient's consent, lest future potential patients be frightened away from seeking care. Each physician is correct in the light of his institutional obligations, and each is concerned about the welfare of the individual patient. Yet when push comes to shove, the two institutional hired hands battle each other with the so-called patient caught in the middle.

Medicine's function as a gatekeeper is a new one and does not apparently represent aggressive behavior on the part of medicine, but rather seduction by society at large. That is, the profession did not seek out its role in validating health or sickness, sanity or insanity, but accepted it when the clergy, the courts, and the civil bureaucracy abandoned it. Modern tort liability has also accelerated this process. A great deal of nonmedical medicine comes from the desire of institutions to protect themselves from lawsuits. In more innocent days a child was sent off to summer camp with a sleeping bag and ten pairs of socks with nametags sewn in. Today he goes off complete with a form from a physician testifying to his robust health. No doubt the camp is genuinely worried that it not get stuck with a child too sick for its capacities. On the other hand, if such a child showed up, he could merely be sent home or, if worse came to worse and pre-existent illness intensified, it could reasonably be believed the parents had assumed this risk when they packed the kid off to camp. No camp director today is going to take this chance or count on the court's assuming that assumption, not with $0.5 million lawsuits a possibility.

No matter how innocently medicine may have assumed its new roles (and there is no doubt that there were aggrandizers in medicine as in other fields), the end result has been a subtle corruption of the physician's role. Increasingly, people encounter physicians, not as helping professionals but as agents of the state or industry. Although Szasz[14] has written most bitterly about the change in the psychiatrist's role, he has also applied his criticism to institutional medicine in general:

The most important economic characteristic of institutional psychiatry is that the institutional psychiatrist is a bureaucratic employee, paid for his services by a private or public organization (not by the individual who is his ostensible client). Its most important social characteristic is the use of force and fraud. The actual client of institutional psychiatry is some social interest and organization (for example, the Peace Corps, a university health service, a state mental hygiene department): its ostensible client is, more often than not, its victim rather than its beneficiary.

One should note, by the way, the manner in which Szasz links the payment for service to the moral impact of the service itself.

One does not have to agree with his "more often than not" phrase to find a disturbing truth in Szasz. Our nation has become so enamored with the power of medicine, so used to thinking of the profession as a gatekeeper, that many of us accept unhesitatingly the idea that presidential candidates should have physical–psychiatric checkups before running. The examples of Senator Eagleton and President Franklin Roosevelt are frequently cited as reasons for this kind of disclosure. When such perceptive men as James Reston overlook the Orwellian implications of a society in which every kind of jobholder would eventually have to have a psychologic seal of approval, then we already have trouble.

SALARIED MEDICAL PRACTICE

Up to now I have tried to sketch the development of payment in medicine and have discussed the problems implicit in physicians hired by a third party to care for a captive population. An entirely different situation exists when patients contract either directly or through a third party to prepay their medical care. There is continued pressure in this country to make that third party the federal government, which, under any one of a number of different plans, would subsidize medical care directly or indirectly.

The major governmental effort in the United States today is toward the establishment of Health Maintenance Organizations (HMOs), which are essentially subsidized prepayment plans. According to Scott Fleming, an advocate of HMOs who helped draft the initial proposal, Paul Ellwood turned to him after a strategy session one day and said, "Now what do we call these things?" Fleming answered, perhaps naïvely, "Why, you call them group practice prepayment plans, of course." Ellwood replied, and I am quoting Fleming, "No, that won't do. Those words are shopworn and they lack sex appeal. We have got to have a better name than that."[15]

Health Maintenance Organization certainly is a better name, but a rose *is* a rose, and prepayment is prepayment, and it's been around a good while. There are frills and flourishes on the various HMO measures, but basically they amount to a federal effort to induce—or force—physicians into prepayment groups. The groups would be organized locally, they would receive a preset amount of federal money each year and then have to stay within budgetary limits, and their costs would be reviewed by the granting agency—the federal government.

While a difference clearly exists between an organization that supplies medical services to an employment group and an organization that people freely join for medical care, similarities exist because organizations are similar. Organizations have a life of their own, as Goffman[16] and Parkinson[17] have detailed, and the larger they become, the less flexible they are and the more they tend to become separated from their clients' concerns. This is not a criticism, but a fact of life, just as an individual professional's inability to offer a complete range of services is a fact of life.

Despite all that has been written about individualism contrasted to institutionalization in medical care, Fields' summary in 1961 remains as dispassionate an explication as exists. Based on interviews with Soviet citizens who had emigrated to either the U.S. or Germany, Fields constructed a model that contrasted the advantages and disadvantages of two systems of medical care, fee for service and third-party. As a practitioner of fee-for-service care, I would initially note that 73 percent of Fields' subjects preferred the Soviet system to the American. His article is hardly a ringing endorsement of fee-for-service medicine. Three quarters of the sample that had experienced both the Soviet and West German system preferred the latter, which was then a state-supported insurance scheme.

Fields found his respondents resented the fact that in the United States they had to choose either paying what they considered exorbitant fees or receiving charity medicine. They preferred the system in the Soviet Union where medical services, even if they were inadequate, were the citizens' right. Analyzing the two systems, Fields[18] wrote,

Stripped of its emotional connotation, there were in the two systems, certain "built-in" flaws that were, actually or potentially, detrimental to the clinical relationship. . . . The third party, whatever its nature or organizational form, is always under some obligation to see to it that the funds for which it is responsible, are expended in what it believes to be the wisest, most economical, most effective, and most honest way possible. In order to carry out this mandate, some kind of review often is exercised over the recipient of funds, in this case, the physician. Institutional safeguards may be built that will reduce such review to the minimum and will allow the physician absolute professional freedom and discretion; on the other hand certain restrictions may be imposed for purposes of economy, as, for example, in prescribing. Further pressure may be imposed in the choice of modalities or treatment and in the assignment of certain standards that must be fulfilled if the physician is to remain in good standing with the third party. Finally, there may be direct interference in, and dictation over, professional matters, coupled with professional or lay disciplinary power over medical personnel, e.g., under certain military, industrial or political situations. Admittedly, the latter is an extreme situation, but it does represent certain implications that can flow from third party medicine, as will be seen below.

Fields then details some of the stresses in third-party medicine in general and within the Soviet system in particular. He notes the ambivalent position of the physician as an employee of the state, certifying whether or not fellow citizens are too ill to work. The problem is not limited to the extreme statism seen in the Soviet Union, for Eckstein[19] writes of the English National Health Service that,

Those doctors who claimed . . . that under a comprehensive public medical service the doctor's loyalty would be torn between his patient and the State were not just talking reactionary nonsense. . . . The chief threat to medical practice in this respect was stereotyping—the gradual replacement of the spontaneous clinical relation by bureaucratic rules and standards.

Eckstein hints at one of the built-in defects of tax-supported welfare programs; i.e., both buyers and sellers are using OPM ("other people's money"), and, in the absence of usual fiscal restraints, a system of auditing or inspection must be imposed to protect the taxpayers' money. A sizeable bureaucracy grows up and additional monies are spent in a very rational effort to save money.

If medical care is believed to be purely an individual responsibility, for example, we need not care if our neighbors spend thousands of dollars a year on chiropractic. It is their money, to spend as they please. If medical services are deemed a right and subsidized by the state, then someone has to define what medical services are and, in this instance, whether tax funds should be used to support chiropractic. If chiropractic, what about naturopathy? scientology? It is obvious from the example of Medicare and Medicaid that any national health insurance scheme will involve protracted and expensive lobbying by unorthodox healing groups in an effort to get their services covered. Furthermore, it is axiomatic that if new healing modalities develop, it will take longer for them to be approved under a major bureaucratic administration than on the catch-as-catch-can basis of individual enterprise. Legislation cannot be amended overnight. One need not be an advocate of unorthodox healing to envision an illness in which an unexpected form of nonmedical therapy appears effective and in which congressional hearings, departmental meetings, and public debate would be required before it is stamped as federally approved.

If medical care becomes totally a tax-supported commodity, will we be forced not only to accept medical care of a certain type but forced to accept some kind of care whether we wish it or not? After all, if each sick person is no longer a burden to himself or to his family but to all of society and if there is a known way of preventing certain illness, does not the taxpayer have a financial stake in his neighbor's health? We used to say that if a man wanted to drink himself to death, it was his own business. Will that be so in the future if we will all be paying each other's medical bills? The example is hardly far-fetched, since society's financial stake in automobile trauma was the major argument in forcing compulsory seat belt buzzers and the no-start seat belt interlock system in the 1974 cars.*

Another decision that will become a societal rather than an individual one will center around the qualifications of the physicians, chiropractors, naturopaths, and others covered by a tax-based health scheme. The medical profession within the United States has developed a fairly extensive and formalized system of specialty associations, a system that is significantly more comprehensive than that found in other professions and most other countries (England may be an exception). Until now, however, the certification of specialty has had only tangential legal import. Any licensed physician can perform an appendectomy if he can find a hospital that will grant him surgical privileges. The hospitals and, of late, the private insurance companies have acted to put limits on either what physicians can do or, as in the case of insurance companies, what they will be paid for (these often work out to be about the same thing). While much criticism has been directed toward medicine because of its supposedly lax standards, it is apparent that no other profession in no other nation has accepted the idea of certification and, now, recerti-

---

*In November 1973, the District of Columbia Medical Society, announcing a symposium on the moral aspects of smoking, told its membership that "the individual has a moral duty to protect his health."

fication so completely as American medicine. Anderson's observation in 1963 that quality of care was under greater scrutiny in the United States than in nations with governmental financing still appears valid.[20] The acceptance, albeit reluctant, of Professional Standards Review Organizations (PSRO) legislation by the medical profession is a new example of this.

The need for some kind of federal standards as to what constitutes a specialist will, predictably, put an emphasis on paper qualifications and overlook performance. This was what Eckstein was referring to when he wrote of "the gradual replacement of the spontaneous clinical relation by bureaucratic rules and standards." The need for paper rather than performance standards is an example of what David Hapgood[21] has termed "diplomaism" and has cited as a restrictive feature of American life. Hapgood's argument is overstated in the case of medicine—we need, I think, exposure to theory and a standard apprenticeship in our surgeons, in addition to good hands and initial competence–but it is particularly applicable to tax-funded medical programs. For some years it has been policy in Veterans Administration and other government hospitals to give additional salary to those physicians who gain specialty certification. While desirable, specialty certification remains a paper yardstick. It represents the result of hard study, knowledge as tested on an examination, and a certain required number of years spent in approved training programs. It says nothing about the physician's actual performance with patients. Since it is easily quantified—either a physician has his Boards or he hasn't—it remains a good bureaucratic measurement. It is significant that there is no other achievement in government medical service that gives the automatic salary increment of certification. That is, no outstanding service to patients, no original discovery, no contribution to scientific knowledge gets rewarded as does the passing of an examination.

Thus we see that when two "reforms" of modern medicine conflict—and they do conflict, despite the fact that many reformers claim to be in favor of both—the issue in a bureaucracy will be settled in favor of "quality of care" (i.e., paper qualifications) over "lateral mobility" (i.e., advancement within the healing arts based on experience and ability).

The effect of the bureaucratic process on the professional himself—especially the physician—has been little studied, though Susser and Watson[22] give a good summary of the literature. Gloria Engel's[23] study of California physicians is one of the few touching on the area. She found that physicians in a moderately bureaucratic organization perceived themselves as having more professional autonomy than those in a highly bureaucratic structure (a government program) or nonbureau-

cratic (solo or small group). The "moderately bureaucratic" practice
was a private, closed-panel group. Engel's findings are qualified both
by the low response rate to her questionnaire (42 percent) and the
process of self-selection. Physicians in solo practice who feel they have
little autonomy may feel they have even less should they switch to a
closed-panel group. Physicians who feel at ease in a group setting voluntarily gravitate toward closed-panel opportunities and may be expected
to feel that they enjoy professional autonomy. More detailed work
needs to be done, including studies on physicians who leave one form
of practice for another, physician attitude toward medicine as practiced
during the required doctor draft, and attitudes of house officers exposed
to different forms of practice. Nonetheless, Engel's work casts some
doubt on the assumption that bureaucracy is incompatible with perceived professional autonomy.

To the effects of government-financed prepaid medicine on the governmental decision-making process and on the physician must be added
those on the patient. Here again research has been singularly scanty. We
have little data about why people who have received fee-for-service care
switched to join prepay groups, how they perceive the quality of care
(as opposed to cost), and why some leave prepayment for fee for service. There has been little curiosity about the amount of "private" care
sought by people already eligible for closed-panel federal, or company
care.

Some early data do exist. Eliot Freidson's study of the Montefiore
Health Insurance Plan group in 1961 indicated that 10 percent of subscribers used non-HIP physicians almost exclusively and another 35–50
percent used them occasionally.[24] A study by Kaiser of Kaiser enrollees
in the late 1960s indicate that 44 percent had used outside medical services on at least one occasion since becoming members.[25] These figures
are skimpy, but suggest that some of the cost-effectiveness of prepaid
groups is merely illusory; the groups do not take care of all actual medical costs for their members, since an unknown percentage of patients
pay for additional care in the marketplace.

Fields cites the temptation to provide fewer services than promised as
a constant problem for prepaid medicine, as the temptation to do more
than necessary is built into fee for service. Just as the unscrupulous physician may operate when surgery is not indicated or have his patient
come back for too-frequent visits, the salaried physician may be tempted
to quit exactly at 5 pm to discourage patient visits and to take protracted coffee breaks. The administrator of such a group will certainly
monitor hospitalizations and make the physician aware if his hospitalization rate exceeds that of his colleagues. After all, the less that is spent

on hospital care, the more there is available to the physicians and other personnel of the group. The pressures may be subtle, but they exist. Proponents of prepayment argue that constant review makes underutilization rare. The same utilization review, of course, is applied to fee-for-service care to limit overuse.

Since this paper is primarily concerned with human values, I will not dwell overlong on the economics of prepayment as opposed to fee for service, except to raise several issues that have been generally ignored. While the Trussell study and studies of the United Mine Workers program showed a marked decrease in hospitalization and surgery when prepayment was compared with fee for service, other, more recent studies suggest that economies of scale drop off fairly soon in medicine. Bailey[26] indicated that some of the apparent efficiency of large group practices came from their tendency to employ laboratory testing instead of physician services. Though critics of medicine seem to believe that physicians operate primarily as economic men, they overlook this aspect in discussing group practice. If group practice were inherently more economic, physicians, as economic men, would naturally flock to it as an opportunity to maximize their incomes. This has not happened, though what has occurred in the context of the marketplace and of the organic development of medicine has been a series of reforms: America is the international leader in group practice, single-specialty groups are increasingly common on the East Coast; physicians no longer practice in their homes but in medical buildings (where ancillary services and other consultants are available) and, increasingly, near their primary hospital; house calls are disappearing; emergency rooms provide a backup office for the physician and a point-of-call for the undoctored patient; etc. All these developments have taken place because they made sense to both patients and physicians, and no government subsidy was necessary. We must ask, "If prepayment's main advantage is in efficiency, why does it have to be subsidized?" If it needs starter money, how much and for how long?

As in fee-for-service medicine, some abuses in prepayment will never show up on a bed utilization audit. Patients with "trivial" complaints can be discouraged by postponing their visits or being made to wait long periods of time. The frequency of elective surgery can be kept down through waiting lists—the patient either learns to live with his hemorrhoids or seeks outside care. One method of dealing with the influx of "the worried well" who innundate Kaiser was described by Kaiser's medical director, Dr. Sidney Garfield, who suggested interposing a machine—the Auto-Analyzer—between patient and doctor to weed out hypochondriacs.[27] Other variations of this strategy are described in the most vicious attack on Kaiser; published in the November 1971 issue of *Ramparts,* this article indicates, as I have suggested, that skepticism about prepayment is not limited to the right wing.

Since we have no way of defining "overutilization," we cannot tell if prepayment encourages it. We do have the analysis of Scitovsky and Snyder[28] of what happened in the Stanford Group Health Plan when a 25 percent coinsurance factor was added for physicians' services that had previously been totally covered. Utilization dropped abruptly, particularly among dependent women and among men of nonprofessional, lower income status. Hospitalization rates, however, did not change significantly. Visits for illness defined as "minor" dropped more substantially than for other diagnoses. Phelps and Newhouse,[32] analyzing the same data from a different statistical approach, concluded that the drop in utilization was independent of the subscriber's income and stressed the change in use of female dependents. They emphasized time costs— the money spent in traveling, baby-sitters, etc.—as affecting utilization. One point that has been overlooked is that the plan was introduced in December 1965, presumably on the basis of detailed academic study and past experience, with all services covered. At the end of 1966, one year later, according to Scitovsky, "the Clinic found that it had seriously underestimated the demand of GHP members for clinic services under the plan." It was this overdemand that prompted—indeed, necessitated—the 25 percent coinsurance.

Experience elsewhere tends to support the empirical belief of physicians that, while most people have no love for medical services and do not seek them out whether paid or prepaid, a small percentage of patients will place a disparate demand on facilities. Physicians who have done their military service, for example, complain commonly that too much of their work load involves unhappy, lonely dependents, and hypochondriacal complaints. While Americans may accept the notion that they have a financial, as well as moral, stake in keeping their neighbors free of catastrophic illness or expense, they may be skeptical about subsidizing their neuroses.

It should be clear that I am skeptical about prepayment. It cannot be repeated too often that even skeptics consider prepayment or capitation valid methods of practice and have respect for what Kaiser has done. Prepayment fulfills the needs of many physicians and patients. No law should limit the development of prepaid practice.

The problem arises when we—the Institute, the profession, the government—decide to encourage prepayment as *the* desirable way to practice. For a while prepayment's enthusiasts claimed it was the only way to practice. Now they claim it is *the* desirable way to structure care.

The enthusiasm of medical academia for prepayment has been matched only by equally strong apathy on the part of the public. Growth of prepayment, particularly in the East, has been very slow. One cannot but help feel that this is a classic example where the planners have decided what is best for the people, but the people ain't buying. The people don't know what's good for them. Faced with this situation, we can damn the people and go full steam ahead, abandon the project totally, or ask ourselves, "Maybe they know something we don't know."

There is evidence that what the people know—and persist in clinging to—is a fairly close relationship to the physician of their choice. Strickland[29] found that while 61 percent of Americans believe basic changes are needed in the medical care system, 84 percent believed they could get good care when they wanted it. The figures are reminiscent of other surveys that indicate that people are somewhat cynical about physicians, in general, but are largely enthusiastic about their personal doctors. (It should be added that the American people put more trust in physicians than any other occupational group except Supreme Court justices; cynicism is a relative term.) People want to pay less for medical care, they would like it to be "free," but there is very little evidence that they want basic changes in the way it is structured.

Rather than continually damning the people for their persistence in obsolescent folkways, perhaps we might re-examine our own assumptions. If we can accept that there are natural shortcomings in governmental or prepaid medicine, we might also learn that the American consumer is not as naïve as we think. It is the conventional wisdom that the consumer has no way of telling which physician is best and that the current system makes the patient an uninformed supplicant. This view finds little support among those who actually practice medicine, for we have seen medical journalism change from an occasional story by Paul de Kruif to a deluge of TV shows, cover stories in *Time*, and newspaper features. I once sat down to watch four weeks' worth of medical shows on TV and came away astounded at the sophistication required of their audiences. One might guess that the American people know more about the workings of the medical profession than they do about any single occupational group, with the possible exception of the Mafia. This is not a false sophistication; the questions that lower middle-class patients ask reflect a real awareness of disease and the techniques available to treatment. Upper middle-class patients, of course, not only have the information, but a relative who is a professor of medicine who can check on the local physician. Since we do not grade journalists on their accuracy each time a by-line appears and since we have no batting averages besides trial attorneys, we are not given a "best buy" rating on local physicians. The

information that the public does have available on physicians exceeds
that in other fields, and the public makes good use of it. Certainly, we
must acknowledge there is no way of rating physicians comparable to
earned run averages for pitchers. Some patients prize technical knowledge above all; others, compassion and humanity. Physicians themselves
often seek care from colleagues who are not as highly trained as might
be expected, thus perhaps maintaining some bargaining power in the
"doctor–doctor-patient" relationship.

As elusive as healing ability is, there is little doubt that any system of
government-subsidized medicine would attempt to quantify it. As I previously indicated, paper qualifications might be expected to become all-
important. It is crucial to remember that whatever the government pays
for, it regulates and, perhaps, controls. In Medicaid programs official
formularies of drugs have been promulgated that, in the interests of
economy and "rational prescribing," deprive patients of badly needed,
long-acting drugs. Amphetamine-based anorexiant pills are prohibited,
despite the evidence that, aside from intestinal bypass, they are the only
effective therapy in a life-threatening illness. Expert physicians may and
do differ in their estimate of anorexiant drugs. The dilemma arises in
tax-supported programs, where bureaucrats are under pressure to make
a decision. Too often this is an either/or decision, handed down by administrative fiat. A drug is approved or unapproved, effective or ineffective.

Do I exaggerate? Not when a distinguished medical thinker[30] writes,
"No procedure should be paid out of public funds, whether it consists
of pills, potions, elixers, surgery or any other form of technologic intervention, until it has been subjected to a random trial."* Note the phrase,
"out of public funds." From the same perspective, he deplores American emphasis on coronary care units, renal dialysis, and coronary bypass
surgery. He suggests that, "there is a larger concern to all physicians, all
health professionals, for the quality of care that is delivered, not just to
the patient whom they serve at the moment, but to the entire population."

Here we are at one of the crucial break-off points. When we think
about it, we realize that the ethic of the legislator and the ethic of the
physician are not merely different but are, in fact, antithetical. The legislator's ethic—and, by extension, that of the conscientious bureaucrat—is
the greatest good for the greatest number. The physician's ethic is the
greatest good for the individual that he is charged with taking care of. A

*This would, of course, exclude psychotherapy, whose most devoted practitioners concede its
value has never been proved.

good physician may lie, cheat, and steal for his or her patient. A good physician, faced with four patients dying of renal failure, salvageable the artificial kidney, does not say to himself, "If we treat these four men and women, we will not have funds for a urine-screening program for children that might ultimately prevent dozens of such cases." He says, "I am going to get treatment for these patients. I want to prevent such cases too, but right now these are my patients." A dedicated but cold-blooded legislator can say to himself, "We will let these people die, because we have limited resources and we need prevention programs." An equally dedicated, equally cold-blooded physician will say, "To hell with the children and to hell with potential disease. I've got four dying patients now. Win today's ball game today."

Each professional is working within the best ethic of his field. Neither is "right" nor "wrong." On the contrary, each is correct and their world views are irreconcilable. Let me pose it this way: You have angina pectoris, it is getting worse, and you cannot walk through an airport lobby without getting chest pain. All medical treatment has failed. There is something called coronary bypass surgery. Its eventual worth is unproved, but it has relieved symptoms in many patients. Do you want to wait until it has been proved effective? Do you want to be told that, although it is effective, it costs the equivalent of 1000 rheumatic fever screening exams in children and therefore is not justifiable? If you do, you are very rare. Most likely, you will, like sufferers from rare tumors or exotic neurologic disorders, search the world for someone who is allowed to perform this kind of surgery. You are not looking for a cost-effective doctor. You are looking for someone who will make your life bearable. Here is where all the background about fee for service, professionalism, and independence come to focus. You do not want an agent of the state, concerned about costs. You do not want someone whose own professional ethic has been subtly distorted by the equally noble ethic of another profession. You do not want someone who is answerable to a committee before he or she can operate. Like a salmon going upstream, like the parents of children with biliary atresia finding their way to Japan, you will find your way to someone who *may* help you.

When we realize that the ethic of the administrator and the ethic of the physician are antithetical, much becomes clear. We see, for example, why no amount of exhortation will ever get the average physician as interested in preventing disease as curing it. Different ethics are involved. While one would like to prevent disease and while most physicians actively work to prevent disease (would that their patients worked equally hard!), the physician is preselected by temperament and reinforced by training to respond to the immediate discontent. This may not be cost-effective, but it is good medicine. Occasionally, the physician may let an individual patient suffer a bit longer so that the underlying disease may become more obvious. Thus delay is for the sake of the individual, not for society. In the long run, the social obligation of the physician is to ignore society. Exceptions to this are so rare that they are specifically written into law; the physician is required to report communicable disease and bullet wounds. That's about where it should stay.

The train of thought may be familiar to atomic scientists and lawyers. The classic legal ethic was that the lawyer did society's work when he represented either side of a dispute with maximum vigor. As contrasted to medicine, however, the law made no attempt to extend this symmetrical doctrine to the poor until the 1870s, and little real effort until the 1960s. As Marks[31] has pointed out, the law has recently revised its ethic in light of the profession's critical decision-making ability in our society. Added to the "gun for hire" concept is the notion that in certain cases the interest of the public might serve to limit action for a client, even though that action was technically legal. Furthermore, with the development of the OEO Legal Services Division, lawyers actively sought out areas of inequality and brought suit to change access or distribution. Often enough, the areas of inequality were in programs of the federal government itself or of the states, resulting in one branch of the government suing another. Congress and the governors had been able to tolerate jurisdictional disputes between government agencies, but solicitation of lawsuits was a different matter. OEO Legal Services today barely exist. The implication is again clear: When the going gets tough, one may count on the bureaucracy not to destroy itself. Gladys Kessler, a Washington public interest lawyer, worked for a firm which, unlike similar groups, did not accept foundation money. Marks quotes her as saying, "I think you are beholden to whoever funds you: We want to be beholden to our clients."

Unlike the law, medicine has always taken special responsibility for the poor. Charity, however, is no longer respectable or even very effective. Medicine must reassert the special obligation that goes with its special privileges. The little-noticed acceptance by physicians of the doctor draft was, one can argue, an example of a unique burden undertaken as a societal obligation. With the doctor draft vanishing and the need for care in isolated areas more apparent, perhaps the profession might assume two years' service in an underserved area as a preconditioning to licensing. This suggestion, which I owe to Victor Sidel, ties the concept of service to the privilege of practice, rather than, as in other programs, the use of a subsidized education. Like recertification, it would be unique to the medical profession and serve to emphasize the unique responsibilities and privileges of the profession.

Note that this does not change the fundamental relationship between the government and profession or compromise the professional ethic, though libertarian physicians would certainly claim "involuntary servitude." As I have tried to make clear, the government's role in medical care should be to prevent financial disaster from medical expenses and to assume direct responsibility for certain groups—Indians, the rural poor, merchant seamen—who fall between the cracks in the current system. The people of the United States are reluctant to see any fundamental change in the way medical care is organized, and only an unethical view would impose such a change. The medical profession is equally unenthusiastic about becoming payees of the government and, in the American context of both the left and right, this resistance appears justifiable. Evolution will continue to occur in the way Americans obtain care, but the evolution will come primarily from social forces outside of governmental programs, programs that we have all too often learned promise more than they can deliver. We need health planning, but we need to forget Daniel Burnham's injunction after the Chicago fire, "Make no little plans." I suggest that we start with some comparatively little plans and, for once, make them work.

REFERENCES

1. Bullough VL: The Development of Medicine as a Profession. Basel, S. Karger, 1966.
2. Sigerist H: A History of Medicine. New York, Oxford University Press, 1951.
3. Bullough VL: *op. cit.*
4. *Ibid.*
5. Boorstin DJ: The Americans: The Colonial Experience. New York, Random House, 1958.
6. Bierce A, Shaw GB, respectively: Familiar Medical Quotations. Edited by M Strauss. Boston, Little, Brown & Co., 1968.
7. Graubard S: The professions. Daedalus, fall 1963.
8. Bullough VL: *op. cit.*
9. Cogan ML: The problem of defining a profession. Ann Am Acad Polit Soc Sci, Jan 1955.
10. Cogan ML: *op. cit.*
11. Goodman P: People or Personnel. New York, Vintage Books, Random House, 1955.
12. Mencken HL: Journalism in America, Prejudices: A Selection. New York, Vintage Books, Random House, 1955.
13. Povich S: A's strategic bombers level it with Orioles. Wash Post, pp D1–D2, Oct 8, 1973.
14. Szasz T (ed): The Age of Madness. New York, Anchor Books, 1973.

15. Fleming S: Chapter in Paying for America's Health Care. Acton, Mass., Publishing Sciences Group, 1973.
16. Goffman E: Relations in Public. New York, Harper Colophon Books, 1971.
17. Parkinson CN: Parkinson's Law and Other Studies in Administration. Boston, Houghton Mifflin, 1957.
18. Fields M: The doctor–patient relationship in the perspective of "fee for service" and "third-party" medicine. J Health Human Behav 2:252–262, 1961.
19. Eckstein H: The English Health Service. Cambridge, Harvard University Press, 1958.
20. Anderson O: Health services systems in the United States and other countries: critical comparisons. N Engl J Med 1963: 269.
21. Hapgood D: Diplomaism. New York, Donald W. Brown, 1971.
22. Susser MW, Watson W: Sociology in Medicine. London, Oxford University Press, 1971.
23. Engel G: The effect of bureaucracy on the professional autonomy of the physician. J Health Soc Behav 10:30–41, 1969.
24. Freidson E: Patients' Views of Medical Practice. New York, Russell Sage Foundation, 1961.
25. Williams G: Kaiser-Permanent Health Plan: Why It Works. Oakland, Calif., The Henry J. Kaiser Foundation, 1971.
26. Bailey RM: Economies of scale in medical practice. Presented at the Second Conference on the Economics of Health, Baltimore, December 5–7, 1968.
27. Garfield S: The delivery of medical care. Sci Am 222:15–23, 1970.
28. Scitovsky A, Snyder N: Effect of coinsurance on the use of physician services. Soc Sec Bull 35(6):3–19, 1972.
29. Strickland S: Chapter in Paying for America's Health Care. op. cit.
30. White K: Chapter in Paying for America's Health Care. op. cit.
31. Marks FR: The Lawyer, the Public and Professional Responsibility. Chicago, American Bar Foundation, 1972.
32. Phelps C, Newhouse J: Effect of coinsurance: a multivariate analysis. Soc Sec Bull 35(6):20–28, 1972.

BIBLIOGRAPHY

Jaco EG (ed): Patients, Physicians, and Illness. New York, Free Press, 1972.
Mencher S: British Private Medical Practice and the National Health Service. Pittsburgh, University of Pittsburgh Press, 1968.
Lewis R, Maude A: Professional People. London, Phoenix House, 1952.
Hughes EC: Men and Their Work. Glencoe, Ill., Free Press, 1958.
Bullough B, Bullough V: Poverty, Ethnic Identity, and Health Care. New York, Appleton-Century-Crofts, 1972.

CARL M. STEVENS
Professor of Economics, Reed College

Selecting Health Care Systems

Many distinctions might be drawn between different kinds of care settings. However, to reduce this discussion to manageable proportions, we may think in terms of a broad, general distinction between two subsets of care settings: (1) conventional fee-for-service settings, most frequently involving sole practitioners, and with care financed with the aid of typical health insurance; (2) health maintenance organization (HMO) settings, comprehensive, prepaid, or group practice.

Many properties of care settings are potentially important in their implications for service to "values." I have thought it useful to direct attention to the following properties: the nature of the (implied) "social contract" between the individual (consumer) and the health care system; and the physician–patient relationship, principally the nature of the physician–patient decision-making process that determines diagnostic and therapeutic events.

HEALTH CARE SOCIAL CONTRACT

It is clear that our national health policy (variously and vaguely articulated though it may be and, one may add, indifferently complied with though it may be) does embody a health care social contract; namely, access by all to adequate health care is a basic right of the citizen in this social order.

253

The nature of the contractual relationship between an individual and the health care system is very different, depending on whether he or she participates in a fee-for-service/conventional insurance setting or in an HMO setting. Under the former, the organization component (the insurer) promises to pay some or all of the health care costs incurred by the individual, who must find and arrange for the requisite care. By contrast, under an HMO setting the organization component arranges for the provision of the requisite care. To put matters starkly, with fee for service, the individual gets care if and when he can find it; with an HMO, the individual knows where to go for access to the care contractually guaranteed to him or her.

Pursuant to compliance with those values inherent in the health care social contract, the distinction I have just suggested between the two kinds of care settings is, in a categorical sense, true. But, we may inquire, how important is it? The short answer is, "It all depends." It all depends, for example, on where you sit in the health care system and on how that system is organized.

Fee-for-service health care markets might adequately serve the social contract values inherent in national health policy under the proper conditions. These conditions would include ample supply of health care resources (manpower and facilities); proper distribution of such resources; and easy entrance by knowledgeable individuals into the health care system.[1]

Given the current organization of the health care sector, these conditions do not generally obtain. For this reason, the fee for service/HMO distinction must be regarded as potentially important for at least some parts of the system. For example, should public policy simply pick up the tab for costs incurred for the medically indigent under Medicaid, when such patients find care? Or should public policy contract with HMOs for the provision of care to such patients? In some states, a movement is under way to go this second route. This usually is rationalized in terms of cost savings, based on the conviction that HMOs will prove more economical. It might be argued, however, that service is as important in the choice as other values. That is, given the present organization of the health care sector, many patients will not enjoy access to care to which they are entitled pursuant to national health policy unless public policy actually arranges for the provision of care (such as by contracting with HMOs).

PHYSICIAN–PATIENT RELATIONSHIP

This dimension is involved with a complex mix of institutional factors, including attributes of the physician–patient decision-making process that determines diagnostic and therapeutic events. It will facilitate exposition to break this topic down into subtopics as follows: (1) "free" choice of physician vs. "closed" panel; (2) the character of the physician's performance *qua* "professional"; and (3) joint physician–patient decision making.

"Free" Choice

All would agree that important values are served if each individual can have as his physicians providers he likes and has confidence in. The question is, "What care settings are most apt to yield such a relationship?" Proponents of the fee-for-service system contend that precisely because it features "free" choice of physician, it facilitates achieving this property of the physician–patient relationship, as contrasted with a group practice HMO in which the patient is constrained to choose his providers from among those physicians who happen to constitute the group. In rebuttal, proponents of group practice HMOs contend that typically in such a care setting the patient is free to select his physician from among those comprising the group and free to change physicians if he wants; typically, the group will afford a range of choice such that eminently satisfactory relationships will be established. How may we evaluate these contentions?

It should be clear at the outset that the actual range of physician choice afforded the prospective patient is not uniquely determined by the type of care setting. Take, for example, a medical service area of 100,000 population in which the individuals, exercising free choice in fee-for-service markets, have distributed themselves among 100 physicians. Alternatively, had these 100 physicians organized themselves as a group practice HMO to serve this population of 100,000, the range of physician choice that could be afforded each member of that population would be exactly the same.

In general, the actual range of choice turns on such features (of any care setting) as the range of manpower resources potentially available and certain properties of the representative consumer. A sophisticated consumer with ready access to information, operating in a large fee-for-service market area, may in fact exercise a wide range of effective choice.[2] On the other hand, an unsophisticated consumer with little access to information, even though in a large fee-for-service market area, may in fact exercise only a very limited range of choice. In some instances, for any of various reasons, such a consumer may have no port of entry into the health care sector other than to repair to a city hospital emergency room. Or, typically perhaps, such a consumer will have identified only a few physicians, by unsystematic and possibly unreliable means, from among whom he makes his "free" choice. For patients of this latter kind, a group practice HMO may present the individual with wider range of effective choice than he would have fending for himself in fee-for-service markets.

It also seems likely that, generally speaking, the probability of the consumer securing high quality care does not depend uniquely on the type of care setting, at least as herein distinguished—HMOs in general vs. fee for service in general.[3]

We conclude that the "free choice" issue is not really concerned with either the actual range of choice, or the objective probability of securing high quality care, so much as it is concerned with the individual's finding a physician he likes and has confidence in.[4] Fee-for-service proponents contend that the kind of choice afforded by that system is most apt to achieve this result. Group practice HMO proponents contend that the kind of choice afforded by that system is just as likely to achieve this result. Generally, this issue does not involve a difference about matters of "principle." It is a matter of empirical generalization— the actual experience of individuals in different care settings, which may be expected to differ between individuals as between particular examples of care settings.

Perhaps all would agree that, however the health care sector is organized (e.g., whatever the mix of types of care settings), and if the situation can be avoided, no individual should be compelled to use physicians he does not like and does not have confidence in. Compliance with this canon probably requires a health care sector made up of several different types of care settings. Also, it probably requires that each type of care setting direct attention to the problem.

The institutional arrangements implied by this canon will depend on the circumstances of each market situation. Some situations, e.g., the one-doctor town, will not afford much scope for adaptation. More generally, however, certain arrangements now commonly in place tend to work in the direction of achieving compliance. For example, HMOs now commonly permit each member to choose his own primary care physician from among those in the group. Also for example, some HMOs follow the rule that their plan may not be offered under a group contract unless the members of the group are afforded an alternative, such as the "Blues." Generally, if one assumes that the fee-for-service setting is in compliance with this canon, then any arrangements that permit individuals the option of seeking care in this setting will be in compliance. Alternatively, in a hypothetical world of 100 percent HMOs, there should be arrangements to facilitate the transfer of membership from one HMO to another.

Physician as "Professional"

We all might agree that high quality professional performance by physicians is necessary if the health care sector is to serve those values we expect it to serve.

The concept "professional" may be defined variously. For present purposes, I define as a good professional performance one in which the physician brings expert, up-to-date knowledge to his tasks, attends carefully and assiduously to his patients' problems, and prescribes only those therapeutic regimens indicated by best-practice standards. In particular, he does not encourage excess utilization of medical services, as by prescribing treatments of dubious merit. Nor does he cut corners, as by failing to provide services indicated by best-practice standards.

Professional workers are accorded extraordinary privileges and responsibilities by the social orders in which they operate. For many jobs and occupations, workplace and other environmental constraints are relied upon to control the quality of work performance. Professionals, on the other hand, are expected to police themselves, to assume direct responsibility for the quality of their work performance. The professional accomplishes this feat in large part by dint of appeal to his sturdy professional superego. There is, in my judgment, no real substitute for professionalism in this sense as a guarantor of the quality of medical practice. Many factors other than the type of care setting in which he operates are responsible for the quality of the physician's professional performance. Consequently, one might expect to find both good and bad professional performance in every type of care setting; indeed, some might argue that the type of care setting should not be regarded as decisive from this point of view.

Nevertheless, the case sometimes is made that the type of care setting may well be important from this point of view. True, there may be no care setting that can by itself guarantee high quality professional performance. However, some care settings may tend to encourage such performance and other care settings may tend to lean in the other direction. In making this case, the features of care settings usually singled out for attention are solo vs. group practice and the nature of the incentives afforded by physician compensation systems.

Proponents of group practice contend that this mode tends to encourage high quality professional performance. Each physician in a group is exposed to some monitoring of his performance by the others in the group. It is harder to hide errors or slipshod work. Moreover, for each physician, the group provides a readily available resource of professional expertise and continuing education. And the group may de-

velop a professional esprit de corps that affords organizational encouragement of excellence. These alleged benefits might derive from various
kinds of physician groups, e.g., prepaid group practice, large conventional clinic groups, medical school faculties, and the staff physicians
in a particular hospital department.

By contrast, the proponents of this view would contend, the representative solo practitioner is at once free of the constraints imposed by
the group practice situation and deprived of the supports and encourage-
ments that stem from the group situation and this is likely to have un-
toward consequences for quality. Only empirical inquiry can validate
these contentions.

Turning to physician compensation, the important distinction is between fee-for-service and capitation–salary arrangements. It commonly
is contended that there is widespread "overutilization" of medical services (including, for example, a distressing amount of "unnecessary"
surgery).[5] It further is contended that a large part of the fault on this
score is to be laid to the fee-for-service system, which allegedly encourages physicians to "create" demand for their services. One way to put
this matter is that the fee-for-service physician confronts a compensation system that tends to introduce an unself-conscious "bias" in favor
of more treatment when making the judgment about appropriate treatment regimens. These judgments come to be reflected in a "style" of
medical practice that encourages overutilization, a style that tends to
become self-reinforcing as physicians generally come to conform to the
medical practice styles they see about them.[6]

The other side of this coin is the alleged salutary influence of physician salary compensation schemes upon utilization and prescribing patterns. For example, it seems to be true that HMOs generally feature
much lower per capita hospitalization rates than those exhibited by the
health sector generally. The explanation of this is frequently found in
the incentive implications of compensation arrangements. In effect,
HMO physicians are usually salaried, meaning that (in any straightforward, short-run sense) their incomes are independent of whether they
do or do not prescribe any given treatment, such as surgery. This circumstance, in this view, results in an "unbiased," best-practice medical
judgment about appropriate prescriptions of treatment, and this in turn,
it is contended, entails less surgery, etc. Collectively, these judgments
come to be reflected in an HMO "style" of medical practice that tends
to become self-reinforcing, for example, as new members of the medical group come to conform to the medical-practice style of the system
of which they are a part.

Under H M O -type financing arrangements, the physicians' incomes over the long run are not independent of whether they do or do not prescribe any given treatment for a given patient, and the incentives afforded may lead to "underutilization" and "under-doctoring." In other words, more time spent with member Paul may preclude making time available for an additional dues-paying member Peter, and in the case of surgery, which demands expensive hospital facilities, it must be reckoned that the more hospital capacity required by the group, the less will be available out of members' dues income to pay physicians' salaries. In this view, it is contended that the physicians are aware of all of this and tend to "under-doctor."[7]

One cannot *a priori* resolve the conflict between these various versions of the performance implications of the financial incentive effects. There is no kind of compensation scheme that can be regarded as neutral in its incentive effects. However, it is hazardous to jump to conclusions about physician performance just on the basis of such financial incentive effects. Financial incentives are only one component of the incentive mix; equally crucial are professional incentives. What is important is whether, as a matter of empirical generalization, there tends to be on average a relationship between these dimensions of quality ("over-doctoring" vs. "under-doctoring"), on the one hand, and different types of care setting on the other. Definitive work to afford this empirical generalization remains to be done.

Important values are served if physicians bring genuine expertise to their tasks and if, armed with this expertise, they attend conscientiously to their patients' problems. "Over-doctoring" in the sense of providing "unnecessary" services (particularly such categories as surgery) surely represents egregious noncompliance with those values we wish to see served in the medical care sector. Similarly, "under-doctoring" can fail to provide those services deemed "necessary" by accepted medical practice standards. Basically, we need to rely heavily on the individual physician's own sense of professional responsibility to secure the desired performance.[8] Nevertheless, those properties of care settings, which tend to bias the performance of the delivery system in the one direction or the other, have potentially important implications for the question of service to values.

Joint Physician–Patient Decision Making

Decisions about medical treatment are properly joint physician–patient decisions. It is of fundamental importance to the conservation of values in the health sector that these decisions result from a process such that both the physician and the patient are, each in his appropriate role, decisive for the outcome. It requires a short chain of argument, undertaken in this section, to show how these considerations relate to distinctions between care settings.

The physician's proper role in this process is technical expert. He assembles relevant data, makes the diagnosis, and identifies potentially efficacious treatments. Then, ideally, he fully informs the patient of the probable advantages and disadvantages of the various treatments (including no treatment). Thus informed, the patient would choose the treatment (if any) to be assayed, depending on his preferences over the probable outcomes, which would include his own attitudes about risk and the like. Clearly, only the patient is in a position to define his own preferences in this sense. A physician–patient relationship of this kind is said to feature "full disclosure."[9]

There are very real difficulties involved with definition of and administration of an adequate standard of physician disclosures.[10] Nevertheless, it seems likely that the development of an adequate standard and adherence to it would afford a substantial assist to promoting and conserving quality and efficiency in the performance of the medical care sector, including service to peculiarly important values.

One might readily agree that the matter of full disclosure is importantly involved with values. At the same time, one might query what all of this has to do with distinctions between "care settings." After all, any given fee-for-service physician may be in default of or may scrupulously observe the duty of physician disclosure. In fact, the same may be said of any given HMO physician.

The answer here turns on problems with the role of "consumer sovereignty" in medical care markets. A decentralized, free-market economy relies heavily on the machinery of consumer sovereignty to map consumer preferences into market performance. A consumer operates the machinery of consumer sovereignty in his role as a marketeer on the demand side of markets. He responds to market opportunities and prices by playing take it or leave it and in this way affords suppliers with information regarding his preferences. Suppliers respond to this information by trying, pursuant to their own interests, to bring market performance in line with consumer preferences thus revealed. Thus, in ordinary markets, the consumer in his sovereign market role influences resource allocation decisions.

There is growing recognition, however, that because of such properties of medical services as product uncertainty, consumer sovereignty may not serve the consumer in medical care markets as well as it generally is supposed to in other markets. The consumer may need somehow to supplement his conventional marketeer role with other institutional roles in order to map his preferences into the performance of the sector. A currently much discussed possibility on this score is what is termed "consumer participation." In broad outline, the concept of "consumer participation" identifies the assignment of the consumer to another role—that of "lay manager," operating as part of the management decision-making process such that there is lay management participation with and lay management constraint upon that professional producer sovereignty that characterizes medical care markets.

It has been argued that a properly defined and properly administered rule of full disclosure is of vital importance to mapping relevant consumer preferences into therapeutic decisions. It may further be argued that if consumers have available to them consumer participation roles (as well as consumer sovereignty roles), the prospects for evolving and properly administering such a role are much better than otherwise would be the case. That is, consumer participation has considerable potential value as a catalyst and synergist to upgrade the potency of the physician's duty of "full disclosure."[11]

As the final link in this chain, it may be argued that certain characteristics of an HMO-type care setting afford a much better prospect for the development of the institution of consumer participation than is afforded by the representative fee-for-service setting. For consumers to serve as participating lay managers, there must be an "organization" to be managed, i.e., a defined constituency to be "represented" and to legitimate the incumbents of the lay management roles, and there must be identifiable management functions and roles. HMO-type care settings afford such an organizational context; the decentralized, fee-for-service sector affords no such organizational context. It may, of course, be possible to contrive various nonconsumer sovereignty modes of consumer intervention in such atomistic fee-for-service markets. Thus, for example, consumers may undertake better to represent their interests through Nader-type "consumer advocacy." Whatever its merits, this mechanism is, however, not at all the same institution as "consumer participation" as defined here.

In sum, the development and administration of an adequate duty-of-full-disclosure rule in the physician–patient relationship is fundamental to the conservation of important values. Because it may potentiate the operation of such a rule (and for other reasons not herein elucidated), "consumer participation" is to be regarded as potentially important to the service of important values. Hence, those care settings that facilitate the development of this institution are, on this ground, to be preferred to those care setting that impose substantial bars to the development of this institution. It has been my contention that the HMO-type care setting has distinct advantages from this point of view.

SOCIETAL STRATEGIES IN SELECTING HEALTH CARE SYSTEMS

Societal strategies in selecting health care systems focus on balancing the advantages of a planned and regulated health care system against those relying more or less on the marketplace model. This language suggests to me the common but misleading dichotomy between "planning" (or "regulation") on the one hand and a "free market" system on the other.

Planning (regulation) of health care markets is a means to an end; namely, those market performance objectives to which regulation is addressed. The regulator or would-be regulator has preferences with respect to sector performance, some of which outcomes are preferred to others. He undertakes regulation (he assays planning strategies) in an effort to increase the probability that the actual performance of the sector will exhibit the preferred outcomes.

Any of various regulation strategies might be resorted to. One might identify the following among categories of implementation strategies:

1. Dissemination of information, e.g., identification of "needs" or perhaps projections of "demands," with the hope that this information will tend to induce other decision makers to undertake desired activities. Manpower "planning" is frequently of this genre, e.g., the physician manpower reports of the late 1950s, which forecast impending severe shortages unless the supply side of the market for physicians' services was altered;
2. Advertising to persuade and influence, admonish, propagandize, etc.; so-called "family planning" programs frequently assume this form;
3. Subsidies of desired activity, leaving the initiative to others to undertake the desired activity. The enrollment–augmentation grants to medical schools were an example of this strategy, providing that if a medical school increased its enrollment, a subsidy would be forthcoming;
4. Financing the demand for medical care (with or without taxes earmarked for the purpose), e.g., Medicare, Medicaid;
5. Government purchase and distribution, e.g., immunization programs in which vaccine is made available to the private health care sector;
6. Legal proscription of unwanted activities, e.g., certificate-of-need

legislation to control additional capacity in the hospital sector;

7. Legal mandating of desired activities, e.g., the promulgation of staffing and equipment norms for health care facilities; and

8. Direct production and delivery by government, e.g., Veterans hospitals, the Public Health Service.

As frequently employed, the term "regulation" applies only to legal control of performance, as by an agency administering definite performance standards. However, as the foregoing discussion suggests, whatever the objectives sought by "regulation," the same objectives *might* be sought by resort to other kinds of implementation strategies; both represent "regulation" in the functional sense of undertaking some kind of intervention with an eye to increasing the probability of preferred outcomes. Given the range of strategical availabilities, it is not fruitful to think in terms "regulation" vs. "free market," as if the system were either "regulated" or "not regulated." Rather, we should think in terms of mixes of implementation strategies with each mix peculiarly tailored to the objectives sought.

It follows from these considerations that it is not fruitful to discuss regulation vs. nonregulation of the health care sector "in general." Rather, such discussion must be directed to particularly identified performance objectives for the sector and to the mix of implementation strategies that might best achieve these. It is not possible to comprehensively survey the health care sector in this way. Consequently, in what follows I undertake to discuss only a few selected points that involve societal strategies in selecting health care systems.

Economic Efficiency of Care Settings

I began this paper with some discussion of the national health care social contract; namely, access by all to adequate health care is a basic right of the citizen in this social order. An important canon contained in this policy dictum is, "No one shall be denied access to medical care because of inability to pay." Central to achieving compliance with this canon is the design of the medical care financing system. Hence this system is importantly involved with service to values. However, most of the issues involved with the overall design of the financing system do not necessarily turn on distinctions among "care settings" as developed above. Consequently, the following does not afford a general discussion of health care financing.

Nevertheless, it is appropriate in this context to direct attention to a couple of related issues. The first is exemplary of the proposition that regulation is the mother of regulation (a special case of the celebrated, more general law that states that invention is the mother of necessity).

Putting a paid-up health insurance policy in everybody's back pocket does not, of course, ensure that all will have adequate access to health care. Whatever the financial terms for access to care, the system cannot meet its access obligations if, in real terms, medical care goods and services are in short supply, either overall or locally (the maldistribution problem). Under such circumstances, financing additional demand may only result in rapidly rising costs and prices. Consequently, once public policy has recognized the legitimacy of the claims to access by implementing a health care financing program, it is necessary to look to the supply side of the market to determine if complementary regulation will be required there.

Such a look to the supply side may well direct attention to the relative economic efficiency of different types of care settings. The more economical the care settings are, the more likely it is that we will be able to comply with access goals, including the matter of holding the line on costs and prices.[12] It is pursuant to such considerations that HMOs have in recent years, because of their apparent economy, attracted considerable attention. For example, it has been much remarked that HMOs generally exhibit per capita hospitalization rates much below the national average. Although less frequently remarked, HMOs use physician manpower at per capita rates (the rate varying with the HMO) considerably below the national average.

The question whether HMOs are, in fact, as some believe, just what the doctor should order to cope with a "crisis" in the nation's health care system is not at issue here. Rather, my intention is to elucidate one particular route by means of which choice among care settings becomes involved with values. The access-to-care goals of national health policy urge that planning (regulation) be assayed on the demand side of the market such as by federal design and sponsorship of health insurance schemes. In this context, relative economy becomes a potentially important differential property of care settings. The more economic types are to be preferred, pursuant to the same right-to-access values that motivated intervention on the demand side in the first place.

Societal Preferences and the Health Care Market

The performance of the health care sector (as does that of the whole economy of which it is a part) will in *some* way reflect the preferences of its constituency. In analyzing the structure of the social decision-making process that accomplishes this preference-mapping function, we may identify two broad roles that individuals may occupy—the "marketeer" and the "planner." These roles will interact in various ways to determine such matters as the rate of resource allocation to the health sector and its various subsectors, the design of various delivery systems, and the mix of these in use.

We may further identify two kinds of consumer marketeer role—consumer sovereignty and consumer choice. In both roles, consumers operate as marketeers on the demand side of markets, responding to prices, and freely decide what to buy and what not to buy. There is a fundamental difference, however. Consumer sovereignty means that consumer market choices have a direct impact on resource allocation; resources flow to the production of those outputs relatively favored by consumers and away from other outputs. In the usual market, this happens because for-profit marketeers on the supply side of the market respond to the cues afforded by consumer choices.

Consumer choice in markets need not have a direct impact on resource allocation, however. Consider a centrally planned economy such that the plan completely determines the mix of goods and services to be produced. With such a system, consumers might still confront prices in markets and freely choose what to buy and what not to buy. Since under such a system planners' decisions have determined the outputs of each of the various economic activities, consumer choice has no direct impact on resource allocation.[13]

To say that under such a system consumer choice has no *direct* impact on resource allocation does not necessarily imply that it has *no* impact on resource allocation. Consumer choices will afford information to the planners about consumer preferences, and the planners might take this information into account in fashioning the plans for the next planning period. In this case, the impact of consumer choice on resource allocation is attenuated; information afforded by the choices is filtered through the planning process and the resulting impact on resource allocation depends on how the planners take it into account.[14]

Turning to planner roles, planning is essentially a political process. The individuals who make up the social order have their impact on resource allocation by participating in that political process that yields legislation to regulate the health care sector in various ways. Thus the difference between a "market system" and "planning" is not that the individual has an impact on resource allocation under the former and under the latter he does not. The individual may serve his consumer interests under either system, albeit the structure of the decision-making process that maps consumer preferences into market performance is very different under the two systems. If one is thinking about "balance

of power" conflicts inherent in resource allocation systems, the market
vs. planning distinction implies a conflict between the consumer (*qua*
marketeer) and the consumer (*qua* planner) role.[15]

How best to contrive the mix between marketeer roles and planner
roles is a perplexing question when designing the resource allocation
machinery for the health sector pursuant to mapping individuals' consumer preferences into market performance. This is so because individuals themselves seem to reach different conclusions about what resource
allocation decisions will best serve consumer interests depending on
which role they are operating out of. And the question becomes even
knottier if (in addition to the "consumer sovereignty" role) we explicitly
take account of the "consumer choice" role and of the various ways in
which the planners might respond to the information thus afforded to
them.

Consumer sovereignty (decisive, direct impact on resource allocation)
and consumer choice (no direct impact on resource allocation) represent
the extreme ends of a spectrum. There may be various degrees of attenuation of consumer sovereignty in between. We suggested that under our
hypothetical consumer choice system, the planners might "load the
dice" by contriving a set of relative prices such that the consumers
"freely" choose to consume just that bill of goods the planners have
decided to produce. More generally, planners might "load the dice" in a
less decisive way, such as by contriving sets of relative prices that influence the pattern of consumer choice while still allowing choice to
have a direct impact on resource allocation. Indeed, this is done—usually
inadvertently—in designing health care financing systems. Depending on
the mix of features in our financing scheme—complete coverage for
some categories of services, no coverage for other categories of services,
deductibles, coinsurance, etc.—we will present the consumer with a certain set of effective relative prices (a partially loaded set of dice) such
that we may expect the consumption patterns and resource use patterns
resulting from his "free" choices to differ from what they would have
been had we presented him with some other set of effective relative
prices.

CONCLUSION

It is perhaps time to return explicitly to the issue to which the last part
of this paper was addressed, namely societal strategies in selecting health
care systems. It must be abundantly clear by now that there is no simple
way to adequately characterize "societal strategies" and the differences
among them, e.g., as by identifying some with "reliance on the market"

and others with "planning and regulation." To characterize a societal strategy adequately, we must identify those decision-making processes and decision roles that collectively map various preferences into market performance, viz.: professional producer sovereignty, variously attenuated versions of professional producer sovereignty, consumer sovereignty, variously attenuated versions of consumer sovereignty, consumer choice, and planners' roles. Then we must specify interactions between these roles. For example, the planners may avail themselves of any of a wide range of planning (implementation) strategies to establish constraints and an incentive structure within which producers and consumers will operate their (thus attenuated) sovereign roles. The planners may in various ways respond to information generated in consequent consumer choice, and so on.

We would all agree that whatever societal strategy we elect to guide the evolution of the health sector, it should be responsive to consumer preferences and it should yield a mix of care settings such as to conserve important values. We might well find it harder to agree just what such a strategy should look like.

Perhaps the best I can do by way of conclusion is to suggest to you the bare-bones outline of what might be regarded as an acceptable strategy. Societal strategies (and the planning and nonplanning they may entail) are means to ends. We need first of all to try to be clear about the objectives we seek. The immediate problem set for this discussion was to achieve an appropriate mix of care settings in the health sector, where the choice has been defined in very general terms as between HMOs and fee-for-service settings. The objective to be achieved in designing the sector in these terms is to conserve values. What values? I cannot here undertake to present an exhaustive list. In the course of this exposition, however, I have made certain suggestions that may be regarded as exemplary:

1. Those values inherent in the proposition that ". . .access by all to adequate health care is a basic right of the individuals comprising the society";
2. That no one should be constrained to use physicians he does not like and does not have confidence in;
3. That the consumer is entitled to high quality care in the sense of a high level of physician performance *qua* professional, including the vital matter of compliance with the physician's duty of "full disclosure."

Value set 1 requires that, whatever other strategies we adopt, we pay due attention to achieving equitable financial terms for access to care.

This no doubt will call for some planning to design the health care financing system adequately. It also requires that we pay due attention to the supply of health services such that access in real terms is guaranteed. This also, no doubt, will require various kinds of planning. More particularly to the point for this paper, compliance with value set 1 *may* involve planning to influence the care setting mix in the health sector. *If* HMOs are more economical than fee-for-service settings (in real terms) and *if* we are unwilling as a matter of public policy to make enough total resources available to meet our access obligations under fee-for-service settings, then as a matter of public policy we may be constrained differentially to favor (as by such planning strategies as subsidies) HMO settings. Beyond this, e.g., some categories of publicly sponsored patients such as Medicaid, we may feel that because of the nature of the contractual relationship between patients and providers afforded by HMOs, we may want, pursuant to compliance with our access obligations, to plan the availability of such settings for such patients.

Turning to value sets 2 and 3, our discussion has shown that arguments pro and con can be made on the score of which care setting best serves these values. On balance, however (and in our present state of knowledge about the performance of each setting), perhaps there is no clear, decisive advantage attaching to either setting. This would suggest to me that, in the evolution of the health care system, HMO and fee-for-service options should be available to each consumer and that care settings of each type should have an equal chance to bid for the consumer's favor. Pursuant to this, our strategy should be to contrive an environment that is as "neutral" as possible, in the sense of not differentially favoring the growth of the one care setting at the expense of the other. Various elements in such a strategy will come to mind and need not be rehearsed here. However, it should be remarked that HMOs frequently require "front end" subsidies from some source to carry them until growth permits them to be self-sustaining, which is analogous to the "infant industry" argument in favor of some tariffs. Planning the provision of subsidies of this sort is not to be regarded as differentially favoring HMOs; it is necessary to "neutralize" the environment in the sense herein intended.

Our societal strategy should include a monitoring system to assemble and feed back to the planners information about the performance of the different care settings, including the information generated by consumer choice behavior in markets. This especially should be the case if, perhaps pursuant to value set 1, we decide to "load the dice" somewhat in favor of HMOs.

REFERENCES AND NOTES

1. We might add an additional proviso, viz: the health care financing system is such that no one is denied access to care because of inability to pay. However, the resolution of most issues involved with health care financing does not turn in any peculiar way on distinctions between types of care settings. (See comment later in this paper.) Consequently, for present purposes, we assume that whatever the type of care setting, the individual can "afford" care and confine attention to those bars to access implied in the text.

2. Some such consumers feel that they can facilitate their choice by, in effect, choosing from among those physicians in a "closed panel" of their own identification—e.g., a medical school faculty, the staff of a prestigious, nationally famous clinic. This suggests that, for some, at least, the problem with the conventional closed-panel arrangement is not just the constraint to choose from among some subset of all of the physicians in the service area. Rather, the problem may be with the particular panel, such as lack of what, to the particular consumer in question, are cues attesting to the quality of the panel.

3. The following section includes more discussion of the quality issue.

4. Another possibility is that (the illusion of?) "free" choice per se is an important source of satisfaction for the consumer, such that he not only wants to find a physician he likes and has confidence in but he also wants to find such a physician via the free-choice route. For such a consumer, a care setting that confronts him with a "closed panel" may be per se unsatisfactory—both *ex ante* any experience with it and even *ex post* any experience he might have with it. For such a consumer, there is really no care setting answer other than a setting he is willing to agree embodies his concept of free choice.

5. What is or is not an "unnecessary" medical procedure of any kind is a complicated judgment that we cannot now explore.

6. Alternatively, physicians under fee-for-service are piece workers, self-conscious of the fact that there is a direct, short-run connection between their treatment patterns and their incomes. Hence, they tend to recommend more treatment than they would otherwise. Fee-for-service physicians generally would deny that their own actual experience conforms to this theory.

7. HMO physicians would deny that their own actual experience conforms to this theory. I have dealt with the question of the operation of incentives in the HMO practice setting at greater length: HMOs—what makes them tick? Health Care Policy Disc Paper Ser No 6. Center for Community Health and Medical Care, Harvard University, Cambridge, Massachusetts.

8. Many observers are, of course, skeptical on this score—feeling that we need to change the structure of the system (e.g., introduce PSROs) to increase the probability of compliance with such professional norms.

9. "Full disclosure" is akin to the traditional "informed consent" doctrine; albeit what I have in mind here is rather more far-reaching in its implications than the usual formulation of the latter doctrine.

10. I have discussed the matter of "full disclosure" at greater length in On "consumer participation" in medical-care markets. Health Care Policy Disc Paper Ser No 5. Center for Community Health and Medical Care, Harvard University,

Cambridge, Massachusetts. Some of the following comments about the role of consumer participation are adapted from this source.

11. Quite apart from the matter of a full disclosure rule, proponents of consumer participation would contend that in various ways this institution affords a necessary assist to efficient discharge of the preference mapping function. I have emphasized the matter of full disclosure because I regard it as centrally important. However, I recognize that consumer participation is a structural feature of care settings that may help to conserve important values in other ways.

12. For health care production activities (as elsewhere) greater economic efficiency means more output per unit of input; in making the calculation, care is taken to count *all* of the relevant output and *all* of the relevant input.

   To avoid misunderstanding, it is perhaps worth remarking that whatever the rate of health care output, more efficient care settings will incur a lower real economic cost and hence are *in general* to be preferred, i.e., quite apart from the particular question of compliance with right-to-access goals implied by national health policy. Nevertheless (and as recent legislative and other events would suggest), it is especially when such goals of national health policy are "taken seriously," as by legislative activity on the national health insurance front, that the matter of the economic efficiency of different care settings seems to have an urgent claim to attention at the central policy level.

13. Such a centrally planned system need not feature consumer free choice. Alternatively, consumers might be issued ration tickets entitling each to a defined share of the planned outputs.

14. The planners need not take consumer preferences revealed by market choices into account in the way suggested. Alternatively, they might adjust the relative prices of outputs so as to clear the market, i.e., adjust relative prices such that consumers "freely" choose to consume just that mix of goods and services the planners had decided to produce.

15. The market vs. planning distinction might also imply a "balance of power" conflict between the consumers (patients) and producers (physicians) if, say, the producers tried to "capture" the planning process and use it to forward their objectives at the expense of the consumers. In the real world of planning and regulation, this is, of course, a lively and important possibility. I abstract from it in this discussion in an effort to hold this topic to manageable proportions and in recognition of the fact that, in any case, this particular problem is the subject of much attention in the regulation literature.

   There may also, of course, be a "balance of power" conflict in the market sector between consumers in their marketeer roles and producers in their marketeer roles. I undertook to draw attention to this earlier in this paper when I discussed the attenuation of consumer sovereignty in medical services markets (e.g., due to product uncertainty) and the physician's role of professional producer sovereignty. I then suggested that if consumers had available to them another role, that identified as consumer participation, it would help with the management of this conflict.

EUGENE OUTKA, Ph.D.
Department of Religion, Princeton University

Commentary

The papers on which I have been asked to comment are in both cases perceptive and illuminating. They are nicely sensitive, for example, to the advantages and disadvantages of the two "subsets" of care settings they consider, namely, fee-for-service and Health Maintenance Organizations (HMOs). When I observe that one can genuinely learn from what Dr. Halberstam and Professor Stevens have written here, I mean this with a seriousness that far exceeds any pro forma opening commendation. Yet my admiration is not unqualified, and for reasons more substantive, I hope, than the general expectation that a commentator must invariably have critical things to say. My principal worry is that important differences between the two papers may be obscured because (1) some of the points are made in an excessively tentative way and (2) the institutional implications of certain values extolled are not always traced relentlessly enough. So casual reader X may draw the misleading conclusion (as it seems to me) that the differences are only, in that flabby phrase, "matters of emphasis." X may point out that while Dr. Halberstam is "skeptical about prepayment," he quickly adds that he considers prepayment or capitation "valid methods of practice"; he respects what Kaiser for example has accomplished; and he repudiates any law that limits "the development of prepaid practice." All that he resists is any decision, whether by the Institute, the medical profession, or the government,

271

"to encourage prepayment as *the* desirable way to practice." And while Professor Stevens is more disposed to stress the advantages of HMOs, he seems not to plump decisively for the decision feared by Dr. Halberstam. Professor Stevens notes that "front end" subsidies for HMOs may be justified simply as a necessary condition in order to *neutralize* the options. So far as many of the most relevant values are concerned (with two notable exceptions, which I shall discuss), no clear advantage obtains for either care setting, he believes, and thus "each type should have an equal chance to bid for the consumer's favor."

Such a thoroughly irenic outcome oversimplifies. To show where, let me consider briefly the respective importance accorded certain pivotal "values" in the two papers and note some specific agreements, puzzles, and misgivings as I go along.

EQUAL ACCESS

The value (or ideal, or societal goal) of equal access to comprehensive health services, irrespective of income or geographic location, has now virtually the status of a platitude. Political leaders on both left and right give it at least verbal endorsement. In Professor Stevens' words, "access by all to adequate health care is a basic right of the citizen of this social order." He goes so far as to call it a "health care social contract." One striking difference between the two papers is that Professor Stevens commends this value far more explicitly and often than does Dr. Halberstam. The latter alludes to it toward the beginning of his paper. Here he construes the notion of medical care as a right to be historically the result of an emergent industrial society. "An ethic grew that saw medical care as a right, subsidized by the state if otherwise unavailable, as an expense that should be shared among the community at large, and as a service that could be organized rationally along the line of an industrial process." He takes no very great pains to applaud this development, for he immediately proceeds to speak of its "inevitable conflict with an equally important concept of the industrial society, the ideal of professionalism." Later he refers in passing to the sense in which Americans may now "accept the notion that they have a financial, as well as moral, stake in keeping their neighbors free of catastrophic illness or expense. . . ." Even here, at least in the context, he seems less than enthusiastic. He is stressing the inordinate demands that a small percentage of patients place on facilities and the way in which freedom from catastrophic expense need not extend to "subsidizing. . .neuroses." Finally, he does indeed make plain at the end that the government's role in medical care should be to furnish safeguards against financial disaster and to assume

direct responsibility for certain groups who currently fall outside the
established system, e.g., "Indians, the rural poor, merchant seamen."
Such provisions do not require, in his judgment, any basic alteration in
the way medical care is presently organized.

The issue then is whether Dr. Halberstam is unduly sanguine about the
prospects of realizing under the established system—at least as well as any
alternative arrangement—the ideal of equal access. He appears to affirm
but not to dwell on the moral relevance of the ideal itself and to be
struck with the ways in which it may clash with other values. Professor
Stevens wrestles more continuously with this question. He allows that
the "social contract" may have implications for our assessment of how
different care settings foster morally relevant human interests. In ponder-
ing these implications, he offers the following argument, which in my
opinion is rather formidable: The more economical the care setting, the
greater the compliance with equal access objectives. HMOs are held to
be less costly per capita in at least two respects: hospitalization rates are
much below the national average and, less often noted, physician manpower is also. There may be an empirical dispute here. Dr. Halberstam
is inclined to doubt some of the claims about the cost-effectiveness of
prepaid groups. Given Professor Stevens's figures, however, I must admit
to some surprise that at the end of this paper his conclusion is so curi-
ously tentative. There he identifies three "value sets," designed as a summary of his paper. The first of these is equal access. Yet when he re-
counts his argument, he puts it now in the hypothetical mood: *If* HMOs
are more economical and *if* we are not, *qua* society, prepared to spend
enough effectively to realize the goal of equal access, *then* we may be
constrained to favor HMO settings via subsidies and planning strategies.
So my query is this, "Does such a conclusion trace with sufficient relentlessness the implications of his own argument?" To put the matter perhaps too crudely," Why should Professor Stevens, in light of his foregoing argument, not actively *press* on behalf of, say, a Kennedy-like
favoritism for HMOs?" The question is reinforced when one observes
that no clear advantage is held to obtain, in Professor Stevens's view, between fee for service and HMOs in regard to the other two value sets.
Why then should the first value set, encapsulated in the phrase "equal
access," not be taken as overriding?

A CLOSE PERSONAL RELATIONSHIP BETWEEN PATIENT AND PHYSICIAN OF HIS OR HER CHOICE

I come now to a value about which there is no apparent disagreement.
All of us presumably concur that such a relationship involves any num-

ber of benefits to everyone concerned. Professor Stevens identifies his
two final value sets along these lines: No one should be forced to seek
the help of physicians one does not like or who fail to elicit confidence;
and every patient should have high quality care as measured by the
criterion of "physician performance *qua* professional."

These contentions too sound platitudinous. Issues arise nonetheless at
two crucial junctures—the meaning of and the priority to be attached to
the provider's distinguishing role, and the character of patient participation. I shall consider the first of these now, and discuss the latter as a
separate consideration.

Dr. Halberstam devotes appreciable space to the vindication of the
physician's role. In so doing he identifies several conflicts between this
role and other commitments the physician and/or the society may have.
I admire Dr. Halberstam's candor here. His refusal to rest content with
the jargon-filled accounts one so frequently encounters that evade the
frank recognition of conflicts. We need to admit explicitly that not all
of the "values" we are prepared to commend separately can be easily
harmonized together. Some of them cut against each other on various
occasions. And when they do, we are forced to set priorities. Yet Dr.
Halberstam neglects perhaps to discuss in as much detail as one would
like (1) the possible relevant differences between the cases he cities and
(2) what criteria might be employed when one is forced to attach priorities. The first sort of case he notes has to do with the conflict between
the physician as an agent of the state or industry or *qua* "gatekeeper,"
on the one hand, and as simply doctor to the individual patient, on the
other. This case warrants the emphasis he gives it, because in general it
seems insufficiently acknowledged. After we have been made duly aware
of some perplexing clashes of interest, however, it is unclear from the
paper what, if anything, might be done. A second sort of case is taken to
be analogous to the first. The dangers that confront the physician whose
patients contract directly or through a third party to prepay for their
medical care are relevantly akin to the former "gatekeeper" kind. Dr.
Halberstam does acknowledge that important differences exist between
the two sorts of situations, yet he believes they overlap enough to en-
danger physician autonomy in either setting. The danger follows because any organization has a life of its own that demands a commitment
from its members. I gather he means to hold that physicians in general
have a *serious* conflict of loyalty in an HMO setting that is absent from
a fee-for-service one. Professor Stevens, it should be observed, appears
not to be similarly concerned. The issues about provider autonomy or
sovereignty do not for him turn decisively on whether the care setting
is fee for service or HMO. So it may be asked whether Dr. Halberstam

makes too much of the overlap between the conflict facing a physician in an HMO and as a member of an employment group. And even if one agrees about the extent of the overlap, other disadvantages to fee for service should be considered if we are to understand the full range of the complexities before us. For physician autonomy is surely corruptible too. Let us remember, for example, this well-known but nevertheless striking point: The United States has twice as many surgeons per capita and twice as many surgeries performed as does England. Fee for service seems not automatically to promote the best interests of every patient, and a close link between the healing art and direct monetary payment seems not always to contribute to a morally responsible medical profession. It should also be admitted that the HMO may be corruptible in the opposite direction; a characteristic temptation would appear to be "underutilization." As Professor Stevens notes, no care setting is entirely neutral with respect to its incentive effects. Perhaps at a minimum we ought to say that each care setting should be available in every region of the country. For if we assume a common freedom to choose between them, each may help to guard against the peculiar temptations to which the other is inclined.

A third sort of conflict case considered by Dr. Halberstam has to do with what he calls the ethic of the legislator and the ethic of the physician. The legislator should be governed by the canon of the greatest good for the greatest number, the physician by the greatest good for the individual patient for whom he or she is responsible. Here is a conflict, Dr. Halberstam alleges, that is implacable. Each canon is justified, but the "world views" they represent cannot be reconciled. So he is led into statements such as the following, which at the very least seem subject to challenge: "In the long run society is best served by ignoring society. The social obligation of the physician is to ignore society." Yet Dr. Halberstam himself later commends something like "two years' service in an underserved area as a condition to licensing." Suppose one agrees with this account of the legislator's responsibility. He or she is required to mesh various value considerations as far as possible for the sake of benefits to as large a number as possible. The overriding commitment is to the "common good" rather than a particular good. In a world of suboptimal alternatives, this will involve difficult choices about the allocation of medical resources overall—choices, if this third sort of conflict is pressed too far, to which the physician by virtue of his ethic seems to have nothing to contribute. Is Dr. Halberstam content to leave it at that? Is there really no place in the physician's ethic for responsibility to society as well as to the individual patient? Especially in light of the widely publicized "new medical humanism," to distinguish without further ado between two incommensurable ethical views may be to oversimplify. At least one hopes that increasing numbers of physicians will come to the aid of legislators and others in devising just criteria for the allocation of scarce resources. On the now well-worn issue of "personalization vs. systematization," is it wholly unrealistic to expect physicians to worry seriously about the latter as well as the former? One relishes those encouraging signs that physicians will not in the name of professional autonomy continue to accept the sheer diffusion of energy and efforts that has characterized so much of American medical practice in the past.

PATIENT PARTICIPATION

Once more we have a value extolled by virtually everyone. Yet the meaning of "participation" needs to be clarified. Professor Stevens distinguishes between different roles "consumers" may conceivably occupy. He maintains in effect that "consumer choice" is not the same as "consumer sovereignty" and cannot be, given the nature of medical care. He also identifies the sense in which "professional producer sovereignty" is crucial and unavoidably so. Dr. Halberstam does not consider similar distinctions, but he does express a basic optimism about the degree of "knowledge" that patients and potential patients possess. Thus he writes, "I would suspect that the American people know more about the workings of the medical profession than they do about any single occupational group with the possible exception of the Mafia." And again, "The information that the public does have available on physicians exceeds that in other fields, and the public makes good use of it."

It seems to me important to distinguish between the public's knowledge of the organizational workings of the medical profession, including an awareness of the phychological nuances of those who practice medicine, from knowledge about assessments of individual illnesses. So far as the latter are concerned, there seems to be a conspicuous limitation to any notion of "consumer choice." On this subject, Professor Stevens's discussion seems particularly helpful (including the clear advantage the HMO possesses here, so far as the organizational context goes). For it seems to remain the case that the public's knowledge in the latter instance is comparatively limited. While we may actively and justifiably seek as much "patient participation" as possible, it should be remembered that the physician makes most of the decisions—about diagnosis, treatment, hospitalization, number of return visits, etc. Some go so far as to contend that:

The consumer knows very little about the medical services he is buying—probably less than about any other service he purchases. . . .While [he] can still play a role in policing the market, that role is much more limited in the field of health care than in almost any other area of private economic activity.[1]

I have argued elsewhere[2] that this kind of restriction on "consumer choice" is one of the special features of health care that renders problematic those efforts to incorporate questions about medical treatments into the usual economic canons of supply and demand. But that is another story.

REFERENCES

1. Schultze CL, Fried ER, Rivlin AM, Teeters NH: Setting National Priorities: The 1973 Budget. Washington, D.C.: The Brookings Institution, 1972, pp 214–215.
2. For the detailed case, see Outka E: Social justice and equal access to health care. J Relig Ethics, spring 1974.

VI

Ethical Problems in the Treatment of the Chronically Ill and the Aged

The chronically ill and aged are potentially large consumers of the resources of the health care system. However, the care of these patients has been ignored because it is often very expensive and limited medical resources are required that could be used to treat the young who might be returned to socially useful lives. The papers in this section examine the ethical implications of social policy regarding the availability of health care to these patients.

JEROME KAPLAN, Ph.D.
Director, Mansfield Memorial Homes, Inc., Mansfield, Ohio

In Search of Policies for Care of the Aged

It has been very forcibly argued that ". . .few, if any, persons are ever 'on their own,' that we are all dependent on people, that we are sustained and shaped through the support of our family, friends, co-workers, and indeed, through the social networks and associations in which we are located."[1] While made in the context of espousing group involvement and support over the methadone approach in treating drug addiction, it is noteworthy that similar interpersonal methods have been successfully used in other situations—such as in alcoholism and obesity—and that they lie at the base of the early moral treatment decisions within our society for the chronically ill and the aging.

In an all encompassing sense, the latter embraces the chronically ill. While simultaneously acknowledging there are variations, a further assumption is that explorations into aging are also explorations with the chronically ill. The largest single grouping of the chronically ill are the aged; hence, the concentration herein of gerontological relationships and content.

SELECT GERONTOLOGY FACETS

Gerontology Defined

There are four related but separate aspects to the study of aging. The biological aspect deals with physical aging—the body's gradual loss of the ability to renew it-

281

self. The psychological aspect deals with the sensory processes, perception, motor skills, intelligence, problem-solving, understanding, learning drives, and emotions of the aging individual. The biological and psychological changes which occur with advancing age, coupled with the social environment of the individual, produce a third aspect—the behavioral. This aspect of aging deals with attitudes, expectancies, motives, the self-image, social roles, personality, and psychological adjustment to the situation. Finally, the sociological aspect of aging deals with the society in which aging occurs, the influence this society has on the aging individual, and the influence he has on it. The older person's health, income, work, and leisure, as these relate to his family, friends, voluntary associations, and religious groups, as well as to society in general, the economy, the government, and the community are all part of the sociology of aging.

These four aspects on aging—biological, psychological, behavioral, and sociological—are all interrelated in the life of any older person.[2]

It has been customary to assume that old age sets in somewhere during the seventh decade of life, and, until recently, much of research and the majority of action programs have focused on the period beginning at or near age 65. It is now recognized, however, that the real turning point comes much earlier. On the basis of present knowledge, it seems possible to identify three stages of advanced adulthood: middle age, later maturity and old age.[3]

Middle Age   Middle age is the period when the individual first becomes aware of the fact that he is growing old. This phase of the life cycle usually occurs during the forties and fifties. At this time the individual becomes aware that he has less energy than he used to, and he often begins to see a need for intellectual activities to replace more physical pursuits as sources of satisfaction.

Chronic illness becomes more prevalent. In the fifties, vision and hearing begins to fail. Women pass through menopause, usually a difficult transition. The work career often reaches a plateau, and the children have left home by the time most couples reach their early fifties.

Later Maturity   Later maturity is marked by greater awareness of aging and by a difficulty in remaining future oriented. Chronologically, it often corresponds to the sixties and seventies. There is a drastic reduction in available energy during this period, and the individual becomes very aware of his failing eyes and ears.

Long-term chronic health problems begin to limit activity during this period. Retirement and the accompanying reduction of income combine with poor health to reduce the individual's personal contacts. Deaths of relatives and friends and movement of children also reduce his social environment. Most people, however, retain a fair measure of physical vigor and obtain freedom from responsibilities.

Old Age   Old age is characterized by extreme frailty, disability, or invalidism. Mental processes slow down. The individual thinks about himself and his past and tries to find some meaning in life. Activity is greatly restricted. Loneliness and boredom are thought to be common.

The above description is based on characteristics not necessarily synonymous with chronological age. While chronological age is related to phases of the life cycle in most cases, this relation is not an absolute. The important point is whether one has the characteristics of old age, not whether one has reached a certain age.

Havighurst[4] raised an important point of definition of old age as it involves work when he suggested that old age is defined more and more by a broad social competence and less and less by narrow work competence. Social competence is seen as relatively independent of biological functioning, which does decline with age. Social competence is not to be understood as synonymous with cognitive and perceptual abilities, which do undergo changes with age. Social competence reflects man's daily interactions and typical responsibilities as distinct from cognitive and perceptual abilities that change with age.

The lawmakers, however, have really defined old age for us. It is 65 years of age. Most people in this country become eligible for retirement with social security benefits at this age, and this legal decision has great import in our lives. Attitudes and expectations are formed on this basis, and it would not be unreasonable to believe that many people become old because they and the world around them have accepted such a definition.

Population and Life Expectancy

The roots of aging as a social problem are complex. Society, though, has not been prepared to receive the large new group of older members who now live the allotted threescore and ten (Table 1).

The number of older people will probably continue to increase rapidly over the next few decades. And the proportion of the population 65 and over may actually increase more than projected in Table 1 as the birth rate decline that began in 1958 continues.[6] Consistent estimates put the 1973 United States population of people 65 and over at 22 million.*

Compared with 1900, males in the United States who are age 45 have an average life expectancy of an additional 27 years, i.e., 72 years' lifespan. For women the life expectancy is nearly 5 years longer.[7]

* H. Brotman, personal communication.

TABLE 1   Percent of Total U.S. Population Age 65 and Over for Selected Years[a]

	1900	1940	1950	1960	1970	2000 (Projected)
Percent age 65 and over	4.0	6.8	8.1	9.2	9.6	11.1

[a] U.S. Bureau of the Census.[5]

Women, living longer than men, constitute a larger segment of older population. This trend appears to be increasing. Figure 1 shows that while in the population of people aged 25 years men outnumber women slightly, the reverse is true after this age and the trend becomes progressive.

Societal Change and Role

Old age is in itself a stigma. This stigma is often the result of stereotypes, but sometimes it results from an adequate evaluation of actual capabilities. Regardless of source, however, the stigma of old age is important because it influences what the aged expect of themselves, and it influences what others think about them. Understanding old people requires an understanding of its stigma and its effects.

By far the most important aspect of the stigma of old age is its negative, disqualifying character. On the basis of their age, older people are usually relegated to a position in society in which they are no longer judged to be of any use or importance. Like most other expendable elements in society, older people are subjected to poverty, illness, and social isolation with subsequent second-class care.

When the pace of change in a society is slow, most people are able to keep abreast of what is expected of them. For the most part, the norms they learned early in life remain appropriate, and unprecedented situations are few enough to not cause major problems.

In a rapidly changing society, however, many people find themselves in unprecedented positions for which norms are not yet specified. These people face the dilemma of having to play an incomplete role.

When changes are few and far between, various parts of society can adjust easily because it is usually necessary to accommodate only a few changes at a time. Rapid change alters this strategy because many changes must be accommodated simultaneously.

Furthermore, the various parts of society do not change at the same rate. Social change usually starts by affecting a subgroup within the

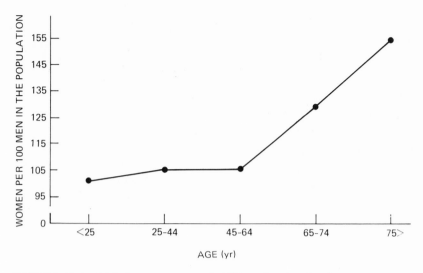

FIGURE 1 Ratio of American women to men in 1970 as a function of age.[8]

whole, and slowly the other parts of society adapt until eventually the entire society feels the effects of the change. A particularly difficult period occurs just after the change begins when the rest of society has not yet recognized or accepted a change within a subgroup. Older people often experience problems because other parts of society have neither recognized nor accepted the fact that chronological age is not even a reliable indicator of an individual's capabilities.[9]

[Several] . . .policies have developed which arbitrarily disqualify people from economic participation once they reach a given retirement age. While most other institutions in society do not phase out older people in quite this rigid a fashion, there are nevertheless norms which downgrade the value of the older person's contribution to the family, the church, the neighborhood, and voluntary associations. Only in politics and government, and in the arts and certain professions like medicine and law, have older people been able to keep positions earned earlier in life more or less intact.[10]

In general, then, American society is not geared to handle certain problems well, like the aged and the chronically ill, since we are a rapidly changing society. Roles are stabilized only in a stable society.

HEALTH PROBLEMS OF THE ELDERLY

Titmuss[11] notes that ". . .we can not inquire about quality standards of family doctoring without taking account of all the facilities and tools, medical and social, which are or might be at the service of the practitioner and the patient's family."

The relationship of the individual to a comprehensive health system includes not only the general environment but the many protective subsystems, such as the family, and, more broadly, the public–private organizations of income maintenance, housing, and health care delivery. The individual's index of health and his ability to rally from insults depend not only on his own capacities but also on the supports necessary and available to achieve optimum functioning. Accordingly, the effectiveness of comprehensive health programs must be measured in terms both of the elderly person's response to the insults to which he is exposed and of the extent to which the health system strives to enable him to function. An acceptable index will be found in the development of scales for evaluating activities of daily living.[12]

Morbidity Statistics

Townsend,[13] in attempting to measure disability, concluded "that the presence of a particular disease does not necessarily indicate for any given person the inhibition of activity which results from it." To follow, the notation that four out of five elderly suffer some chronic condition insult does not necessarily indicate the extent of impairment of function.[14]

While 81 percent of those over 65 suffer some chronic illness, 33 percent have no physical limitation on their activities; 7 percent have some limitations, but not on their major activity; 26 percent have limitations on major activity; and about 16 percent are unable to carry out their major activity. Thus, approximately half of the elderly are somewhat disabled because of a chronic illness.[15]

The specific level of mobility is of particular importance. Eight percent of the noninstitutionalized elderly are bedfast or housebound. In addition, 6 percent have limited physical ability to move in the community. Overall, more than 30 percent report difficulty in walking stairs.[16] Physical disability as a correlate of aging has been extensively documented.

Limitations of function are also imposed through mental impairment. Estimates of the incidence of mental impairment among the elderly vary from 10 to 25 percent.[17] Rates of psychosis, symptoms experienced as physical illness and organic mental disorders, as with physical disabilities, rise with advancing age.

There is mounting evidence of the rehabilitation potential of the elderly by practitioners in the field. Yet somehow this has not been translated into practice. Considerable research has dealt with negative attitudes that permeate the area of geriatrics.

It was found that both administrative and treatment staff inappropriately fear that the elderly are unresponsive and unrehabilitatable. Popular misconceptions about treatability often delays seeking help until a crisis develops.[18]

A system of comprehensive health care delivery should provide medical, health, *and* support services to enable the elderly who are physically disabled and/or impaired to utilize those resources.

Parsons points out the importance of ideological aspects of American society with respect to the health goals. The valuation of the "achievement" is heavily emphasized in our society, an "attitude which asserts the desirability of *measuring* the problems of health, and from that, for the individual sick person, the obligation to cooperate fully with the therapeutic agency, that is to work to achieve his own recovery."[19] The elderly are a part of the same cultural scene.[20]

By any of the measures of physical, mental, and environmental disability, older people in our society are a high risk group. The nature and number of their problems are beyond individual and family resources, thus requiring public coordination and support. Shanas[21] estimates that the target population of elderly needing services to maintain them at home is one in seven. The Baltimore Chronic Illness Study noted that when considerations of mental impairment and environmental hazards are added to those of physical disability, the need for services is one in three.[22] I would bend in this direction.

Chronic Illness and the Older Aged

Brotman's report based on the 1970 Census that the rate of increase of those 75 and over has escalated to three times as great as that of the 65–74 age group is an important consequence.

In other words, of the 3.5 million increase in the total older population between 1960 and 1970, only 1.4 million of the increase was in the 65–74 group with 2.1 million in the 75+ group. The 7.6 million people now aged 75+ make up 38 percent of the total older population (65+), a substantial jump from 33.6 percent in 1960 and 31.4 percent in 1950.[23]

The 75 and over group is significantly more vulnerable to the mental, physical, and environmental insults and assaults. While 35 percent of those 65–74 with chronic illness were subject to significant impairment of function, 53 percent of those over 75 were similarly limited.[24] Riley and Foner's[25] summary of research findings indicate that rates of all types of psychosis rise steadily by age. Given a functional approach to needs for comprehensive health services, more than a third of the elderly may require support services.

SOCIAL IMPLICATIONS OF AGING, VALUES, PUBLIC AND SOCIAL POLICY

Concern with the service needs of older people has grown greatly in a period of a few years due in large measure to federal government involvement. This does not negate citizen concern at a local level, which is interrelated with governmental concern at all political levels.

The attempt of the usual organization and profession, with rare exception, is to serve the aged when the old become problems that an individual or a family is unable to successfully resolve. And while it is necessary to be prepared to serve in this manner, an even more significant challenge of planning at all geographic and political levels is to educate and motivate those in the direct service to ferret out individuals and families before their situations become problems of such magnitude that the agents of society cannot adequately cope with them. Simultaneously, the planning agents would be gearing themselves to redefining services, refining goals, and effecting coordination and synthesization in an evolving society to cope with changing demand at the proper time instead of a decade or two later when needs and methods of resolving them have already been modified.

Goal Development and Interaction with Policy

Do we have a national goal for older people or multiple goals? Should we have them? Are we working in a cohesive manner to attain these goals? As we move into the fuller acceptance of separate planning bodies such as for "comprehensive health, mental health and retardation," among others, are we next going to move into a planning entity to coordinate the planning entities?

The responsibility for leadership in the field of aging is that of providing for the development of adaptive responses among the many social institutions, agencies, and organizations of society to the facts and realities of aging. Such adaptive responses must be predicated on a recognition of the generalized requirements of a society with increasing percentages and numbers of older persons in order that there be resources mobilized, allocated, and utilized to meet the individualized needs of the older person. Such adaptation to both the generalized requirements of society and the more specific requirement of the individual, his family, and community must encompass our economic and occupational policies and practices; our housing and living arrangements; our medical, health, welfare, and educational services; our recreational, cultural, and leisure programs; and our basic social institutions of education, family, government, and religion.

The development of social policies, and the movement of such policies into practice, requires the formulation of a philosophy based on scientific knowledge. Such a philosophy reflects one's conceptions of aging as it relates to the individual, his family, community, and society. The services to older people, in turn, reflect value orientations of administrative and organizational policies and practices that also, in turn, relate the values of our society.

To serve the elderly, the philosophical base should be one of understanding aging as an interacting, interrelated behavioral, biological, psychological, and sociological process. It should recognize the rigidities inherent in the concept of chronological aging and the traditional orientation of societal practices and policies to such a stereotyped view. Further, it must be based on knowledge of the changing form of society and the environments within which the human aging takes place. Such a philosophy must concern itself with the implicit moral connotations of related knowledge as it affects our reappraisal of traditions of behavior and usage that may no longer be valid. It must reflect the commitment of leadership as well as both the already tested and emerging methods essential to the development of policies and practices.

Too often, the goal has been to provide a service or plan a community program for the older person as an end in itself. For example, our perception may be the provision of a safe nursing home for an aged individual. While good in itself, specific needs of older persons must be put within a broader concept of providing networks of living arrangements and health services to permit alternatives of choice based on present and predictable changing individual requirements and preferences. To date, the majority of our services have failed to view the essential unique and individual characteristics of older individuals.

Planning and the formulation of policy intertwine. Neither exist without altering each other. The balancing of interests and concerns alter what our policies turn out to be just as they affect when and how we undertake planning toward whatever goals appear to be dominant at that moment of time.

Effect of Values on Policy

Public policy, as a balancing of interests for whatever time period—until the interests are out of balance again which, by itself, is almost a constant—are a reflection of societal values. Gross[26] has identified 15 major value belief clusterings salient to the American culture as follows:

1. Activity and work
2. Achievement and success

3. Moral orientation
4. Humanitarianism
5. Efficiency and practicality
6. Science and secular rationality
7. Material comfort
8. Progress
9. Equality
10. Freedom
11. Democracy
12. External conformity
13. Nationalism and patriotism
14. Individual personality
15. Racism and related group superiority

Almost two thirds of these value beliefs belittle the elderly. To test the latter, it is suggested that one may personally compare these value clusters of the elderly with the population as a whole within the American culture. Gross[27] further states that ". . .running through these complex orientations. . . is an emphasis on the worth of active mastery rather than a passive acceptance of events. . . and a high evaluation of individual personality rather than collective identity and responsibility." If the Gross formulation is accurate, and it is one with which I concur, then the aged are excluded from high value considerations.

Social Policy and Public Policy

Social policy is a reflection of values. Public policy is a deliberate effort to either modify social conditions or restructure society to prevent undesirable conditions. The latter has obviously not taken place. The former has had sporadic limited effort, but no concentrated cohesive effort has taken place.

Public policy becomes dependent on social policy. The latter is reflected in the synthesization of organizational and individual energies often in competition, sometimes in cooperation, and in other instances competitive cooperation. Such energies operate within a philosophy of values.

Since effort is undertaken within a culture not yet willing to value the aging—regardless of the energy expended by those concerned—social policy, which is more closely guided by values than is public policy, is unable to sufficiently influence public policy.

Without an "upward bound" value change for aging Americans, social policy will be hampered. To give a favorable outlook or at least one of equality of opportunity compared with other age and problem groupings commensurate with the risk level, aging Americans would have to be accepted as a risk group. As such, special treatment becomes a necessary goal to attain equality in the American culture. The special treatment via public policy will have to be molded first, then, by a social policy that will make feasible the acceptance of the high risk group known as the Aging American.

As values evolve, social policy changes. As social policy changes, public policy evolves. To those who would argue that public policy is an important part of social policy, instead of social policy setting the tone in America, one only needs to be reminded of how the Vietnam conflict developed and continued on the American side to recognize the power of a public policy. It took a decade for a social policy to evolve and alter the public policy. In another sense, one may recall the American World War II public policy in allowing the armies of the Soviet Union to advance in Europe, not necessarily in consonance with a then possible American social policy of concern about communism.

The essential ingredient of a public policy is the acceptance of a social policy that is reflected in our social philosophy. The fulfillment of the dignity of man may give us the beginnings of such a social philosophy. But why is it that aging man in America needs to so be dignified as others and, in an important way, perhaps even more dignified than others?

Public Policy and Aging Research

One of the best of possible answers lies in aging research. The major problem here is that we have not yet evolved a social public policy about gerontological research. We have come closer in our social policy insofar as research per se is concerned, but we are considerably less advanced with our concern about gerontological research.

To change values about aging, on the assumption this is by itself a high value, research into operative value standards relative to aging Americans is necessary as a base in diagnosing, planning, and treating the societal problem therein as it reflects on both the millions of aging people as a group and on each one as a person with resultant differing personal effect.

But what is a research public policy on the aging and the aged? Is it:

1. Earmarked funds for both fundamental and programmatic research on an approximate equal basis?
2. To support fundamental research primarily?
3. A national planning agency need to establish guidelines for research fund utilization?

4. A Presidential Commission Task Force to comprehensively study aging towards the evolvement and implementation of a research policy?
5. To support specific research centers throughout the United States under a National Gerontological Research Institute?
6. Necessary to insert a research component in every specific, major gerontological program in the United States?
7. That we cannot agree on which areas of research hold priority?
8. That we should invest the same percentage of aging expenditures for aging research as business and industry does with their available funds?[28]

These questions make it clear that we do not have a national public policy on aging research. But, do we need only one public policy or do we need several?

Public Policy in Gerontology

Since we do not have a public policy on gerontological research, we lack the basis for a sound public policy on aging practice. And, just as the question may be raised as to whether or not *a* research public policy or a series of policies is to be considered, the same query is logical relative to the service arenas of gerontology. Public policy on aging obviously has not emerged in the absence of sufficient sound research and sound analysis that are the keys to effective planning.

What do these areas consider? Do they include:

1. A desire to learn what success in retirement really is?
2. A goal to eliminate loneliness?
3. An effort to insure self-mastery by the aged?
4. An acceptance that education may continue throughout life?
5. The basis for individual variance to allow for work and to allow for early retirement?
6. The opportunity for choices to enable one to select that which fits him rather than being pushed into a selection which denigrates?[29]

Research, training and practice constitute an integrated gerontological professional concern. As public policy in gerontology develops, an overall policy will set the tone for the remainder. And, if no cohesive policy appears to evolve, then we may even argue that the lack of a public policy is a reflection of our social concern as it is affected by our values, and this public policy lack has become our public policy.

A main feature of aging research and training is its sparcity. A main feature of practical or applied gerontology is its "hit and miss" character, more often than not unrelated to knowledge we already have. The old person or a family of an old person more often than not receives "improper" services at a time when a "proper" service is required.

Public Policy and Aging Training

The field of gerontology is a relatively new field, an infant in terms of structured theory about the processes of aging, professional development, and organized training and research programs. Its infancy is all the more startling when compared with the immense population toward which it is directed and the amount of knowledge yet to be.

To demonstrate the newness of this field, one need only be reminded that organized training programs in gerontology were first supported by the National Institute of Child Health and Human Development in 1965 and by the United States Administration on Aging in 1966.

TREATMENT RESOURCES AND THEIR APPLICATION

The treatment of chronic illness and aging has two general levels: the provision of treatment resources and the application of those resources. Even a third level might be distinguished; namely, the reception or assimilation of treatment resources on the part of those being treated.

Treatment Resources

The provision of treatment resources for the chronically ill and aged refers most obviously to the federal government, to public and private agencies and institutions, and to professional personnel. Not to be overlooked, of course, are families and the patients themselves. Ultimately, all taxpayers are involved on this level of treatment and in a particularly critical sense so too are the entire socioeconomic and sociophilosophical orders, both national and local, which the mainstream of people participate in, embody, and represent.

With respect to the application of treatment resources, at least four points of reference can be distinguished. First, there are the categorical groups for which respective treatment resources are intended and/or designed. Second, there are the categorized individuals within those groups. Third, there is the application of treatment resources by means of institutional methodologies, the hospital, the home for aged, the nursing home, the residence. Fourth, and perhaps of particular significance for the future, is the application of treatment resources via parallel methodologies, both structured—such as in the case of visiting nurses associations, personal care organizations, homemaker/health-aide services, meals-on-wheels—and the nonorganized—such as family, neighborhood, church, and civic initiatives.

Treatment Assimilation

On the level of treatment reception or assimilation, such measurable factors as personal need, individual and group psychology, patient involvement, and auxiliary supports have to be distinguished. Similarly, such intangibles as patient or client willingness, individual life-style, coping resources, spiritual well-being, the ebb and flow of relationships, and environmental influences must be attended.

Fortunately, not all the problems to be met within the treatment of chronic illness and aging are ethical problems. Some are merely technological, methodological, procedural, or logistical. Some, however, are essentially ethical in nature, entailing decision making that has direct, and, at times, irreversible repercussions on the well-being of persons. Others have only an ethical facet or dimension, dealing substantially with the manipulation of nonhuman entities but having implications or consequences for persons touched in some way by that manipulation.

Ethical Base

For present purposes, an ethical situation is one involving human decision, human repercussion, and an evaluation of both in terms of human well-being. According to the classical Western tradition, an ethical act requires the measuring of human decisions and consequences against the essential expectations or requirements of human nature. To undertake and meet that measure, through the process of judgment called conscience, is to act ethically and well; it is to perform a good action. By derivation, it is to be a good person, at least in terms of what one has done. To decline that measurement, on the other hand, or to decide against its imperative, is to act unethically and badly: It is to perform an evil action and, by derivation, to be an evil or bad person, at least in terms of what one has done or failed to do.

There never has been unanimity on the conceptual structure of human ethics. Even the core concept of the Western tradition (namely, the evaluation of human actions against the requirements of human nature, to say nothing of the logical derivatives of that concept) has repeatedly been the subject of debate. The Western tradition is challenged in part as it affects the aged and chronically ill, and clues as to the import of why some challenge is necessary have already been indicated.

To employ general, undifferentiated humanness as the measure of human interaction is certainly to indicate, if not demonstrate, the basic humaneness (or inhumaneness) of human actions. According to that measure, human decision making must always be humane. It must be in keeping with the dignity of both the person deciding and the person or persons decided about. Failing that measure, one faults both himself and whoever is to experience the effects of that fault.

Moral Actions in Treatment

Thus it is possible to establish an extensive catalog of moral and immoral actions with respect to the treatment of the chronically ill and aged. Such actions as the following illustrate this:

1. Negotiation or imposition of treatment options;
2. Provision of adequate or inadequate nutrition;
3. Maintenance or disregard of patient privacy;
4. Promotion or restriction of unnecessary institutionalization;
5. Therapeutizing or dehumanizing treatment methodologies;
6. Processing or neglect of patient care, including the inability of a physician to visit a nursing home patient;
7. Servicing or exploitation of patient deficits;
8. Provision or disregard of safety and security measures;
9. Professionalizing or desensitizing treatment personnel;
10. Unifying or compartmentalizing related treatment resources;
11. Liberation or prolongation of patient dependencies; and
12. Provision or withholding of related treatment supports or resources.

This assertion is seen most vividly in dramatic instances. Two particular instances are cases in point. The State of Ohio reported in September 1973 that a woman has been "discovered," as it were, by a newly appointed superintendent, to have been committed to a mental hospital over 60 years ago, with no record or prognosis of why she was there at all; as the superintendent noted, this is a case of a wasted life.[30] In Florida, at about the same time, two welfare clients died in wheelchairs in a hospital hallway during a three- or four-day waiting period for admission to a neighboring nursing home; even assuming that these persons received food and other care while waiting, this instance in its total social context is grossly demeaning and inhumane.[31] Both situations, in a word, are immoral, serious departures from the norm of humaneness.

In our culture some of the more gross immoralities regarding mistreatment of the chronically ill and aged are also crimes, actions specifically prohibited by statute or legal precedent. In this respect public law is another repository of consent to the substance of the Western ethical tradition.

Any departure from the classical ethical norm should note two operative accompaniments. (1) As there are gross immoralities in the treatment of the chronically ill and aged, so there are also dramatic instances of morality, that is, instances of superlative correspondence with the norm of humaneness. (2) By no means are all instances encompassed by the catalog of illustrations listed previously dramatically clear in their rightness or wrongness. There may well be situations and facets of situations inferred in that catalog that defy clarification, whose resolution at best may lie only in a selection of the lesser evil and at worst in an opaque and often heartrending, "damned if you do and damned if you don't" tossup.

Moral Actions in Provision

The illustrations cited earlier deal mainly with the application level of treatment resources. Similar illustrations of moral and immoral actions can be noted on the provision level of treatment resources; for example:

1. Assurance of adequate or inadequate income supports;
2. Provision or denial of feasible care options;
3. Provision or disregard of the social components of care;
4. Enacting or impeding of adequate protective laws;
5. Processing or neglect of cost control mechanisms;
6. Application or detouring of categorical care allocations;
7. Setting or inhibiting of relevant public priorities;
8. Renewal or endorsement of entrenched resource and treatment systems;
9. Correction or perpetuation of categorical myths;
10. Correction or perpetuation of entrenched vested interests;
11. Provision or prohibition of spiritual well-being resources; and
12. Compensation or requirement of competitive inequalities.

It is here that a legislator's decision, for example, can have repercussions on millions of chronically ill and aged persons, and a subsequent presidential or gubernatorial decision can change it all. Prior to such decision, however, one must note the entire sociopsychological context that contributes to their evolvement. In a sense it relates to corporate responsibility, including merit and guilt, a concept reappearing of late in certain Christian theologies.[32]

On the provision level of treatment, then, one meets interlocked value systems, degrees of social consciousness and social conscience, overlays of previous ethical fallout, surges of ethical evolution, entrenched inhibitors of change and growth, and whatever other factors are operative in the process that gives a body politic its ethical identity.

On this provision level, in a word, the gigantic problem of public policy formulation is met interfaced by our social policy evolvement, the matrix ethical problem involved in the treatment of the chronically ill and aged.

Classical Norm

To approach this problem, it is necessary to take issue in part with the basic ethical norm of the classical tradition. The problem at hand is too critical to be processed through the prism of general, undifferentiated humanness; the problem is one of very specialized humanness, requiring a measure of unique rather than general humaneness.

Morality is measured, according to the classical Western norm, by the compatibility or discrepancy of human decisions with all the requirements that are essentially rooted in or related to human nature. An intellectually sophisticated construct, this norm provides the weights and measures of ethics for general human behavior on the part of the general run of persons.

The classical ethicists are not to be faulted for any failure to give due consideration to categorical and individual differences in general human nature. By an elaborate and multifaceted doctrine of circumstances, they interpreted general humanness as distributed through a multiplicity of categorical and individual variations, out of which were drawn the ethical implications. The weak of mind, for example the senile, were thus seen as accountable only in proportion to the strength and scope of their lucid moments.

Nor are the savants of ethics to be held responsible for what the beneficiaries of their legacy would do with it. How were they to perceive nuances of a democratic society, destined to arise long after their theorizing, whereby general nature is ascribed to the general run of men, to the majority, and restricted nature to minorities? Or, if that be too harsh, how were they to know that socially, politically, economically, militarily, educationally, and even religiously, general human nature would repeatedly support the claims of the established order, and with the same persistence urge the denial of the claims of subgroups?

What the classical ethicists bequeathed to us is an abstruse norm albeit a humanizing development beyond the ancient Greek *hubris* and the Roman paternalism. It is a great improvement also over the primitive revelation of the Hebrews synopsized, in caricature, by the doctrines of "an eye for an eye" and the "doom" for national enemies. Further, it is a convincing alternative to the "Superman" pattern of Nietzsche and the Nazis and the organized racism of the Ku Klux Klan.

In spite of its credits, the classical norm suffers a variety of intrinsic and extrinsic deficiencies. For example, it has a tendency to support restricted social systems. With respect to that tendency, the fault in question may ultimately be more attributable to the moral weakness of its devotees and followers than to the deficits of the norm itself. If the historical odyssey of that norm, or of any moral norm for that matter, teaches us anything it is that a schedule of moral goals or requirements, no matter how accurately drawn, is not of itself an effective instrumentality for its own achievement. If morality were solely science, would not then our generation and times be the most moral of all eras?

Morality requires, in addition to a clear schedule of goals, corresponding and harmonious behavior, decision making and followthrough compatible with those goals. It is at this point that human initiative chronically breaks down. A norm of moral truth and fidelity is perhaps not as attractive as the things that rival it and is less tangible. On the other hand, there is an attractiveness about truth and moral goodness that is not unfamiliar to the mainstream of men. My point is that the classical norm fails to exploit that attractiveness. This is its external deficiency.

As I read contemporary commentators on the classical norm, its originators had at their disposal only an insight into the static and consummately constituted facets of human nature.[33]

Intuitions of differentiation, particularity, and change they certainly had, but nothing akin to the fuller view of humanness now available in synthesis of modern psychological, sociological, philosophical, and even biological insights.[34] This is its intrinsic difficulty. Today, for example, the mainstream of thinkers, scientists, and practitioners are as comfortable with an evolutionary view of humanness as were the classical ethicists with their absolute view. The very mutuality of this comfort would suggest that a more adequate and operative view of humanness would involve a pairing of the two perspectives. Both, I believe, are true, as far as they go. Neither, however, is of much long-term help in isolation.

Change in the Classic Norm

Human nature is essentially developmental; with this construct, human nature is essentially aging. Further, chronic illness is a constitutive component of humanness, certainly as to its developmental implications, whether progressive or retrogressive, and perhaps also as to its very being. Maves has observed the following:

I submit the hypothesis that the nature of religious experience may be different at different stages of adult life because of the way in which the Holy and the Unconditioned is customarily encountered. Therefore, the forms of religious expression will need to be different to take account not only of the experience itself but also of the changed capacities and needs of the person. Thus, the institutionalized expressions of religious experience and faith need to be examined to see whether or not they are adequate to deal with the new length of years that medical science has added to us.[35]

Implicit in what Maves perceived as the developmental roots of religious experience, expressions, and needs is the deeper perception, I believe, of the developmental roots of aged persons themselves. Such persons are versions of embodiments of processive human nature. As such, they represent not general, undifferentiated humanness, but specialized and, to a unique degree, actualized and finalized humanness. Furthermore, the norm of humanness demanded by their unique being is one not of general dignity and morality, such as the traditional norm established for all persons, but of uncommon and wholly specialized responsibility. If it be sound, as Maves suggested, that the institutionalized aspects of religion need to be re-examined in light of a developmental theory of religious experience, it seems even more sound that institutionalized treatment resources for the aged, on both the application and provision levels, demand re-examination if developmental theory is pertinent to humanness itself.

There is an attractiveness to the construct. Moreover, implications for responsibilities and actions are far more clearly directed and specific than disclosed by the classical moral norm. Ultimately, there are stronger grounds for a more insistently humane psychology and public policy regarding categorical groups than are to be found with the classical ethical norm.

Chronology alone, however, is not necessarily an operative measure of the humanizing process. We all know that comprehensive human development issues from a concurrence of a multiplicity of stratified vitalities, some normally following a chronological age and quite independent of absolute age correlation. We know, too, that developmental vitalities often fail to materialize or they materialize unequally or at least unevenly, thus spawning the whole gamut of personality and psychosocial variations among people.

Proposing an expanded and fuller humanness in the elderly, therefore, means the elderly are more fully human not solely for what has actually developed within them but also for their potential development. In some instances they are marked mainly by actualization: Some older persons are richly endowed with abilities, great in their social achievements, and noble in moral stature. In other instances they are marked mainly by potentiality. Usually, though, older persons are marked by a combination of both.

Whether aged or not, humanness touched congenitally, accidentally,

or pathologically by chronic disability is a uniquely intensified humanity. Thwarted in normal channels of expression, at times even frustrated
entirely, the vitalities of a chronically ill person must necessarily be re-
grouped, redirected, and compensated in an intensive, alternative way.

This construct of the chronically ill and aged is attractive. There is
an objective dignity and order of entitlement here, perhaps both clearer
and stronger than that offered us in the Western ethical tradition.

Ethical Implications

What are some of the specific ethical implications of this construct? If
the chronically ill and aged are, indeed, uniquely specialized and intensified embodiments of human nature, the humaneness owing them, in
terms of the provision and application of treatment resources, must reflect the following sensitivities:

1. They are persons of ontological stature *at least equal* to all the
rest of us and are not to be paternalistically acknowledged and supported.

2. Social policy regarding the aged, including allocations and services,
is adequately framed and oriented only when it is cognizant of their
priority rather than minority status on the continuum of ontological
personal worth. This scale accords them a very high, not very low rank
after the common or collective needs of the body politic.

3. Public policy regarding the aged, including allocations and services, will be also ethical only when it is comprehensive, adequate, uni-
fied, and facilitated, geared not to separable categorical needs but to
separable categories of persons defined in terms of uniquely related
needs.

4. Home and neighborhood is one's primary habitat, the cultural
setting affecting individual worth; the first and mandatory focus, then,
for assistance, care, and support.

5. Alternative treatment forms are alternatives, then, to home forms,
rather than vice versa, and the ample and suitable provision and application of alternatives humanely follows on their free choice and/or real
need rather than by the imposition of tradition or vested interests.

6. Spiritual well-being is a goal of all treatment forms rather than
vice versa, and the spiritual components of care accordingly are given
due professional and structural rank in the treatment construct.

There should be critical hesitation before one attempts to define the
needs of old people in terms of absolute rights. If we ever aim solely at
an order of justice, to paraphrase the late European theologian Guardini,

we are bound to fail, to culminate in an order of relentless demand, counterdemand, and recrimination; whereas if we aim at an order of love, perhaps we can hope to culminate in an order of justice. Perhaps the only concepts of love large enough to carry the issue at hand are essentially theologically based: I am thinking of the Hebrew *hesed* (compassion) and the Christian *agape* (charity).[37]

The social implications of aging in America are inherently related to the values of our society. Apart from an occasional, unusual planner and practitioner, what we create and how we utilize what we create will depend on how we value the chronically ill and the aged in the years ahead. While sporadic public achievements may take place without an upward social value change, permanent progress will eventuate only when the value base becomes firm and solid. Such firmness is dependent on our willingness to provide the chronically ill and old at least what we provide others. This will not take place unless exceptional consideration is practiced. This, though, is not the contemporary norm, and it remains unclear as to whether or not it is an evolving norm.

A variation of the Western classical norm, a full acceptance and backing of research into the chronically ill and the aged, a stress on the uniqueness of the chronically ill and the aged, and an intensification of a comprehensive system of care allowing at least for equal if not preferential treatment are interwoven in any discussion on the ethical value issues in health care of the chronically ill and the aged.

REFERENCES

1. Lennard HL, Epstein HJ, and Rosenthal MS: The methadone illusion. Science 176:883, 1972.
2. Atchley RC: The Social Forces in Later Life. Blemont, Calif., Wadsworth Publishing Company, 1972, p 5.
3. Tibbits C: Handbook of Social Gerontology. Chicago, University of Chicago Press, 1960, p 9.
4. Havighurst RJ: The sociological meaning of aging. Address given at the general session of the International Gerontological Congress in Merano, Italy, July 15, 1957.
5. U.S. Bureau of the Census, 1970 tabulation.
6. Sheldon HD: The changing demographic profile, Handbook of Social Gerontology. Edited by C Tibbits. *op. cit.*, p 41.
7. Brotman H: Facts and Figures on Older Americans. No. 2. SRS-AOA Publ 182. Washington, D.C., Department of Health, Education, and Welfare, 1971.
8. AOA Publ No. 5, 1971, p 4.
9. Atchley RD: *op. cit.*, pp 14, 15.
10. *Ibid.*, pp 15, 16.
11. Goldberg E: Helping the aged, National Institute for Social Work Training Services. No. 19. London, Allen and Unwin, Ltd., 1970, p 13.

12. For discussion of activities of daily living research see Lawton MP, Brody EM: Assessment of older people: self maintaining and instrumental activities of daily living. Gerontologist 9 (3):179–186, 1969; Brody EM, Kleban MH, Lawton MP: Excess disabilities of mentally impaired aged: impact of individualized treatment. Gerontologist 11 (2):124–133, 1971.

13. Townsend P: Measuring incapacity for self-care, Processes of Aging. Edited by RH Williams, C Tibbits, W Donahue. New York, Atherton Press, 1963, Vol II, p 83.

14. McMullan JJ: The prevention and management of disability in general practice. J R Coll Gen Pract 17:83, 1969.

15. National Center for Health Statistics: Chronic Conditions Causing Activity Limitations, U.S., July 1963–June 1965. Ser 10, No. 51. Washington, D.C., Department of Health, Education, and Welfare, Feb 1969, p 19.

16. Shanas and Associates: Old People in Three Industrial Societies. New York, Atherton Press, 1968, pp 22 ff.

17. Brody BJ: Prepayment of medical services for the aged: an analysis. Gerontologist 11 (2):156, 1971.

18. Brown BS: Where do we go from here? Address at the Governor's Conference on Aging, Nashville, Tennessee, September 26, 1973; reproduced in Congr Rec, Oct 3, 1973, p S 18504.

19. Parsons T: Definitions of health and illness, Patients, Physicians and Illness. Edited by EG Jaco. New York, The Free Press, 1958.

20. Brody EM: Long-term care for the elderly: optimums, options, and opportunities. J Am Geriat Soc 19 (6):487, 1971.

21. Shanas E: Measuring the home health needs of the aged in five countries. Paper presented at 8th International Congress of Gerontology, Washington, D.C., August 1969.

22. Commission on Chronic Illness: Chronic Illness in a Large City, The Baltimore Study, Chronic Illness in the U.S. Cambridge, Harvard University Press, 1957, Vol IV, Table 16, p 16.

23. Brotman H: *op cit.*

24. National Center for Health Statistics: Age Patterns in Medical Care, Illness and Disability, U.S., July 1963–June 1965. Ser 19. Washington, D.C., Department of Health, Education, and Welfare, 1966, p 46.

25. Riley NW, Foner A, et al.: Aging and Society. Vol I. New York, Russell Sage Foundation, 1968, p 370.

26. Gross BM: Individual and group values. Ann Am Acad Polit Soc Sci 371, 1967.

27. Gross BM: *ibid.*

28. Kaplan J: Social Implications of Aging: Values, Public Policy and Social Policy. Triad of papers for a Mt. Angel College symposium. Private printing, 1971.

29. *Ibid.*

30. Mansfield News Journal, Sept 25, 1973, p 11.

31. Mansfield News Journal, Oct 1, 1973, p 1.

32. Hartman LF: Retribution, Encyclopedic Dictionary of the Bible. New York, McGraw-Hill, 1963, Col. 2032-2036.

33. Dupré L: Natural end and natural law, Contraception and Catholics: A New Appraisal. Baltimore, Helicon, 1964, pp 37–52.

34. Curran CE (ed): Absolutes in Moral Theology. Washington, D.C., Corpus Books, 1968.

35. Maves PB: Research in religion in relation to aging, Proceedings of Seminars— 1961–65. Durham, N.C., Council on Gerontology, Duke University, 1965, pp 69–79.
36. Guardini R: The Lord. Chicago, Henry Regnery Co., 1954, pp 81–82.
37. Hartman LF: *op. cit.*, Love, Col. 1377 ff.; Love in the OT and NT, The Interpreter's Dictionary of the Bible. New York, Abingdon Press, 1962, Vol 3, pp 164 ff; Spicq C: Agape in the New Testament. St. Louis, Herder, 1963–66, 3 Vol.

SISSELA BOK, Ph.D.
Fellow in Medical Ethics, Harvard University

Commentary

Dr. Kaplan eloquently documents the failures of research and treatment
to cope with the problems of the chronically ill and the aged. He stresses
the importance of increasing the assistance given to them, while avoiding their dependency and exploitation.[1] I fully share these goals. In this
paper, I would like, however, to explore a possible conflict between
helping others and preserving autonomy. When these goals conflict,
some form of paternalistic coercion often results. Those who suffer
from severe illness in old age are, I believe, especially vulnerable to such
coercion; they will be the focus of my paper.

The papers of this volume have shed much light on all the difficulties
that beset a fair allocation of good health care to all who need it. If
these problems are confronted, great strides can be made. But for the
aged and the chronically ill, the very provision of adequate help is itself
problematic. Is the common good sought by medicine the same for these
patients as for others? What is really "good" for them? What does "help"
really mean in caring for them? A conflict often arises between doing
what is thought to be good for them and doing that which preserves
their autonomy and their dignity to the greatest possible extent. When
there are such conflicts, it should be an urgent responsibility for medical
ethics to consider how they ought to be resolved.

Many are now disturbed about the denial of dignity at the end of life.

A Swedish editor has compared the emaciated elderly encountered in nursing homes and hospitals there, who are given the very best of medical care, to the inmates of concentration camps encountered at the end of World War II.[2] But these patients are not, as were the inmates of the camps, the victims of persecution. Rather, they bear witness to a benevolent concern to help them—to help them live on and, if possible, recover.

Montaigne held that in order to learn how to live, men have to think about death and be prepared for it.[3] Approaching one's death should give the chance to reflect on the life that is drawing to an end. Thus the concern for dignity and autonomy goes far beyond the wish to make isolated personal choices; it is a desire to be able to consider one's life as a whole, with a beginning, a duration, and an end. In society's magnificent effort to help the ill to survive, the severely ill and aged often are brought past the point where such reflection is still possible; in pressing medical care for them to such a level, society may reflect the fears of those who are still well—fears of coming up against questions about the meaning of one's life and the inevitability of death. Undue *authority* may then be exercised to carry through such assistance for survival, even at the price of defeating and belittling those so assisted.

At one time, authority was taken for granted. Slavery, the power of rulers over their subjects, of parents over their children, and husbands over their wives were rarely questioned. Hobbes listed three ways in which a person can become subjected to another: through voluntary offer, through captivity, and through birth.[4] Only when the unquestioning acceptance of this subjection was seriously challenged did the need for justifying it arise. It became necessary to ask, "When *can* authority be justly exercised over a person's purely private decisions?"[5] The answer given by paternalism is that such authority is justified when it is exercised over persons for their own good. But such intentions have guided innumerable offenses. Men, women, and children have been compelled to accept alien religious practices, have been institutionalized against their own will, or suffered from wars alleged to "free" them—all in the name of what has been declared to be their own interest.

Yet no one would hesitate to keep a child from playing with matches in dry grass. Parents, health professionals, and trustees are all in positions where they are expected to exert authority over others and held accountable for failing to do so. How, then, should we distinguish between unjustified and justified authority in all those many cases where those who use force over others claim to be acting in the interest of those persons? The law of torts specifies that two conditions must hold: The individual whose personal integrity is violated, as in surgery, must be "physically or otherwise incapable of giving consent"; the intervention must be so manifestly in his interest that a reasonable man would want to be thus interfered with.[6]

Using these criteria, it is possible to distinguish justifiable from unjustifiable paternalism in a rough way. But there is a difficult borderline region of unclear cases, where one or both of the criteria is disputable. The person coerced may be marginally rational and marginally able to give consent. Or the intervention may be such that reasonable men would differ as to the benefits achieved, even, as to whether benefit or harm actually results.

Nowhere are there more difficult borderline cases than in the care of those who suffer from severe chronic illness in old age. While some of them are in fact incompetent to make decisions for themselves, others are able to do so at times, but not always. Some are in such discomfort or depression that it is difficult to know the extent to which their choices reflect their long-term wishes. When they are compelled by others to accept procedures they do not wish—operations for example—reasonable men can and do differ as to whether they themselves would wish to be so treated.

VULNERABILITY TO PATERNALISM

Since it is exceptionally difficult at times to know whether paternalism is justified with respect to chronically ill and aged persons, the mere fact of belonging to these groups greatly increases the vulnerability to control by others. The fear of being helpless in the face of such control has grown in strength in our century, as a result of very real changes in the ways in which people now spend their last years.[7] The ability to protect one's freedom of personal choice shrinks with weakness and prolonged illness; and the incidence of such illness has greatly increased. At the beginning of this century, the major communicable diseases were the leading causes of death, and the average life expectancy was around 47 years. Now, the average life expectancy is around 70 years, and chronic degenerative diseases cause most of the deaths at that age. Dying is now more prolonged and more often associated with mental degeneration.

While this period of dependency and weakening has lengthened, the nature of the care given has shifted dramatically toward institutionalization. The family units have shrunk, and many elderly live alone; when they need help, institutional help is overwhelmingly more frequent. Patients who are severely ill often suffer a further distancing and loss of control over their most basic functions. Electrical wiring, machines, intravenous administration of liquids create new dependency, and at the same time new distance between the patient and all who come near.

They sometimes even lead to what has been called the "intensive care syndrome," characterized at times by acute psychological and behavioral disturbances. These may result from sleep deprivation, mechanization, unfamiliar and impersonal surroundings, and a Kafkaesque uncertainty about one's predicament.[8]

Such a degree of distance and distress is often worth enduring for the curable patient. But for the severely chronically ill patient in old age, these procedures create the distress and the human distance and the sense of impotence without providing any cure. In fact, they then become a substitute for comforting human acts. Yet those who suffer in this way often fear to seem troublesome by complaining.

Another factor that makes it difficult to protect the autonomy of the aged and the chronically ill is that they are largely out of sight. Whether they live alone or in institutions, they cannot easily call attention to themselves. Even so, it is just possible that our society will respond to their predicament sooner than to others. For most people have witnessed at least a few relatives or friends go to a death they would fear for themselves. The privileged are as vulnerable as all others to prolonged chronic illness and slow deterioration. Money can buy exemption from many health problems, but not from these. Already, there is greater unity of concern and publicity about these problems. And the trust, which Dr. Hellegers and Dr. Jonsen so rightly stressed as the cornerstone of the doctor–patient relationship, is endangered as more and more people become concerned about what will befall them should they be ill in later life.

EFFECTS OF PATERNALISM ON INDIVIDUAL DECISION MAKING

The severely ill are especially vulnerable to paternalistic coercion. In what specific ways does paternalism affect their ability to make decisions concerning their life?

To make a rational decision for oneself, one must have access to the available information regarding one's situation and the alternatives that are open. One must be aware of the different possible outcomes associated with the alternatives and be able to formulate a subjective estimate of the likelihood of these outcomes, as well as of one's own preferences regarding them.

All of these elements are absent to some degree in a paternalistic relationship. But the denial of information is at the root of the harm of paternalism. Without information a person cannot begin to choose reasonably. Depriving him thereof not only limits his present choices, but also affects the choices he will be able to make in the future. He cannot, for example, make the important decision of whether or not to enter a hospital in a case of terminal illness. This decision depends on knowledge about his condition, the kinds of help available, the possible discomfort and suffering associated with hospital versus home stay, and the expenses to be expected. Lacking such information, someone may slip unwittingly into prolonged patienthood at the end of life, where death is held at bay through one operation after another, using increasingly broad life support measures.

Yet it has long been accepted medical practice for physicians to control the amount of information available even to their competent patients. All or part of the truth may be withheld. At times the truth is even distorted and placebos are frequently prescribed.[9] Oliver Wendell Holmes[10] advised physicians beginning their careers in the last century as follows:

Some shrewd old doctors have a few phrases always on hand for patients that will insist on knowing the pathology of their complaints without the slightest capacity of understanding the scientific explanation. I have known the term "spinal irritation" serve well on such occasions, but I think nothing on the whole has covered so much ground, and meant so little, and given such profound satisfaction to all parties, as the magnificent phrase "congestion of the portal system."

The chances of a patient's learning the truth are especially low when he suffers from a terminal condition. Studies indicate that most doctors do not tell their patients of their chances of impending death, even though they themselves would, if ill, wish to be told the truth.[11]

When information about the condition of a patient is denied to him or distorted, all the other aspects of decision making are also undercut. There is no way of thinking about alternative courses of action, or of forming a coherent estimate of personal preferences. Whether or not to go to a hospital, whether or not to have an operation, whether or not to put one's affairs in order—all such choices become chancy and tinged with arbitrariness. Tolstoy has given an unforgettable description of the bewildered fears and sense of abandonment of a man thus kept in the dark, in *The Death of Ivan Ilych*.

Yet the physician's choice is not always an easy one. He is influenced by generations of accepted medical practice inclining him to alter the truth for the good of his patient. He is aware of the benefits that can flow from the use of placebos and may not even clearly view such usage as a form of dishonesty.[12] He is acutely aware of the uncertainty under which he operates and of the difficulty of giving correct and meaningful answers to patients. He knows that disclosing his uncertainty or his pessimistic prognosis can diminish those benefit to the patient's health that depend on faith and the placebo effect. He dislikes, as do all of us, to be the bearer of bad news. And sitting down with a patient to discuss an illness truthfully and sensitively may take much needed time away from other patients. Finally, there are many patients who might not believe the truth. Some are unwilling to confront the possibility of illness and death and expressly ask their physicians not to let them know. Others, to the contrary, won't believe that nothing is wrong with them and demand to have an ailment diagnosed and some form of treatment prescribed.

Despite these difficulties, I believe that, with a very few exceptions,[13] honesty is the best policy, both for physicians and for patients, but most of all for the entire institution of medicine. For it is impossible to look on each incident of distortion or withholding of the truth as taking place in a watertight compartment, between a physician and a patient, with no ripples reaching the outside. I have already spoken of the harm that I believe comes to a patient thus kept in the dark. But other patients and other physicians are also harmed by such a practice.

First, whenever there is an accepted practice of altering the truth, the practice has a tendency to *spread.* More and more patients will tend to be misled, and some will come to be dependent on drugs or placebos that they cannot know that they do not need.[14] At present we are witnessing the dangerous spread from the prescription of harmless placebos to the prescription of antibiotics and other harmful drugs where they are not needed. This development reinforces the effects (described by Dr. Maccoby) that the media have in increasing the number of people who want to resort to medication or other forms of therapy for any real or imagined complaint. The most insidious form of spread, however, is perhaps that which occurs when a physician departs from the original intention of deceiving patients for their own good to the point of deceiving experimental subjects for the good of his research project and society. This spread is facilitated by the fact that many patients are simultaneously subjects in investigations.

Second, in addition to this danger of the spread of dishonest practices once they are tolerated for what seem to be altruistic motives, knowledge about the dishonest practices inevitably filters out and is often biased by suspicion and fear. I believe that even those many doctors who do not mislead their patients are thus harmed by those who do. The crisis of confidence between physicians and patients is profound, and many physicians are now needlessly suspected. The whole institution of medical care is therefore threatened by such practices, however harmless they may seem in individual cases.

Truthfulness is the foundation for meaningful communication between human beings. The temptation often arises to abandon it, for the good of a person or the good of the state. But once it becomes known, as will usually happen, that truthfulness has been compromised, then trust is lost, and the imagined benefits shrivel by comparison to the loss we all suffer.

Yet individual physicians alone cannot combat this failure in trust. The shift must also be an institutional one. The policy of promoting an informed public, of helping each patient to understand his health problems, and of combating measures of concealment, must be defended by consumers groups, set forth in Bills of Rights for patients, stressed in medical and nursing schools, and supported by the government.

But even where a patient has all the necessary knowledge, and has decided upon a particular course, his ability to carry through his choice may be very limited, and once more thwarted by paternalistic policies. Most often, these policies impose on the patient something that is thought to be good for him—medication, surgery, or a change in his life.[15] This problem may seem to have been circumvented by the strict requirements for consent, which is the most obvious and common safeguard against coercion. I have tried to show, however, how difficult it is at times to decide whether a patient should be considered capable of making judgments about consent for himself, and how easy it is for abuses to slip in. But consent may also be ignored at times even when the patient is quite lucid and able to express his wishes. All too frequently, those who choose to refuse medical treatment at the end of their lives as a result of an illness they consider intolerable are not heeded. There are indications that resistance is growing to such practices of overriding the wishes of patients. Recent court cases have upheld the right to refuse treatment.[16] And Bills of Rights put out by the American Hospital Association and a number of hospitals provide for such refusals.[17] But much remains to be done to give force to these rulings and standards.

Under our present standards, it is quite possible that one of the most lucid men who ever lived—the Roman stoic thinker Seneca—would be declared irrational in our hospitals if he showed the desire to act upon the following thought[18] :

Few have lasted through extreme old age to death without impairment, and many have lain inert. . . . I shall not abandon old age, if old age preserve me intact for myself . . . but if old age begins to shatter my mind, and to pull its various faculties to pieces, if it leaves me, not life but only the breath of life, then I shall rush out of a house that is crumbling and tottering.

When a child is held back from a dangerous highway, or a temporarily depressed adolescent is rescued from suicide, it is not only their lives but also their chance to shape their own lives in the future that have been preserved. But in terminal or severe chronic illness, no such future is preserved by forcing a patient to stay alive. Where there is no future or hypothetical consent, the whole rationale for paternalism collapses; interfering with a person's wishes then becomes itself unreasonable, no matter how irrational or self-destructive these wishes may appear. For the very *meaning* of rationality shifts as a person's perceived future shrinks. The paternalist looks to the future and will sacrifice present desires for future benefits. But present desires—for comfort, for relief from distress, for human companionship, and for recognition as a person—must be foremost in caring for the severely ill in old age.

CONCLUSION

I have sought to describe some of the ways in which aging and chronically ill patients can suffer from the very benevolent policies intended to *help* them. And I have tried to show how this word "help" may have a different meaning for such patients. More than for other patients, "help" ought to be what *they* wish and what *they* consider helpful, not what others decide is best for them. I share Dr. Kaplan's view that our society now fails to take their best interests into consideration in a human way.

One way to focus on this problem is for research to be devoted to what people actually hope for and fear as they approach old age. A recent article by the Swedish internist Dr. Gunnar Biörck documents the preference for a quick death rather than one that comes slowly and for a death that comes before mental deterioration sets in.[19] If this preference is further documented in different societies, what effects could it have on the allocation of research and therapy efforts—between illnesses, for example, and between age groups? What effects might it have with respect to the attitude toward suicide, which, among the elderly and the chronically ill, is such a different matter than among other groups?

In treatment, the greatest possible openness and accountability must be advocated. Dr. Kaplan lists a number of moral and immoral actions in the provision of treatment; they could serve as a focus for inquiry and standard setting. Consumers' organizations, patient advocates, Bills of Rights may seem cumbersome and bureaucratic to physicians and hospital personnel, but they are essential for the safeguards required by patients and for the visibility that alone will prevent abuses.

There are problems in medical ethics of agonizing difficulty; some of them will perhaps always remain insoluble. These are problems where claims or rights conflict sharply—where to satisfy one legitimate claim or right, another claim has to be sacrificed. No ethical theory has yet been clearly applied so as to resolve such problems. One of the most essential procedures in medical ethics must therefore be to winnow out these problems, to isolate them, and to reduce their scope as much as possible. They must be set apart from those many other problems that are more easily resolved.

Foremost among these more soluble problems are, I believe, those where only one person's welfare is at stake; problems of whether that person should *know* about his situation, and whether others should be able to coerce him for his own benefit. What is at stake in such conflicts, and what is denied by paternalism, is perhaps the most basic feature of moral relationships between human beings: the recognition, in Kant's[20] words, that:

Man . . . exists as an end in himself, not merely as a means for arbitrary use by this or that will. . . .

REFERENCES AND NOTES

1. Throughout his paper, Dr. Kaplan also voices the hope that the aged and the chronically ill will come to be valued at least equally, but preferably more highly than others. I fully share his hope for equal valuation, and do agree that our society fails grievously to provide it. But I would not wish to go beyond equality to maintain that the aged, or the young, or members of some race or other group rank higher than others on any scale of personal worth or merit.
2. Olof Lagercrantz, personal communication. Compare also May Sarton's superb recent novel, *As We Are Now*. New York, W. W. Norton, 1973.
3. Montaigne: Que philosopher, c'est apprendre à mourir, Essais. Garnier Freres, Book I, ch XX.
4. Hobbes T: de Corpore Politico, Vol II, ch 4, p 1.
5. In this paper, I am considering the clear cases of decisions that affect the lives of primarily one person. It is not, however, always easy to distinguish such cases from those where several persons' interests and rights enter in.
6. Prosser WL: Law of Torts. St. Paul, Minnesota, West Publishing Company, 1971. For discussions of paternalism, see Mill JS: On Liberty, The Philosophy of John Stuart Mill. Edited by M Cohen. Cleveland, The World Publ. Co., 1965; Hart HLA: Law, Liberty, and Morality. Stanford, Calif. Stanford University Press, 1963; Dworkin G: Paternalism, Morality and the Law. Edited by R Wasserstrom. Belmont, Calif., Wadsworth Publ. Co., 1971; Rawls J: A Theory of Justice. Cambridge, Harvard University Press, 1971, pp 209, 249.
7. See Lerner M: When, why, and where people die, The Dying Patient. Edited by O. Brim et al. New York, Russell Sage Foundation, 1970, pp 5–29. See also four articles in BioScience 23(8), 1973: Bok S: Euthanasia and the care of the dying; Meyers D: The legal aspects of medical euthanasia; Crane D: Physicians' attitudes toward the treatment of critically ill patients; Cassell E: Permission to die.

8. McKegney F: The intensive care syndrome. Conn Med 30: 633–44, 1966; Hackett T, Cassem N, Wishnie H: The coronary care unit. An appraisal of its psychologic hazards. N Engl J Med 279:1365–1370, 1968.
9. For a still unrivaled discussion of the intricacies of withholding and distortion of truth, unintentional and intentional deception, and other aspects of lying, see St. Augustine, Contra Mendacium *and* De Mendacio, in Treatise on Various Subjects. Edited by R Deferrari. New York, The Fathers of the Church, 1952, p 172.
10. Holmes OW: Medical Essays. Cambridge, H. O. Houghton, 1883, p 388.
11. Oken D: What to tell cancer patients: a study of medical attitudes. J Am Med Assoc 175:1120–1128, 1961. For an overview of the subject of information in medical situations and a challenging thesis, see also Waitzskin H, Stoeckle J: The communication of information about illness. Adv Psychosom Med 8:180–215, 1972.
12. Beecher KK: The powerful placebo. J Am Med Assoc 24:1602–1606, 1955; Shapiro AK: A contribution to the history of the placebo effect. Behav Sci 5:109–35, 1960.
13. The exceptions are those where there is *justified* paternalism—the incompetent, children, and those who refuse to know about their condition. In all these cases, however, I believe that distortion should be kept to a minimum as well.
14. Vinar O: Dependence on a placebo: a case report. Br J Psych 115:1189–1190, 1969; Cabot R: Teamwork of doctor and patient through the annihilation of lying (an exceedingly thoughtful examination), Social Service and the Art of Healing. New York, Moffat, Yard & Co., 1909; Buffet EP: A popular medical error to be corrected by the physicians. Medico-legal J (New York), 1898.
15. The question of euthanasia and that of suicide will be virtually untreated in this short paper. I have discussed them in Voluntary Euthanasia. PhD dissertation. Cambridge Harvard University, 1970.
16. Robitscher J: The right to die. Hastings Cent Rep 2(4):11–15, 1972; Kantor N: A patient's decision to decline life-saving medical treatment: bodily integrity vs. the preservation of life. Rutgers Law Rev 26(2):228–264, 1973; Crane D: *op. cit.,* p 474.
17. Bill of rights for patients. The New York Times, Jan 9, 1973.
18. Seneca: Epistles, epistle LVIII. Cambridge, Loeb Classical Library, Harvard University Press, 75:407, 1967.
19. Biörck G: How do you want to die? Arch Intern Med, pp 605–606, Oct 1973.
20. Kant I: Groundwork of the metaphysics of morals, in The Moral Law. Translated by HJ Paton. London, Barnes & Noble, 1948.